HANDBOOK OF PEDIATRIC INFECTIOUS DISEASES

Allan D. Friedman, M.D.

Associate Professor of Pediatrics/Adolescent Medicine
St. Louis University School of Medicine

Attending Physician
Divisions of Ambulatory Pediatrics and Infectious Diseases
Cardinal Glennon Children's Hospital
St. Louis, Missouri

Ishiyaku EuroAmerica, Inc.
St. Louis •Tokyo •1987

Ishiyaku EuroAmerica, Inc./Medical Series
Allen D. Soffer, M.D., Editor
Carlo P. Caciolo, M.D., Editor
Antonio M. Salvador, M.D., Editor (Pathology)
Book Edited By: Lisa A. Meyers
Book Designed By: Joan Evers

Ishiyaku EuroAmerica, Inc.
11559 Rock Island Court, St. Louis, Missouri 63043

Library of Congress Catalogue Card Number 86-081376

Allan D. Friedman, M.D.
  Handbook of Pediatric Infectious Diseases

ISBN 0-912791-29-2

Ishiyaku EuroAmerica, Inc.
St. Louis ● Tokyo

Composition by Pulsar Publishing, St. Louis, Missouri
Printed in the United States of America

TABLE OF CONTENTS

PREFACE

Infectious diseases account for a large percentage of sick visits to pediatricians, a significant percentage of hospitalizations of pediatric patients, and a significant amount of school absences by children. Important advances have been made in the prevention and treatment of infections, yet infections remain a major cause of morbidity in the pediatric population. A solid understanding of pediatric infectious diseases is therefore essential to those who care for infants and children.

This book is designed to provide the medical student and non-M.D. child-care provider with an introduction to pediatric infectious disease, and the intern and resident with a convenient source for information needed to diagnose and treat children. Rather than attempting to comprehensively cover all pediatric infections, the book is designed to cover the practical essentials for the diagnosis and treatment of major infections and to give a "taste" of some of the less frequently seen infections. As must be the case in a handbook of this size, only selected topics are covered. In addition to chapters that deal with diagnosis and treatment of specific diseases, additional chapters have been included to provide practical information on antimicrobial use, immunizations, prevention of infections, and the usefulness and limitations of laboratory tests.

It is hoped that this concise and practical book will provide a solid introduction to prediatric infectious diseases to the student and will be a manageable and valuable reference and guide for the intern and resident.

I am grateful to Harold A. Conrad, M.D. for valuable comments and suggestions. My special thanks to Sally A. Fuqua for her tireless and efficient secretarial assistance.

1

INFECTIONS OF THE EAR, NOSE, THROAT AND ORAL CAVITY

ACUTE OTITIS MEDIA

Clinical Manifestations

Symptoms of acute otitis media often include ear pain (infants may rub or tug at the ear), otorrhea, and fever. The presence of fever is not required for the diagnosis of AOM. Hearing loss, vertigo and disturbances of balance are less common symptoms in children. Infants may have very non-specific symptoms such as restlessness, irritability and lethargy.

Etiology and Epidemiology

The majority of children have had AOM at least once by the age of 2 years. There may be a relation between early onset and later difficulty with relapse, recurrences, and reinfection. AOM is more common in whites than blacks and in boys than girls. It is more common in winter than summer. The frequency of AOM generally decreases with increasing age and may be associated with improved eustachian tube function and improved immunity and host defense. In patients with unrepaired cleft palate and in patients with Down's Syndrome, AOM is very common.

Over half of AOM is caused by either *Streptococcus pneumoniae* or *Haemophilus influenzae*. *S. pneumoniae* is more commonly found than *H. influenzae* and accounts for an increasingly large percent of AOM with increasing age. Recently *Branhamella catarrhalis* (was *Neisseria catarrhal-*

is) has been identified with increasing frequency as an etiologic agent of AOM. Many of the *B. catarrhalis* found have been β-lactamase producing. (The implications of this will be discussed under Therapy.) *Staphylococcus aureus* and group A β-hemolytic streptococcus have also been reported as pathogens in AOM. In infants under six weeks of age, enteric bacteria and group B β-hemolytic streptococcus are also found. In about 1/5 of the cases of bilateral AOM the results of culture from one ear will differ from the other ear. It appears that anaerobes (as the primary pathogen), viruses, and mycoplasma play a relatively small role as etiologic agents.

Diagnosis

Diagnosis of acute otitis media (AOM) is made by visualization of the tympanic membrane (TM). A red or yellow-white TM, inability to see the bony landmarks behind the TM and bulging of the TM are all hallmarks of AOM. Decreased mobility of the TM is the most sensitive sign of fluid behind the TM. Mobility can be demonstrated only when there is a good seal of the otoscope within the external ear canal. *REMEMBER:* The normal TM is pearly gray, translucent with a good light reflex, and will move with air pressure unless restricted by fluid or scarring and adhesions. Crying may make the TM appear red but usually not to the extent that is seen with AOM. Intense or localized redness of the TM means inflammation.

Who should have a diagnostic tympanocentesis? Although relatively easy to do with practice, and fairly safe, diagnostic tympanocentesis is generally reserved for four circumstances:

1. The neonate with otitis or the infant with symptoms suggesting serious disease.
2. The immunocompromised/immunosuppressed child with otitis.
3. The child with AOM unresponsive to the commonly used antibiotics. (Unless the child is getting worse, allow 48-72 hours to observe improvement.)
4. The child with AOM and major complications such as meningitis, cerebral abscess or mastoiditis.

Tympanocentesis can be accomplished by insertion of a 20 gauge spinal needle attached to a syringe through the inferior portion of the TM and applying negative pressure. The external canal should be cleaned and sterilized (alcohol will work) prior to insertion of the needle.

Treatment

AOM is analogous to an abscess. It is a confined pocket of pus. Spontaneous cures can occur when the abscess drains either through the eustachian tube or by spontaneous rupture of the TM. Nevertheless, antibiotic therapy remains the accepted mode of treatment.

There are several antibiotics available to treat otitis. Ampicillin (or Amoxicillin), trimethaprim-sulfamethoxazole (TMP-SMX), erythromycin-sulfisoxazole, penicillin G plus a sulfonamide, and cefaclor all seem to be reasonably effective. In populations where the incidence of ampicillin resistant *H. influenzae* is high or where *B. catarrhalis* has been reported (*B. catarrhalis* is frequently 6-lactamase producing), one of the other choices of therapy may be more appropriate. 6-lactamase inhibitors, such as clavulonic acid, are available in combination with amoxicillin (Augmentin[R]). When given to the patient, clavulonic acid will prevent 6-lactamase from inactivating amoxicillin and thus will make amoxicillin-resistant (or ampicillin-resistant) bacteria sensitive to these antibiotics. REMEMBER: Penicillin V is less active against *H. influenzae* than Penicillin G. If a penicillin is chosen to treat otitis, the appropriate form is Penicillin G. Also, remember that in patients where Group A beta hemolytic streptococcus is suspected, TMP-SMX will *not* be effective.

Amoxicillin (or ampicillin) remains the preferred initial therapy since it still covers the majority of pathogens involved in otitis and is relatively inexpensive. In areas where the incidence of ampicillin resistant *H. influenzae* is high or where *B. catarrhalis* has been recognized as a frequent pathogen, or in patients with allergy to the penicillin, alternative antibiotics should be used. Therapy should be continued for 10 to 14 days.

Caution should be used in using sulfa compounds in children. Serious cases of erythema multiforme major (Stevens-Johnson Syndrome) in association with administration of sulfa drugs have been reported. Use of TMP-SMX has also been associated with lowering of the white blood cell count.

The value of other medications in the treatment of AOM is questionable. Clinical studies do not provide any strong evidence that decongestants or antihistamines have any beneficial affect on AOM.

It is not yet clear whether administration of the currently available pneumococcal vaccine or administration of experimental *H. influenzae* vaccine will have any long term beneficial effect in preventing AOM.

Sequelae and Complications

The list of complications is large, but with the early institution of therapy, the risk of developing complications is small. Complications include meningitis, encephalitis, central nervous system abscesses, lateral sinus thrombosis, petrositis, labyrinthitis, mastoiditis, facial nerve involvement, cholesteatoma and osteomyelitis. Delayed speech and language development is seen in some patients.

KEY POINTS

1. Children should demonstrate some clinical improvement within 48-72 hours. If there is not improvement or if the patient has gotten worse, consider:
   A. tympanocentesis
   B. change of antibiotic regime
   C. the possibility of spread of the infection to include other structures outside of the ear.
2. The presence of fluid in the middle ear at the end of the therapy does not necessarily mean failure of the therapy. Forty percent of children may have an effusion at one month after AOM. There is no evidence that steroids are effective in treating middle ear effusions.

REFERENCES

1. Fosarelli PD, Deangelis C, Winkelstein J et al: Infectious illnesses in the first two years of life. Pediatr Infect Dis 1985; 4:153-159.
2. Klein JO, Bluestone CD. Special Series: Management of Pediatric Infectious Diseases in Office Practice. Acute Otitis Media. Pediatr Infect Dis 1982; 1:66-73.
3. Mackinin ML, Jones PK: Oral dexamethosone for treatment of persistent middle ear effusion. Pediatrics 1985; 75:329-335.
4. Paradise JC, Otitis Media in infants and children. Pediatrics 1980; 65:917-943.
5. Pelton SI, Whitley P. Otitis Media: Current concepts in diagnosis and management. Pediatric Annals 1983; 12:207-218.

SINUSITIS

Clinical Manifestations

The clinical diagnosis of sinusitis is frequently difficult. The best known symptoms of tenderness and swelling over the affected sinuses are often absent. The presence of periorbital edema upon awakening is a helpful clue. The edema may lessen during the day. Other more common but less specific symptoms include headache, fever, nasal discharge (usually purulent), cough and a "bad" cold. *REMEMBER:* Most viral colds (upper respiratory infections) last about 1 week. In a patient with prolonged symptoms of a cold lasting at least 10 days without significant improvement, think sinusitis.

Etiology and Epidemiology

Most sinusitis in children is in the maxillary sinuses. The ethmoids may also be involved in these children. In adolescents, infection of the frontal sinus becomes increasingly common. Children with allergies have a high incidence of sinusitis.

The majority of sinus infections are caused by *Streptococcus pneumoniae* and *Haemophilus influenzae* (mostly non-typable). Recently, *Branhamella catarrhalis* has been isolated in patients with sinusitis, and in some studies, equals or exceeds the frequency of *H. influenzae*. Anaerobes also appear to play a role in some cases. Group A beta hemolytic streptococcus, alpha hemolytic streptococcus, staphylococcus and viruses seem to be responsible for a small percentage of acute sinusitis. *REMEMBER:* It appears that bacterial cultures of the nasopharynx and throat are poor predictors of bacteria recovered from the sinus and do not aid in choosing appropriate antibiotic coverage in any individual patient. In patients in whom sinus aspiration will not be done, antibiotics should be choosen based on the most recent bacterial epidemiological data available. Anaerobes, staphylococci, and streptococci seem to play a larger role in chronic sinusitis than acute sinusitis.

Diagnosis

Sinus x-rays may be useful in confirming a clinical diagnosis of sinusitis. Lateral, occipitomental, and antero-posterior views are needed. Caution must be exercised in interpreting these films, especially in infants. Normal non-infected sinuses may not appear identical when contralateral sinuses are compared. To make the x-ray diagnosis of sinusitis, look for air-fluid levels in the sinuses, mucosal thickening, or opacification of the sinus. A negative set of sinus x-rays does not role out sinusitis. Positive findings help confirm your clinical impression.

Other less frequently used aids in diagnosing sinusitis include transillumination of the sinuses. To transilluminate the frontal sinus, place the light source under the superior orbital ridge (must be done in a dark room with the light shielded from the observer). To examine the maxillary sinuses place the light source in the mouth. This method has been evaluated in adults but its usefulness in children is still not resolved. Ultrasonography appears useful in finding fluid in sinuses. False positive ultrasound examinations are rare but false negatives are not uncommon.

When are we justified in doing an aspiration of a sinus? In routine practice, sinus aspiration is rarely done. Antibiotic choices are based on those pathogens commonly seen in acute sinusitis. Nevertheless, certain specific circumstances argue for aspiration. These include the immunocompromised or immunosuppressed host, lack of response to appropriate therapy, life-threatening disease in association with sinusitis and severe facial pain or headache. The procedure, which should be done by someone experienced with it, involves puncture below the inferior turbinate, through the lateral nasal wall, into the maxillary sinus.

Treatment

Therapy is directed at sterilizing the infected sinuses, preventing spread of the infection, and aleviating symptoms. Since the spectrum of organisms causing acute sinusitis in children is similar to that which causes acute otitis media, the same antibiotic regimens may be used. In locales where ampicillin resistant *H. influenzae* and *B. catarrhalis* are prevalent alternatives to ampicillin or amoxicillin should be sought. Cefaclor, trimethoprim-sulfamethoxazole, and erythromycin-sulfisoxazole are alternatives. When possible at least two weeks of therapy should be given to reduce chances of recurrences.

The potential value of decongestants and antihistamines remains controversal. Their potential value in opening obstructed sinuses must be weighed against their potential (especially decongestants) of inhibiting ciliary motility, thus delaying clearing of infected matter. In addition, they may decrease local blood flow and thus restrict delivery of adequate amounts of antibiotic to the area.

Irrigation and drainage are effective procedures in treating sinusitis, but are in general reserved for refractory cases or patients with spread of their infection to orbital or central nervous system (CNS) sites.

Sequelae and Complications

Most commonly, acute sinusitis resolves without any problem. Not infrequently however, children may develop preseptal cellulitis (inflammatory edema) resulting from impedence of local venous drainage. (There is not actually soft tissue infection.) Appropriate therapy of the sinusitis will result in resolution of the edema. The swelling is usually soft, non-tender and most severe in the morning.

Other complications are infrequent but result from spread of the infection. They include CNS abscess, frontal or maxillary osteomyelitis, orbital cellulitis, subdural empyema and sinus thrombosis (cavenous or saggital). *REMEMBER:* Sinus infection appears to aggravate chronic reactive airway disease (asthma). Successful treatment of sinusitis will often enable discontinuation of bronchodilator use.

KEY POINTS

1. Typical symptoms of sinusitis in adults, such as tenderness and swelling of the infected sinus, may be absent in the pediatric patient.
2. Periorbital edema that decreases during the day may be a helpful clue to acute sinusitis.
3. Acute sinusitis is caused by the same organisms that cause otitis media in children and antibiotic choice should therefore also be similar.
4. Sinus infections may aggrevate asthma in children.
5. Staphylococci, streptococci, and anaerobes are commonly found in chronic sinusitis.

SELECTED REFERENCES

1. Brook IB: Bacteriologic features of chronic sinusitis in children. JAMA 1981; 246:967-968.
2. Jazbi B, Ritter FN: Sinoscopy and sinus disease in children. Otolaryngologic Clinics of North America 1977; 101:71-80.
3. Kovatch AL, Wald ER, Ledesma-Medina J, et al: Maxillary sinus radiography in children with nonrespiratory complaints. Pediatrics 1984; 73:306-312.
4. Nelson JD: Eye and parnasal sinus infections. Pediatr Infect Dis 1983; 2(3suppl):528-532.
5. Rachelefsky GS, Kate RM, Siegel SC: Chronic sinus disease with associated reactive airway disease in children. Pediatrics 1984; 73: 526-529.
6. Wald ER: Special series: Management of Pediatric infectious diseases in office practice. Acute sinusitis in children. Ped Inf Dis 1983; 2:61-68.
7. Wald ER, Reilly JS, Casselbrant M, et al: Treatment of acute maxillary sinusitis in childhood: A comparative study of amoxicillin and cefaclor. J Pediatr 1984; 104: 297-302.

PHARYNGITIS AND TONSILLITIS

Clinical Manifestations

The diagnosis of pharyngitis/tonsilitis is made by carefully visualizing the throat. Erythema, exudate and swollen tonsils are all signs of infection. In small children pharyngeal examination may be difficult. Use of a tongue blade may be necessary, and assistance may be required to immobilize the head to enable a good examination. In older children, asking them to stick out their tongue, and pant rapidly, "like a dog", will often give you an adequate view without resorting to the use of a tongue blade. In younger, more obstinate children who clench their teeth as soon as they see a tongue blade or a light, pinching their nose forcing mouth breathing will often result in unclinching their teeth and opening their mouth to facilitate breathing.

Etiology and Epidemiology

Although there are many causes of pharyngitis and tonsilitis, beta-hemolytic streptococci, Epstein-Barr virus, adenovirus, parainfluenzae and influenzae viruses, probably account for the majority of cases. Less commonly enteroviruses, *Neisseria gonorrhea, Treponema pallidum, Mycoplasma pneumoniae, Corynebacterium diptheriae* and *Francisella tularensis* are also responsible for pharyngitis. Of the more common etiologies, only streptococcus requires pharmacological intervention.

In unusual cases viral throat cultures can be done for common viral pathogens. Group A streptococci are predominantly spread by airborne droplets and hand contamination. "Strep throat" is a self-limited disease. Prevalence of the asymptomatic carrier state in children is in the range of 10-20%. Bacterial pharyngitis tends to be more common in the summer months. Pharyngitis in infants is more likely to be viral. *REMEMBER:* Streptococcal pharyngitis is rare in infancy.

Diagnosis

The only way to accurately diagnose "strep throat" is by culture technique or antigen detection techniques. Throat cultures should be obtained from the posterior pharyngeal wall on the tonsils. Streptococci infections cannot be diagnosed on physical examination alone without risk of misdiagnosis. Pharyngitis due to EBV infection can be diagnosed by heterophil antibody test (or Monospot) or by specific EBV serology. Mycoplasma serology and culture can be done to diagnose mycoplasma. Diphtheria and gonococcal pharyngitis can be cultured and syphilis and tularemia serologies are available. *REMEMBER:* Not all throats that look like "strep throats" are, and "viral looking" throats may grow streptococci.

Treatment

Of the most common etiologies, only streptococcal pharyngitis is routinely treated. Penicillin therapy for streptococcal pharyngitis is primarily for prevention of rheumatic fever, however, some recent evidence contradict previous held belief and indicates that penicillin may also reduce the duration of symptoms. Commonly used alternatives to penicillin are erythromycin cin, clindamycin, and a cephalosporin. In treatment failures on penicillin alone, the combination of penicillin plus rifampin may be valuable. Penicillin may be given as benzathine penicillin 600,000 to 1,200,000 units intramuscularly or oral penicillin G 800,000 to 1,000,000 units divided in three or four doses for 10 days. Gonococcus and treponema are treated with penicillin. Tularemia can be treated best with streptomycin.

Sequelae and Complications

Acute rheumatic fever appears to be decreasing in frequency. It has been described in 0.5% to 3.0% of individuals untreated for streptococcal infection. The risk of acute post streptococcal glomerulonephritis appears to vary with the strain of streptococcus. It is uncertain that penicillin prophylaxis will decrease the risk of glomerulonephritis. Glomerulonephritis is more commonly associated with streptococcal skin infections. Prompt therapy can prevent suppurative complications of streptococcal pharyngitis. These complications include otitis, sinusitis, mastoiditis, and peritonsilar abscess.

KEY POINTS

1. Not all "streptococcal-looking" pharyngitis is due to streptococcus.

2. Strep throats in infants are rare. Adenovirus is a more common etiology of pharyngitis of this age.
3. Treatment of strep throat helps prevent rheumatic fever and may speed up recovery from the pharyngitis.
4. Streptococcal pharyngitis relapses should be treated with alternatives to penicillin if the patient really did have good compliance with the initial penicillin course.
5. Gonococcal pharyngitis can be seen in association with gonococcal arthritis.

REFERENCES

1. Brian JH, Bass J: Streptococcal pharyngitis: Optimal site for throat culture. J Pediatr 1985; 106:781-783.
2. Chaudhery S, Bilinsky SA, Hennessy JL, et al: Penicillin V and rifampin for the treatment of group A streptococcal pharyngitis: A randomized trial of 10 days of penicillin vs 10 days penicillin with rifampin during the final 4 days of therapy. J Pediatr 1985; 106:481-486.
3. Kaplan EL, Top FH, Dudding BA, et al: Diagnosis of streptococcal pharyngitis: Differential of active infection from the carrier state in the symptomatic child. J Infect Dis 1971; 123:490-501.
4. McCraken GH: Diagnosis and Management of group A streptococcal pharyngitis. Pediatr Infect Dis 1982; 1(3 suppl): 530-532.
5. Peter G, Smith AL: Group A streptococcal infections of the skin and pharynx. NEJM 1977; 297:365-370.
6. Randolph MF, Redys JJ, Cope JB, et al: Streptococcal Pharyngitis: Post-treatment carrier prevention and clinical relapse in children treated with clindamycin palmitate or phenoxymethyl penicillin. Clinical Pediatrics 1975; 14:119-122.
7. Rowe RT, Stone RT: Streptococcal pharyngitis in children: Difficulties in diagnosis on clinical grounds alone. Clin Pediatrics 1980; 16:933-35.
8. Schwartz RH, Wientzen RL, Grundfast KM: Sore throats in adolescents. Pediatr Infect Dis 1982; 1:443-447.
9. Stillerman M, Isenbery HD, Moody M: Streptococcal pharyngitis therapy: Comparison of cephalexin, phenoxymethyl penicillin, and ampicillin. Am J Dis Child 1972; 123:452-461.

CERVICAL ADENITIS

Clinical Manifestations

Cervical adenitis needs to be distinguished from other causes of swelling about the head and neck. A detailed history may be helpful, as is a careful physical examination. Often the presence of associated symptoms may be helpful. Typically, involved lymph nodes are 2-6 cm in diameter. Tenderness is often present, and the overlying skin may be erythematous and warm. Fever and systemic symptoms may or may not be present. Suppuration may be present. The nodes involved may be unilateral or bilateral, single or multiple. Diffuse edema around the nodes may be present.

Etiology and Epidemiology

There are many infectious and non-infectious causes of cervical adenitis. The table (p. 13) includes many of the infectious etiologies that should be considered. When infection is not proven, non-infectious causes must be considered. Malignancies, drugs, collagen-vascular diseases, hygromas, and cyst need to be considered.

Most bacteria associated with cervical adenitis are normal flora of the respiratory tract and skin. *Mycobacterium tuberculosis* and group A streptococcus are the exceptions and are a result of person-to-person spread. Staphylococci and streptococci account for 60-80% of all cervical adenitis. These bacteria have no sexual or seasonal preference. Mycobacterial cervical adenitis has distinct features (see chart).

Diagnosis

The specific etiology often determines what associated symptoms are present. Diagnosis of inflamed lymph nodes is best made by aspiration of the node for culture. If aspiration fails to yield an organism, then node excision biopsy should be considered. Additional diagnostic tests include: PPD, heterophil, VDRL, ASO, and serology for specific fungi; viruses; toxoplasma or Epstein-Barr titers.

Treatment

Treatment depends on the etiologic agent. If no aspiration is attempted and no cultures done, antistaphylococcal therapy should be tried empirically. Lack of response to therapy necessitates further investigation. The table lists therapies for some of the more common pathogens.

Sequelae and Complications

Complications and sequelae depend on the etiologic agent. Early diagnosis and institution of appropriate therapy usually insures a benign course. Most complications are rare. Complications include dissemination of disease (especially *M. tuberculosis*), abscess formation (bacteria) and sinus tracts (*mycobacteria*). Glomerulonephritis has been associated with streptococcal adenitis.

Cervical Adenitis

Organism	Characteristics	Therapy
Staphylococcus aureus	Often unilateral; fever-mild or absent; suppuration can occur; can cause adenitis in newborn; symptoms last about 10 days.	semisynthetic penicillins; first generation cephalosporins; clindamycin; erythromycin; vancomycin.
Group A beta-hemolytic streptococcus.	often unilateral; fever-mild or absent; suppuration can occur; occur; symptons last about 4 days.	penicillin; first generation cephalosporins; clindamycin; erythromycin.
Group B beta-hemolytic streptococcus.	cellulitis-adenitis syndrome; age 3-7 weeks; male greater than female; fever, poor feeding bacteremia common, otitis often seen.	penicillins
Viral (Epstein-Barr, Herpes Simplex, Cytomegalovirus, enteroviruses, rubella, adenoviruses, and others).	often bilateral; secondary to respiratory infections; nodes-small, often rubbery, may not be tender; gingivostomatitis-herpes simplex; herpangina-entero-viruses; posterior cervical adenitis-rubella.	
Cat Scratch Disease (bacteria)	onset 5-60 days after inoculation; often solitary node; tender node may be large; suppuration often occurs; systemic symptons usually mild.	

Cervical Adenitis

Mycobacteria	M. Tuberculosis—all ages; unilaterial but occasionally bilateral; PPD greater than or equal to 10 mm; black; abnormal chest x-ray; urban residence; usually painless nodes; firm gradually become softer. **Atypical**--less than or equal to 5 years old; unilateral; PPD less than 10 mm; white; usually normal chest x-ray; rural residence.	**M. tuberculosis** rifampin plus isoniazid. **Atypical**-surgical excision.
Kawasaki syndrome	often only 1 node involved; node firm; slightly tender; with suppuration; usually subsides with defervescence; -lymphadenopathy not a universal finding.	Aspirin and supportive care.
Toxoplasmosis (toxoplasma gondii)	node-nontender, usually posterior cervical area; most patients are asymptomatic.	pyrimethamine (controversial)

Miscellaneous Causes of Adenitis

Anaerobic bacteria
Gram negative bacteria
Diphtheria
Tularemia
Brucella
Treponema pallidum
Haemophilus influenzae
Yersinia pestis
Actinomyces israelii
Histoplasma
Cryptococcus
Aspergilla
Candida
Coccidioides

KEY POINTS

1. Most cervical adenopathy is due to either staphylococci or streptococci.
2. Tuberculosis adenopathy requires anti-tuberculosis chemotherapy, atypical mycobacterial adenopathy can frequently be treated with surgical excision.
3. Failure to achieve a clinical response to antibiotics directed against staphylococci and streptococci should result in further investigation including either node biopsy or excision.
4. If mycobacterial infection or malignancy is suspected, node excision is preferred over aspiration.

REFERENCES

1. Barton LL, Feigin RD: Childhood cervical lymphadenitis - A reappraisal. J. Ped. 1974; 84:846-852.
2. Brook I: Aerobic and anaerobic bacteriology of cervical adenitis in children. Clin Ped. 1980; 19:693-696.
3. Ginsburg CM: Cat-scratch adenitis. Pediatr Infect Dis 1984; 3:437-439.
4. Knight PJ, Mulne AF, Vassy LE: When is lymph node biopsy indicated in children with enlarged peripheral nodes. Pediatrics 1982; 69:-391-396.
5. Lake AM, Oski FA: Peripheral lymph adenopathy in childhood: Ten year experience with excisional biopsy. Am J Dis Child 1978; 132:-357-359.
6. March SM: Infections of lymph nodes of the head and neck. Pediatr Infect Dis 1983; 2:397-405.
7. Saitz EW: Cervical Lymphadenitis caused by atypical mycobacteria. Pediatric Clinic of North America 1981; 28:823-839.
8. Zitelli BJ: Neck Masses in children: Adenopathy and malignant disease. Pediatric Clinics of North America 1981; 28:813-821.

ORAL INFECTIONS

There are a wide variety of infections that affect the oral cavity. This section will briefly describe some of the more common oral infections.

Herpes Simplex

Primary infection with Herpes simplex often presents as gingivostomatitis in children. The incubation period is usually 2 days to 2 weeks. Systemic symptoms frequently occur. Headache, fever and malaise may precede the oral eruptions. The infection is characterized by numerous vesicles on the perioral region and on the tongue. The vesicles rupture and ulcerations form. The affected area is often erythematous. The mouth is usually painful. Healing begins at the end of the first week with resolution usually complete by the end of the second week.

The infection remains latent, usually in the trigeminal ganglion and in some patients, will reactivate frequently presenting as cold sores (recurrent herpes labialis). Stress frequently is the precipitating factor for recurrences. Recurrences can also occur internally resulting in small ulcers on mucosa that overlays bone.

The infection is usually self-limited. Routine use of acyclovir is therefore not recommended. Patients with lesion should protect against contact of their lesions with other people to avoid spread of the infection.

Candida Albicans

Thrush is a common oral infection in infants. Thrush is an acute pseudo-membraneous candida infection on mucosal surfaces. The lesion is a white plaque which, if scraped off, will often leave a bleeding lesion. If there is a question of the diagnosis, a potassium hydroxide wet mount can be done to visualize the fungal elements.

In neonates the infection is frequently acquired from the maternal vaginal mucosa which is frequently colonized with yeast. Outside the neonatal period, oral candida infections are usually limited to immunocompromised patients or patients on antibiotic therapy. In most cases, localized treatment is sufficient. Topical antifungal medications such as nystatin, miconazole, or clotrimazole are frequently used.

Coxsackie Virus

Coxsackie viruses, especially group A, frequently infect the oral cavity causing herpangina. The patients usually present with fever, sore throat, anorexia, and malaise. The lesions are usually found on the palate, tonsillar pillars, tonsils, and on the pharyngeal wall. The typical lesion is a vesicle which ruptures leaving a small eroded area. The infection usually occurs in summer, is usually mild, and is self-limited.

Coxsackie viruses can also cause hand-foot-and-mouth disease. Vesicles are found on the soles and palms and oral lesions may occur anywhere in the mouth. Fever frequently is present. The illness is self-limited.

Aphthous Ulcers

Aphthous ulcers are not thought to be infectious but are frequently confused with infectious lesions. These lesions usually occur on the lip, soft palate, tongue, and cheek. The lesion is a white fibrous exudate with a erythematous border. No vesicles are present. The lesions are painful. The lesions heal spontaneously.

Aphthous ulcers are thought to be an autoimmune phenomenon. It is most common during childhood and early adult life, and is more common in higher socioeconomic groups.

KEY POINTS

1. Primary Herpes simplex infection frequently presents as gingivostomatitis.
2. Herpes may reactivate causing cold sores (fever blisters).
3. Thrush (Candida) usually occurs in infants after passing through an infected vaginal area.
4. Coxsackie viruses can cause oral lesions. Herpangina typically occurs in the posterior pharynx. Hand-foot-and-mouth disease involves the palms and soles, as well as the oral cavity.
5. Aphthous ulcers, although not due to infection, are frequently confused with an infectious process.

REFERENCES

1. Evans AS: *Viral Infections of Humans.* New York, Plenum Publishing Corp, 1982; pp 253-271.

2. Fiddan AP, Yeo JM, Stubbings R, et al: Successful treatment of herpes labialis with topical acyclovir Br Med J 1983; 286:1699-1701.
3. Wright JM, Taylor PP, Allen EP et al: A review of the oral manifestations of infections in pediatric patients. Pediatric Inf. Dis. 1984; 3:80-88.

REVIEW QUESTIONS

1.) Criteria for tympanocentesis include: (4)

2.) The diagnostic hallmarks of AOM are: (4)

3.) True or False

   1. Fever is a required criteria for diagnosing AOM.

   2. Pneumococcus and *H. influenzae* are responsible for the majority of AOM in children.

   3. All forms of penicillin are equally effective against *H. influenzae.*

   4. TMP-SMX is very effective against Group A beta hemolytic streptococci.

   5. The spectrum of organisms sensitive to ampicillin, amoxicillin, and Augmentin(R) are identical.

4.) True or False

   1. Periorbital edema is a clue to the presence of sinusitis.

   2. Tender sinuses may be seen in children with sinusitis.

   3. There is a relationship between the presence of sinusitis and the severity of asthma in children.

   4. Bacterial cultures from the nasopharynx are useful in determining the etiology of acute sinusitis.

5.) Common etiologies of pharyngitis include: (4)

6.) Antibiotic therapy appropriate for the treatment of streptococcal pharyngitis includes which of the following?

   a   penicillin

   b   trimethoprim - sulfamethexazole

   c   clindamycin

   d   erythromycin

7.) Match patient and organism

   A. 4 month old with pharyngeal injection and tonsilar exudate.

   B. 3 year old with pharyngeal injection and tonsilar exudate.

   C. 12 year old with pharyngeal injection, tonsilar exudate, and palpable spleen.

   D. 16 year old with pharyngeal injection and arthritis.

   1 Epstein-Barr Virus

   2 Group A streptococcus

   3 Adenovirus

   4 *N. gonorrhea*

8.) Match patient and organism

A. Onset up to 2 months post-inoculation solitary node usually tender node.

B. 5 years old, white child, usually rural resident, PPD 10mm, cervical node.

C. Associated with rash, conjunctivitis, cracking lips, peeling skin and cardiac abnormalities.

D. Black child, urban, abnormal chest X-ray, cervical node.

1. Epstein-Barr Virus
2. Atypical Mycobacteria
3. Kawasaki Disease
4. M. tuberculosis

9.) Match lesion in column A with associated disease in column B.

A. White painful fibrinous exudate with erythematous border.

B. Vesicles on tongue and perioral region that ulcerate.

C. Vesicles in posterior oral cavity, frequently occurring in summer.

D. White plaque on mucosal surfaces that have an erythematous or bloody base.

1. Aphthous ulcers
2. Thrush
3. Herpangina
4. Herpes Simplex infection

2

OCULAR INFECTIONS

BLEPHARITIS

Clinical Manifestations

Blepharitis is a recurrent, chronic inflammation of the eyelids. Symptoms include: scaling and itching of the lids, redness, and sometimes loss of eyelashes. Keratoconjunctivitis and thickened eyelids are reported. Occasionally, the infection may be localized to the angle of the lids (angular blepharitis). Preauricular adenopathy may be present. Commonly the disease begins as seborrhea and is then secondarily infected.

Etiology and Epidemiology

Blepharitis occurs fairly commonly in childhood. It is particularly common in patients with underlying diseases such as diabetes, debilitated patients, and patients with underlying skin disease.

Staphylococci (aureus and epidermitis) are the most common pathogens. Angular blepharitis is often caused by *Hemophilus duplex.* Herpes, molluscum contagiosum, warts, yeast, fungi, and a variety of other bacterial organisms have also been reported.

Diagnosis

Diagnosis is made by clinical appearance and culture of material from the lid. This condition needs to be distinguished from lice infection of the lids and from contact dermatitis involving the lid. When there is a viral etiology, there is frequently skin lesions which may suggest the diagnosis.

Treatment

When the etiology is bacterial, therapy usually consists of the use of topical antibiotics in association with warm compresses and scale removal. Antibiotics may be administered as ointment or drops, or both. Use of antiseptic soap for cleaning may help avoid spread. Topical IDU (idoxuri-dine) has been used for treating *Herpes simplex* blepharitis. If warts are present they must be carefully excised, and molluscum can be treated with incision of the lesion and expressing the contents. Prevention is best achieved by early institution of antiseborrhea treatment (selenium sulfide) and good hygiene.

Sequelae and Complications

Untreated, the patient can develop keratoconjunctivitis, hordeolum, or chalazia. Occasionally scarring may occur. Most viral lid infections are self-limited.

CHALAZIONS AND HORDEOLUMS

Clinical Manifestations

Hordeola are infections of hair follicles, meibomian glands or sebaceous glands near the margins of the lids. These are purulent infections. They usually appear as tender, painful swollen areas of the lid margin. A yellowish head usually forms. Hordeolums are frequently preceded by blepharitis.

Chalazia are chronic lipogranulomas of the meibomian gland. There is usually no inflammation and the lump develops slowly.

Etiology and Epidemiology

Hordeola are usually the result of staphylococcal infection. Usually the etiology is *S. Aureus*. Obstruction to drainage of the gland or follicle seems to predispose to the development of hordeola or chalazia.

Diagnosis

The typical clinical manifestations can usually make the diagnosis. Cultures from the lesion can be attempted; although they are frequently negative.

Treatment

Warm soaks to the hordeolum is usually sufficient therapy and results in drainage of the lesion. At times, surgical incision and drainage may be necessary. If there is an associated conjunctivitis or blepharitis, topic antibiotics should be used.

Chalazia that do not regress spontaneously need incision and curettage.

Sequelae and Complications

Recurrences are common. Good hygiene, control of seborrhea, and treatment of associated blepharitis can reduce the chances of recurrence.

DACRYOADENITIS AND DACRYOCYSTITIS

Clinical Manifestations

Dacryoadenitis is inflammation of the lacrimal gland. It is a relatively uncommon pediatric disease. Pain and swelling occur in the area of the gland. A discharge, conjunctivitis, and cellulitis may be present. Rarely, there is restriction of extraocular movement.

More common in pediatrics is dacryocystitis. This is inflammation of the lacrimal sac. Edema, swelling, and erythema are usually present. Discharge from the puncta is seen, and a secondary conjunctivitis may develop.

Etiology and Epidemiology

There are multiple etiologies for these two diseases. *Staphylococcus aureus* is the primary pathogen associated with dacryocystitis. Streptococci have also been reported. Dacryoadenitis is seen with Epstein-Barr infection in infectious mononucleosis. Staphylococci, chlamydia, and herpes zoster have also been associated with acute infection. Chronic dacryocystitis or dacryoadenitis is often associated with syphilis or tuberculosis.

Diagnosis

The diagnosis is made by clinical manifestations and culture results. If bacterial cultures are negative, appropriate chlamydial and viral cultures and serologies should be done.

Treatment

Dacryoadenitis should be treated with hot compresses and appropriate systemic antibiotics. Dacryocystitis requires the same treatment regimen. In mild cases of dacryoadenitis the use of local antibiotics may be sufficient. When obstruction of the nasal lacrimal duct persists surgery may be necessary to establish drainage.

Sequelae and Complications

When appropriately treated, complications are rare. The resolution of cases associated with systemic diseases (T.B., syphilis, mononucleosis, etc.) depends on adequate control or resolution of the systemic illness.

CELLULITIS

Clinical Manifestations

Cellulitis in the region of the eye can be divided into two types: orbital and preseptal. Orbital cellulitis involves the orbit and the area behind the orbital septum. Preseptal cellulitis is inflammation in periorbital tissue that is preseptal.

Orbital cellulitis is usually unilateral and is characterized by lid edema and erythema, orbital pain, proptosis, conjunctival injection, and chemosis. Eye motion is decreased and can be painful. Leukocytosis, fever, and in severe cases, decreased vision are present. Patients with orbital cellulitis often have an associated sinusitis, and therefore may have additional symptoms associated with the sinus infection.

Preseptal cellulitis may also have fever and a leukocytosis. Lid edema is frequently more mild than in orbital cellulitis. Conjunctivitis may be present although proptosis is usually absent. Decreased eye motion and pain on motion are usually not seen. Adjacent areas of skin near the eye may also be involved with the cellulitis.

Etiology and Epidemiology

Preseptal and orbital cellulitis are seen in children throughout the world. In children less than 3 years old *Haemophilus influenzae* is a common cause. In patients with debilitating disease, fungal sinusitis and orbital cellulitis have been reported.

In patients with preseptal cellulitis secondary to trauma, *Staphyloccus aureus* is most frequently recovered. *Streptococcus pyogenes* is also seen. *H. influenzae type b* is a frequent cause of preseptal and orbital cellulitis, especially in young children. *H. influenzae* infection is associated with hematogenous spread, and may be associated with *H. influenzae* infections at other body sites. Orbital cellulitis usually results from spread from contigous sites and most often is due to staphylococci, streptococci, pneumococci, or *H. influenzae* infection. Anaerobes are also found, especially when the sinuses are also involved.

Diagnosis

In patients with the symptom complex suggestive of orbital or preseptal cellulitis, attempts should be made to recover the organism. Blood cultures and cultures of adjacent skin lesions can be helpful. When a well demarcated leading edge of cellulitis is present on the skin adjacent to the orbit, an attempt should be made to aspirate the leading edge using a syringe with some nonbacteriostatic saline and a small gauge needle. This aspirate can then be sent for culture. If purulent conjunctivitis or sinusitis is also present, culture of the purulent material may also be of help in identifying the pathogen. If an orbital abscess is suspected, computed axial tomography may be of assistance.

Treatment

Initial therapy should cover the most likely organisms based on the age of the patient, associated findings, and possible mode of infection. Once culture results are available antibiotic therapy can be appropriately adjusted. Initial therapy, especially in young children, should include a penicillinase-resistant penicillin and chloramphenicol. Certain second and third generation cephalosporins will also provide adequate coverage. In older children with obvious skin trauma or impetigo, a penicillinase-resistant penicillin alone may be adequate. If there is concommitant sinusitis, improved anaerobic coverage will be attained by using penicillin G in addition to the antistaphylococcal coverage.

When *H. influenzae* is the etiology, a careful examination is necessary to rule out additional sites of infection. In infants, a lumbar puncture should be considered to rule out a meningitis. Occasionally, surgical drainage of orbital abscesses or paranasal sinuses is necessary.

Sequelae and Complications

With appropriate, high dose antibiotic therapy, complications are not frequent. Infrequently there may be extension into the CNS. Cavenous sinus thrombosis may develop. These patients may develop nausea and vomiting as well as papilledema and retinal vein engorgement due to the thrombosis. Increased ocular pressure or optic nerve involvement may lead to loss of vision.

CONJUNCTIVITIS

Clinical Manifestations

Symptoms vary somewhat depending on the etiology. Bacterial conjunctivitis usually is manifested by watery irritated eyes. The patient may then develop redness of the eyes and matting of the lids. Blurry vision and photophobia may also be present. Bilateral involvement is common. Conjunctiva are usually hyperemic. The appearance of small petechial hemorrhages suggests pneumococcal or hemophilus infection. A membrane or pseudomembrane can be seen in streptococcal or diphtherial conjunctivitis.

When the inflammation is severe, gonococcal infection is frequently seen. There is usually a large amount of pus. The eyes and lids are painful and tender. Chemosis, hyperemia and preauricular nodes may be present. Without treatment, corneal perforation and endophthalmitis may result.

Staphylococci can produce a chronic mucopurulent conjunctivitis. Small yellow or gray follicles may appear in the conjunctiva with viral or chlamydial infection.

Etiology and Epidemiology

Bacterial conjunctivitis is common in all pediatric age groups. It can be found throughout the world. Pneumococcal conjunctivitis is often the cause of "pink eye" which is frequently seen in school children and among family members. Crowding and winter months are frequently associated with outbreaks. During the summer months, *H. aegyptius* is a common cause of "pink eye." Ophthalmia neonatorum is conjunctivitis during the first three weeks of life as a result of inoculation of the neonates' skin and eye with either chlamydia or gonococcus as the child passes through the birth canal. Staphylococcus and herpes have also been implicated as etiologic agents. Besides causing conjunctivitis in neonates, gonococcus causes infection in adults and adolescents. The infection is primarily the result of sexual contact.

Pharyngoconjunctival fever and epidemic keratoconjunctivitis are usually due to adenovirus infection. Outbreaks are common, and both air droplet spread and fomites have been implicated in the spread.

Chlamydia trachomitis causes trachoma, a chronic follicular conjunctivitis with pannus formation. Conjunctival scarring may result. Trachoma is spread eye-to-eye and is found in India, Northern Africa, and the Middle East as an endemic infection. In the U.S., trachoma is seen among American Indians and Mexican Americans. Most chlamydial eye infections in the U.S. are inclusion conjunctivitis, frequently found in infants, and are spread from the genital tract. Worldwide, the incidence of trachoma is decreasing, but it remains the major cause of blindness in the world.

Other etiologies for conjunctivitis include: moraxella, pseudomonas, *Corynebacterium diphtheriae,* Epstein-Barr virus, *Herpes simplex,* varicella zoster virus, Newcastle virus, cat scratch disease, *Fransicella tularensis,* mycobacteria, and *Treponema pallidum.*

Diagnosis

The diagnosis can frequently be made on clinical grounds. Therapy depends on an accurate determination of the pathogen involved. Obtaining a smear and culture of the infection is important. Gram stain for bacteria and Giemsa staining for chlamydial inclusions can be helpful if properly done. Bacterial, viral and chlamydial cultures can also be of value.

Treatment

Bacterial conjunctivitis is usually self-limited but therapy can lead to a more rapid resolution of symptoms. Topical therapy (ointment in infants, drops in older children) are usually adequate therapy for pneumococcus, staphylococcus, hemophilus (non-*H. influenzae type b*) and chlamydial infections. In some other bacterial conjunctivitis infections, systemic therapy should also be included. This is particularly true of gonococci, pseudomonas, streptococci and *H. influenzae* type infections.

Sulfacetamide, a topical sulfonamide, is adequate therapy for conjunctivitis due to chlamydia, hemophilus species, pneumococcus and moraxella. Staphylococci can be treated with topical bacitracin. Erythromycin topical preparations can be used for pneumococcus and moraxella. Other infections should be treated based on sensitivities.

Prophylaxis against ophthalmia neonatorium can be accomplished with topical silver nitrate, tetracycline, or erythromycin. The latter two may be effective against chlamydia as well as gonococcus.

Sequelae and Complications

Treated appropriately, most bacterial conjunctivits resolve without sequelae. Untreated, neiserria and hemophilus infections may progress to corneal ulceration and, occasionally, to endophthalmitis. Systemic spread of these infections may also occur. Ophthalmia neonatorium may lead to blindness if not treated. Most viral conjunctivitis is self-limited, although recurrences, especially with herpes, occur. The prognosis of conjunctivitis associated with systemic diseases depends on successful therapy of the underlying systemic infection.

KERATITIS

Clinical Manifestations

Pain, irritation, tearing, edema, blurred vision, corneal vascular congestion, and occasionally photophobia are present in patients with keratitis, an inflammation of the cornea. There is usually an accompanying conjunctivitis which is responsible for many of the symptoms. Additional clinical manifestations are related to the specific etiology. Other symptoms include punctate infiltrates and superficial to deep ulcerations of the cornea. In severe cases, perforation of the cornea and the development of a pus pocket in the anterior chamber of the eye (hypopyon) may occur.

Etiology and Epidemiology

Many different organisms have been associated with keratitis. In children, the infection is usually superficial and is associated with staphylococcal infection, but many other organisms can also be responsible for keratitis. A partial list includes: *Herpes simplex,* varicella-zoster virus, *N. gonorrheae,* chlamydia, and adenovirus.

The epidemiologic pattern is dependent on the etiologic agent. Poor hygiene and malnutrition are associated with recurrent chlamydial infections; chronic eczema with staphylococci; immunodeficient, immunosuppressed, or oncology patients are predisposed to *Herpes simplex* keratitis; and neonates will sometimes contract herpes (type 2) while passing through the birth canal. In Africa, Mexico, Venezuela, and Guatemala, onchocerciasis occurs which may lead to blindness in as many as a third of the patients.

Diagnosis

Clinical manifestations usually suggest the diagnosis. Culture and cytology of scrapings of corneal lesions or accompanying conjunctivitis will aid in determining the specific etiology. If bacterial cultures are not diagnostic, then cytologic exam for multinucleated giant cells or inclusion bodies might suggest likely etiologies.

Treatment

The specific therapy depends on the etiologic agent. Antiviral therapy is available for herpetic lesions. Idoxuridine, trifluridine (1% solution), and Vidarabine (3% ointment) are available to treat herpetic eye infections. Bacterial infection will frequently respond to topical antibiotic preparations, however, in severe cases, especially due to pseudomonas, parenteral therapy may be needed.

Sequelae and Complications

Most keratitis that is superficial heals with little or no residual problems. More serious forms of keratitis may lead to scarring with associated loss of vision, perforation, secondary glaucoma, or cataracts.

UVEITIS

Clinical Manifestations

Uveitis refers to inflammation of iris, ciliary body, or choroid. It is frequently found in connection with retinitis. Pain, photophobia, decreased acuity and tearing are typical clinical manifestations. Often symptoms are more subtle and uveitis may present simply as decreased vision. Uveitis is frequently a component of systemic disease and is discovered as part of the workup to determine the extent of involvement of the systemic disease.

Etiology and Epidemiology

Uveitis is fairly rare in children but is often quite serious. Seven percent of all pediatric eye enucleations are due to uveitis. The most common cause of anterior uveitis (iris or ciliary body) is juvenile rheumatoid arthritis. Posterior uveitis (choroiditis) is often due to toxoplasmosis. The list of etiologies for uveitis, however, is huge and includes viruses such as the herpes group, adenoviruses, rubella, and mumps; bacteria including staphylococcus, Neisseria, and Listeria; fungi-like coccidioidomycosis, candida, cryptococcus, histoplasma; and assorted other organisms like the mycobacteria; spirochetes; and parasites like toxocara, toxoplasma, and onchocerca.

Diagnosis

Symptoms, associated findings, and systemic symptoms may suggest a differential diagnosis. Appropriate serologic tests (syphilis, rubella, CMV, toxoplasmosis, etc.) may be useful. Viral cultures from appropriate sites, and bacterial cultures may also prove helpful.

Treatment

The therapy depends on the underlying etiologic agent. In severe cases, adjunctive therapy using steroids, topical mydriatics and cycloplegics may be necessary. (Appropriate therapy for various underlying etiologies can be found in other section of this book.)

Sequelae and Complications

In severe cases, enucliation may result. In less severe cases, the extent of involvement is influenced, at least in part, by the etiology. Early intervention usually aids in limiting the extent of damage.

KEY POINTS

1. Blepharitis is a recurrent, chronic infection of the eyelids, frequently caused by staphylococci and treated with topical antibiotics.
2. Hordeola are infections of hair follicles, meibomian glands, or sebaceous glands near the margins of the eyelids, usually caused by staphylococci and treated with warm soaks.
3. Chalazia are chronic lypogranulomas of the meibomian gland and often regress spontaneously.
4. Dacryoadenitis is an inflamation of the lacrimal gland due to a variety of organisms. It is treated with warm compresses and appropriate antimicrobial therapy.
5. Dacryocystitis is inflamation of the lacrimal sac, primarily due to staphylococci and will usually respond to compresses and antibiotics (local or systemic).
6. Cellulitis (orbital and preseptal) is frequently due to *H. influenzae, S. aureus* or streptococci. Careful evaluation for extension of this infection is important. Initial therapy frequently includes chloramphenicol and an antistaphylococcal antibiotic.
7. Conjunctivitis can result from infection by a wide variety of organisms. Common symptoms include red, watery eyes, blurry vision and photophobia. Usually a self-limited infection, treatment will often speed recovery and prevent complications.

REFERENCES

1. Barrett-Conner E: Gonorrhea and the pediatrician. Am J Dis Child. 1973; 125: 233-238.
2. Boger WP: Late ocular complications in congenital rubella syndrome. Ophthalmo 1980; 87:1244-1252.
3. Dawson C, Darrell R, Hannal, et al: Infections due to adenovirus type 8 in the United States. N Engl J Med 1963; 268:1034-1037.

4. Grayston JT, Wang S: New Knowledge of Chlamydia and the diseases they cause. J Infect Dis 1975; 132:87-105.

5. Jones DB: Microbial preseptal and orbital cellulitis in Duane, T.D. (ed): *Clinical Ophthalmology.* Vol. 4. Hagerstown, Md., Harper and Row, 1976, Chapter 25 pp 1-19.

6. Londer L, Nelson DL: Orbital cellulitis due to Haemphilus influenzae. Arch Ophthalmo. 1974; 91:89-91.

7. Meisler DD, Bosworth DE, Krachmer JH: Ocular infectious mononucleosis manifested as Parinaud's oculoglandular syndrome. A, J. Ophthalmo 1981; 92: 722-726.

8. Patriarca PA, Onorata IM, Sklar VE, et al: Acute hemorrhage conjunctivitis. Investigation of a large-scale community outbreak in Dade County, Florida. JAMA 1983; 249:1283-1286.

9. Shackelford PG, Smith M: Ocular infections in *Textbook of Pediatric Infectious Diseases* Cherry J and Feigin R (eds); 1981, Saunders, Philadelphia, pp 661-683.

10. Thygeson P: Complications of staphlococcal blepharitis. Am J Ophthalmo 1969; 68: 446-449.

11. Wilhelmus KR: Ocular involvement in infectious mononucleosis. Am J Ophthalmo 1973; 117-118.

12. Wilkinson CP, Walch RB: Introcular Toxocara. Am J Ophthalmo 1971; 71: 921-930.

REVIEW QUESTIONS

1.) Match the infection with the appropriate description:

A. Conjunctivitis	1. recurrent, chronic inflamation of the eyelids.
B. Orbital Cellulitis	
C. Blepharitis	2. infection of hair follicles or glands near the lid margins.
D. Hordeolum	
E. Dacryocystitis	3. inflamation of the lacrimal sac.
F. Uveitis	
	4. lid edema, orbital pain, proptosis, chemosis, erythema, decreased eye motion.
	5. when caused by chlamydia may result in pannus formation and conjunctival scarring.
	6. often associated with juvenile rheumatoid arthritis.

2.) Match the organism with the appropriate description:

A. Adenovirus	1. Ophthalmia neonatorum
B. Chlamydia trachomatis	2. "Pink Eye"
C. H. influenzae	3. Pharyngoconjunctival fever
D. N. gonorrhea	4. Chronic follicular conjunctivitis.
E. H. aegyptius	5. preseptal cellulitis.

3

RESPIRATORY INFECTIONS

Clinical Manifestations

Cough, fever, tachypnea, rales, ronchi, and wheezes are all associated with lower respiratory tract infections. Flaring of the nares, pleural chest pain, and increased sputum production are also seen. The presence of any or all of these signs and symptoms should suggest the possibility of lower respiratory tract infection (LRTI).

While it is often difficult to distinguish the cause of LRTIs based on clinical criteria alone, certain characteristics of the presentation may suggest a specific etiology.

Adenovirus - Frequently presents with an acute onset. Fever, cough, dyspnea, tachypnea, and wheezes are often present. The presence of conjunctivitis in this clinical setting is often a helpful clue. These children may appear quite ill. The presentation may be suggestive of a bacterial etiology.

Respiratory Syncytial Virus (RSV) - This is responsible for much of the bronchiolitis we see. Occasionally it may result in pneumonitis. Fever, wheezes (especially expiratory), dyspnea, cough, and mild cyanosis are commonly present. RSV infections tend to be seasonal, the incidence being highest during the winter.

Chlamydia trachomatis (CT) - A major cause of pneumonitis in infants (especially during the first 6 months of life). CT infections are usually prolonged afebrile illnesses. Cough, congestion and tachypnea are commonly seen. About half the cases are associated with conjunctivitis. The cough is frequently described as staccato in character. More serious cases may mirror pertussis. *REMEMBER:* In infants with an afebrile pneumonitis, think chlamydia.

Streptococcous pneumoniae (Pn) - The major bacterial cause of pneumonia in children, Pn usually presents with an abrupt onset. Shaking chills, fever, cough and pleural pain may be present. Pn pneumonia may occur anytime during childhood. As the child's age increases these classic symptoms become more likely.

Hemophilus influenzae (HI) - HI is more likely to cause infection in preschool age children than in older children. Clinically it is not readily distinguished from Pn pneumonia.

Mycoplasma pneumoniae (MP) - This is usually a mild pneumonitis. Fever, cough, rales, and sore throat are commonly seen. MP infection is rare in preschool age children. It is associated with an exanthem, headache and malaise. *REMEMBER:* If the chest x-ray findings appear more severe than the clinical state of the patient, think mycoplasma.

Mycobacterium tuberculosis (MTB) - Infections with MTB still occur in children in the U.S. Infants and adolescents seem to be particulary susceptible. The onset is usually insidious and cough and night sweats are seen. The presentation may be very similar to some fungal pneumonitis clinical presentations. *Histoplasma capsulatum* and *Coccidioides immitus* are responsible for pneumonitis in children living in those parts of the country in which these organisms are endemic.

(For Respiratory Infections in the neonate see the chapter on Neonatal Infections.)

CMV, pneumocystis, Epstein-Barr virus, Staphylococcus, group A Beta-hemolytic streptococcus, and varicella zoster are some of the other causes of common respiratory tract infections in children.

Etiology and Epidemiology

Most respiratory infections in children are non-bacterial. The specific causes of a respiratory infection is age related, but there is considerable overlap. RSV, CT, and adenovirus are all seen during the first year of life. After 9 months of age, CT becomes uncommon. Most cases of adenovirus are seen by 18 months of age, and RSV is most common in children under 2 years of age and frequently occurs in the winter. *H. influenzae* is seen throughout childhood but decreases in frequency after 4 years old, and *S. pneumoniae* is seen throughout childhood. Mycoplasma is usually first seen in school age children, and tuberculosis is found most commonly in infants and adolescents.

Diagnosis

The diagnosis of a lower respiratory infection can usually be made on clinical ground (see symptoms) in conjunction with a chest x-ray. Determining the specific organism responsible for the infection may be more difficult. Blood cultures for bacterial pathogens are helpful if they grow an organism, but a negative blood culture does not rule out bacterial pneumonia. *S. Pneumoniae* pneumonia is associated with a negative blood culture at least 50% of the time. Sputum cultures are of questionable value and are difficult to impossible to obtain from infants and young children. In older children where sputum may be obtainable, Gram stain of the specimen may be helpful. In seriously ill children, pleural fluid, lung aspirate fluid, or lung biopsy specimen may yield a pathogen. Antigen detection methods such as counterimmunoelectrophoresis and latex agglutination can also be useful.

Viral etiologies can be identified by culture of throat, nasopharyngeal (NP), and stool specimens. Florescent antibody staining of exfoliative cells or respiratory secretions may also be helpful. Serial antibody determinations to adenovirus can make a retrospective diagnosis.

Chlamydia trachomatis can be diagnosed by isolation of the organism from nasopharyngeal (NP) aspirate, swab of the NP, or tracheal aspirate. In addition, antibody to CT can be detected in serum, tears, or NP.

Mycoplasma can be cultured in laboratories equipped for this. Specific antibodies against mycoplasma can be obtained. Cold agglutinins may be present in mycoplasma infection, but are also sometimes present in viral disease, and therefore the test is not specific.

Suspicion of TB can be confirmed by doing a PPD. Sputum cultures, acid fast staining, and gastric aspirate (usually in the morning prior to eating) for culture and acid fast staining are additional diagnositic aids. Fungal infection may be diagnosed by serology and by culture. Skin testing for histoplasmosis is not recommended.

Radiologic findings are quite variable. Lobar consolidation is more common in bacterial pneumonia than in non-bacterial pneumonia. It is important to attempt to distinguish consolidation from atelectasis, which is sometimes seen in non-bacterial pulmonary infections. Effusion, when present, usually suggest bacterial infection. Fungal pulmonary infections may cause a nodular, lobar or interstitial pattern on x-ray. Cavitary or mass lesions may also be seen radiologically in fungal infections. Perihilar lesions may make it difficult to distinguish fungal infection from tuberculosis. Chest x-ray findings in patients with tuberculosis are variable. Hilar or mediastinal adenpathy, pulmonary infiltrates, calcifications, and evidence of pleurisy should suggest the possibility of tuberculosis. *REMEMBER:* Primary tuberculosis lesions in the lung may occur in any lobe, not just lower lobes. Interstitial and alveolar patterns are frequently seen in viral pneumonitis. Hyperinflation and patchy atelectasis is often seen in RSV infection. In immunocompromised patients who are infected with *Pneumocystis carinii,* chest x-rays reveal interstitial and alveolar patterns. Chlamydia infection may cause hyperinflation, peribronchial thickening and occasionally focal consolidation or an interstitial pattern may be present. *Mycoplasma pneumoniae* pneumonia is characterized by either lobar or alveolar involvement. *REMEMBER:* There may be very poor correlation between the severity of symptoms and the extent of mycoplasma disease seen on the chest x-ray.

Treatment

An initial decision to institute therapy must be based on how ill the patient appears and on available clinical, radiological, and laboratory data. In seriously ill children, the initiation of antibiotic therapy is usually indicated pending the results of cultures and other diagnostic laboratory aids.

Bacterial pneumonia - *S. pneumoniae* and *H. influenzae* are the two most common bacterial pathogens in children. Ampicillin and/or chloramphenicol are appropriate initial coverage. In mild disease, oral amoxicillin is appropriate initial therapy. A decision to use ampicillin alone must be based on the frequency of *H. influenzae* resistance in your area and on the seriousness of the child's illness. In older children, *H. influenzae* decreases in frequency and penicillin alone may be sufficient treatment. Second generation cephalosporins such as cefuroxime are alternatives to the use of ampicillin and chloramphenicol. Continued deterioration or lack of response within 48-72 hours should result in further efforts to determine the organism and/or a change in therapy. Antibiotic coverage may need to be expanded to cover staphylococcal infection.

Chlamydial pneumonia - Erythromycin or sulfonamide therapy will improve symptoms usually within one week and eliminate shedding in 2-3 weeks. Tetracycline is also effective but should not be used in children.

Mycoplasma pneumonia - Both erythromycin and tetracycline are effective for treating *Mycoplasma pneumonia.* Tetracycline is not recommended for use in children. The effectiveness of therapy is related to early initiation of therapy.

Tuberculosis - Therapy for TB pneumonia is usually isoniazid plus rifampin. In serious or extensive disease, streptomycin is also added for the initial 4 weeks. Therapy is usually 12 - 18 month. Is it desirable to obtain drug sensitivities for the patients' organism, if available. This is especially true for patients who may have acquired their infection from outside the United States.

Viral Pneumonitis - Adenoviral pneumonitis is usually managed with supportive care. Gammaglobulin may be valuable in life-threatening infection. Respiratory syncitial virus pneumonitis is also managed with appropriate supportive measures. Ribavirin appears to be of value in shortening the course of the disease and decreasing viral shedding. Its use has so far been reserved for serious and life-threatening infection. Interferon therapy may play a role in the treatment of RSV in the future. Most other viral respiratory infections are handled with supportive care.

Fungal pneumonias - The antifungal agent chosen depends on the specific fungus isolated and drug sensitivities when available. Antifungal agents available include amphotericin-B, 5-flurocytosine and miconazole. In addition, ketoconazole, an oral preparation may be appropriate for some fungal infections.

Sequelae and Complications

Most lower respiratory tract infections in otherwise healthy children resolve with few sequelae or complications. Occasionally pleural effusions and empyemas occur. Clinical findings may suggest their presence, and x-ray can help confirm it. Thoracentesis is usually advisable to distinguish pleural effusion from abscess. The distinction may be important therapeutically.

Lung abscesses are rare and are usually diagnosed on x-ray. Pneumatocele and pneumothoraces can also complicate lower respiratory tract infections.

KEY POINTS

1. Chlamydia pneumonitis often presents as an afebrile illness with cough, tachypnea, hyperinflated lungs and conjunctivitis.
2. Mycoplasma pneumonia is seen infrequently in preschool age children.
3. Mycoplasma pneumonia is seen infrequently in preschool age children. pin. In the southwest part of the U.S., coccidioides infection may

Miscellaneous Other Causes of Lower Respiratory Tract Infections in Children

Organism	Comments
Staphylococcus aureus	Often rapidly progressive infection in neonates and immunocompromised patients.
	Associated with pneumatoceles, abscesses, and pleural effusions.
	Treatment with anti-staph. penicillins
Varicella-Zoster virus	Usually in immunocompromised or infants.
	May respond to ARA-A or Acyclovir treatment.
Herpes simplex virus	Neonate, immunocompromised
	High mortality - often associated with disseminated disease.
	May respond to ARA-A or Acyclovir treatment.
Pneumocystis carinii	Neonate, immunocompromised patients rapidly progressive - uniformly fatal without treatment.
	Treatment [with TMS/pentamidine*]
	Pentamidine side effects - abnormal renal function, decreased calcium, rashes, decreased BP, hematologic abnormalities.
Toxocara Canis (VLM)	Symptoms - cough, wheeze, enlarged liver, pulmonary infiltrates-often greater than 30% eosinophils, increased IgE.
	Diagnosis - History, percipitant Ab's-of larvae on biopsy. ELISA/RIA also used.
	Treatment - Thiabendazole.
Legionella pneumophilla (Legionellosis)	Rare in children. Symptoms - **low grade fever, weakness, malaise, anorexia, cough**, diarrhea, shaking chills, bradycardia. Chest x-ray - patchy alveolar infiltrate. Lobar consolidation.
	Diagnosis - culture-positive in 5-7 days. FA staining on pleural fluid, sputum, or lung tissue - serology.
	Treatment - erythromycin x 3 weeks.
Cytomegalovirus	Primarily a disease of neonates and immunocompromised patients.
	Causes a diffuse interstitial pneumonitis.
	Diagnosis made by urine or saliva culture, by serial sera for antibody titers, or by fluorescent staining of biopsy specimen.
	Most CMV infections are asymptomatic.

*TMS=Trimethoprim-sulfamethoxazole

resemble tuberculosis. Histoplasma may also mimic tuberculosis. Histoplasmosis is endemic to areas of the Ohio and Mississippi Valleys, Panama, Mexico, and to a lesser extent is found in areas of Australia, the Philippines, South America, Europe, and South Africa.

4. RSV, CT and adenovirus pneumonitis are primarily seen during the first year of life.

REFERENCES

1. Asher MI, Spier S, Beland M, et al: Primary Lung Abscess in Childhood. Am J Dis Child 1982; 136:491–494.

2. Dworsky ME, Stagno S: Newer agents causing pneumonitis in early infancy. Pediatr Infect Dis 1982; 1:188–195.

3. Fosarelli PD, Deangelis C, Winkelstein J, et al: Infectious illnesses in the first two years of life. Pediatr Infect Dis 1985; 4:153–159.

4. Glezen WP, Denny FW: Epidemiology of acute lower respiratory disease in children. N Eng J Med 1973; 288:498–505.

5. Grossman M, Klein JO, McCarthy PL, et al: Consensus: Management of presumed bacterial pneumonia in ambulatory children. Pediatr Infect Dis 1984; 3(Suppl):497–502.

6. Krasinski K: Severe respiratory syncitial virus infection: Clinical features, nosocomial acquisition and outcome. Pediatr Infect Dis 1985; 4:250–257.

7. Lorin ML, Hsu KHK, Jacob SC, et al: Treatment of tuberculosis in children. Pediatr Clin North Am 1983; 30: 333–348.

8. Odio C, McCracken GH, Nelson JD: Disseminated adenovirus infection: A case report and review of the literature. Pediatr Infect Dis 1984; 3:46–49.

9. Radkowski MA, Kranzler JK, Beem MO, et al: Chlamydia pneumonia in infants: Radiography in 125 cases. Am J Roentgenology 1981; 137:703–706.

10. Stagno S, Brasfield DM, Brown MD, et al: Infant's pneumonitis associated with cytomegalovirus, Chlamydia, Pneumocystis and Ureplasma: A prospective study. Pediatrics 1981; 68:322–329.

11. Storey DD, Dines DE, Coles DT: Pleural effusion - A diagnostic dilemma. JAMA 1976; 236: 2183–2186.

EPIGLOTTITIS AND CROUP

Epiglottitis

Clinical Manifestations

Epiglottitis is an infection of the supraglottic region with associated edema. The edema can result in airway obstruction. Typically, the patient presents with a febrile illness with an abrupt onset. The patient is in respiratory distress and frequently sits leaning forward with his neck hyperextended to facilitate breathing. Drooling and restlessness are also seen. Commonly, the patient complains of a sore throat. The peripheral white blood cell count is usually elevated.

Etiology and Epidemiology

The overwhelming majority of cases of epiglottitis are caused by *H. influenzae* type B. Rare cases due to *Streptococcus pneumoniae, H. parainfluenzae* and *Staphylococcus aureus* have been reported.

Seventy-five percent of patients with epiglottitis are between 1 and 5 years of age. Infection is most common in winter months with an occasional smaller peak in the summer. Epiglottitis is primarily seen in temperate climates.

Infection is most likely the result of direct invasion by *H. influenzae* with a secondary bacteria. Some evidence exists for a genetic predisposition to epiglottitis.

Diagnosis

Epiglottitis is a life-threatening infection. It is therefore important to consider the diagnosis in patients presenting with appropriate symptoms, and then rapidly confirm the diagnosis so that treatment can be started.

Diagnosis is made by visualizing the epiglottis. The typical appearance is that of a cherry red, swollen epiglottis. Visualization of the epiglottis should be done under controlled circumstances so that if airway obstruction occurs, intubation or tracheostomy can be done. At many medical centers, the direct visualization of the epiglottis is done in the operating room with an otolaryngologist and an anesthesiologist present to assist if necessary. A lateral neck radiograph will show a swollen ("thumbprint") epiglottis. If visualization of the epiglottis is to be done, the radiograph is unnecessary and may waste valuable time. Cultures of the epiglottis and blood should be obtained.

Treatment

Once the diagnosis is made, the airway must be secured. In most medical centers, intubation is the preferred mode of maintaining an airway. Frequently a nasotracheal (NT) tube can be placed. Complications with a nasotracheal tube appear to be rare. Tracheotomy is an alternative to intubation. Nasotracheal tubes need stay in place an average of about two days before extubation can be attempted safely.

Antibiotic therapy should be initiated after the airway has been secured and cultures obtained. Chloramphenicol should be started. Therapy can be altered once the organism is identified and antibiotic sensitivities are obtained.

Sequelae and Complications

Acute airway obstruction is the major complication to be feared. Promptly securing the airway and good care in maintaining the airway can greatly reduce the risk of this problem. Infrequently bacteremic spread to other sites occurs. Meningitis, arthritis, and pericarditis have infrequently been reported.

CROUP

Clinical Manifestations

Croup is a term used to describe an illness that is characterized by hoarseness, a barky cough, and inspiratory stridor. Although the term croup is used to describe a variety of entities all characterized by obstruction in the laryngeal area, this section will primarily deal with acute laryngotracheitis, an infection usually of viral origin causing subglottic narrowing of the airway.

These patients are often febrile but are not dysphagic, nor do they usually appear toxic. Pharyngitis, if present, is minimal, and the epiglottis appears normal. Frequently upper respiratory symptoms precede the onset of croup.

Etiology and Epidemiology

A variety of viruses are responsible for causing croup. Parainfluenzae viruses are the most common etiologic agent. Influenzae viruses, respiratory syncytial viruses, and adenoviruses cause croup less frequently than does parainfluenza.

Most cases of croup occur during the first three years of life. The illness is seen more frequently in boys than in girls. Many outbreaks of croup occur during the late fall and winter months.

Diagnosis

The diagnosis of croup is usually made on clinical grounds. Subglottic narrowing of the airway can be seen on posterior-anterior (PA) views of the neck. Occasionally croup must be differentiated from epiglottitis. This can usually be done by direct visualization of the epiglottitis under controlled circumstances (see diagnosis of epiglottitis section) or by obtaining PA and lateral neck films. If identification of the specific viruses is desirable, nasopharyngeal or throat cultures can be obtained for viral identification.

Treatment

Therapy is supportive. Mist therapy is the hallmark of croup management. Mild hypoxia is frequently seen, and these children should also receive oxygen. There is no clear evidence that steroid therapy benefits a child with croup. Racemic epinephrine provides acute but transient improvement in patients, although rebounds occur requiring repeat treatment. Racemic epinephrine, therefore, should not be used on outpatients.

Sequelae and Complications

Complications including pulmonary edema, respiratory failure, pneumothorax and death are infrequently seen today. Secondary bacterial infections may occur and should be appropriately treated.

KEY POINTS

1. Distinguishing croup from epiglottitis is critically important so that appropriate life-saving intervention can be made, especially in the case of epiglottitis.
2. Typically, epiglottitis has a sudden onset of respiratory distress, fever, and a toxic appearance. Dysphagia, hyperextension of the neck and a swollen epiglottitis seen on lateral neck radiograph or on direct visualization are classically present.
3. Croup usually has a gradual onset with fever, hoarseness and a barking cough. Frequently upper respiratory symptoms antedate the croup. Posterior-Anterior films of the neck show subglottic narrowing.
4. There is enough similarity and overlap of clinical presentations of croup and epiglottitis that the diagnosis should be made cautiously.

SELECTED REFERENCES

1. Holdaway MD: Croup and epiglottitis: Diagnosis and action. Drugs 1977; 13:452–457.
2. Molteni RA: Epiglottitis: Incidence of extra epiglottic infection, Report of 72 cases and review of the literature. Pediatrics 1976; 58:526–531.
3. Rapkin RH: Nasotracheal intubation in epiglottitis. Pediatrics 1975; 56:110–112.
4. Westley CR, Cotton EK, Brooks JG: Nebulized racemic epinephrine by IPPB for the treatment of croup. A double-blind study. Am J Dis Child 1978; 132:484–487.

PERTUSSIS SYNDROME

Clinical Presentation

There are three stages of the syndrome. The first is the catarrhal stage during which non-specific upper respiratory symptoms occur. This lasts one to two weeks and is followed by the paroxysmal stage. This stage is characterized by progressively severe coughing which is often followed by a high pitched whoop. This stage usually lasts two to four weeks and is followed by the convalescent stage. Recovery may take one or more months. Lymphocytosis is common and is usually quite marked in patients whose illness is due to *Bordetella pertussis.*

Epidemiology and Etiology

The pertussis syndrome can be caused by either *Bordetella pertussis* or *Bordetella parapertussis.* The role of other etiologic agents in causing the pertussis syndrome remains controversial. B pertussis is highly contagious, especially during the catarrhal stage. In general, B pertussis causes more serious disease than does B parapertussis.

The pertussis syndrome can occur in both adults and children. In adults, symptoms may be very atypical and mild. Partially immunized children may also have an atypical presentation or milder symptoms. Unimmunized infants usually have the most serious course with the highest morbidity and mortality. The infection is spread by the respiratory tract.

Diagnosis

Clinical diagnosis should be confirmed by laboratory studies. Culture of the organism is the most specific method of diagnosis. Late in the disease there are a significant number of false negative results, however. An alternative method of diagnosis is immunofluorescent antibody staining (IFA). This method is rapid and very sensitive. Efforts should be made to have experienced personnel read the slides in order to reduce the number of false positive results. Serologic methods are available for retrospective diagnosis.

Treatment

Adequate antibiotic therapy for pertussis does not exist. Erythromycin therapy within a few days of exposure to pertussis may help prevent clinical disease, however, once the paroxysmal stage begins, antibiotics appear to do little to alter the clinical course. Erythromycin or trimethoprin sulfamethoxazole therapy for 7 to 14 days will reduce the infectivity of the patient.

Pertussis can be prevented by use of vaccine. It is 80-90% effective in preventing acquisition of the organism and the prevention of symptomatic disease. Despite occasional serious side effects from the vaccine, the risk of serious disease from *B.pertussis* outweighs the risk of the vaccine in infants and young children.

Sequelae and Complications

Death can occur as a result of pertussis. Mortality rates are highest in infants. Apneas, seizures, hypoxia, intracerebral bleeding from coughing, subconjunctival hemorrhages and pneumonia are among the reported complications.

KEY POINTS

1. Pertussis can be prevented by immunization.
2. Erythromycin given soon after infection occurs can abort or modify the disease. Once classic pertussis symptoms begin, erythromycin may decrease length of time the patient is infectious, but will not significantly modify symptoms.
3. Diagnosis can be confirmed by culture or immunofluorescence.

REFERENCES

1. Donaldson P, Whitaker JA: Diagnosis of pertussis by fluorescent antibody staining of nasopharyngeal smears. AM J Dis Child 1980; 99:423–427.
2. Geller RJ. The Pertussis Syndrome: A persistent problem. In Nelson JD, McCracken GH (eds). Clinical Reviews in Pediatric Infectious Diseases. Phila: B.C.Decker, Inc., 1985: 187–192.

3. Henry RL, Dorman DC, Skinner JA et al: Antimicrobial therapy in whooping cough. Med J Australia 1981; 2:27–28.
4. Hinman AR, Koplan JP: Pertussis and pertussis vaccine: Reanalysis of benefits, risks, and costs. JAMA 1984; 251: 3109–3113.
5. Nelson JD: The changing epidemiology of pertussis in young infants. AM J Dis Child 1978, 132: 371–373.

REVIEW QUESTIONS

1.) Match illness with description.

A. Pertussis	1. Positive cold-agglutinins, school age children, CXR more severe than symptoms suggest.
B. Chlamydia pneumonitis	
C. RSV bronchiolitis	
D. Croup	2. Peak pediatric incidence in infants and adolescents, insidious, night sweats.
E. Epiglottitis	
F. Tuberculosis	
G. Pneumococcal pneumonia	3. Whoop, preventable with vaccine, erythromycin, lymphocytosis.
H. Mycoplasma pneumonia	

4. Afebrile pneumonitis, infant, conjunctivitis.
5. Abrupt onset, febrile, drooling, hyperextended neck, usually due to *H. influenzae.*
6. Subglottic narrowing, viral etiology, mist therapy.
7. Most common bacterial etiology of pneumonia.
8. Fever, wheezing, mild cyanosis, may respond to ribavirin.

2.) True or False
1. Most epiglottitis can be treated with chloramphenicol.
2. Lateral x-ray of neck is helpful in diagnosing croup.
3. First priority in suspected epiglottitis is securing the airway.
4. Croup usually has a gradual onset with fever, hoarseness and a barking cough.
5. Pertussis is usually a mild illness and immunization is no longer recommended.

3.) The 3 stages of pertussis are:

4.) List the steps in the evaluation and treatment of epiglottitis.

4

GASTROINTESTINAL INFECTIONS

ACUTE INFECTIOUS NON-BACTERIAL GASTROENTERITIS (AING)

Infectious gastroenteritis is a major cause of morbidity and mortality throughout the world. In the late 1970's, the annual incidence of diarrhea was in the billions, and mortality was estimated to be in the millions. Mortality in infants in third world nations from diarrhea is high. Some of the most important and common ones will be discussed here.

The most common symptom complex includes vomiting, diarrhea, fever and malaise. The result is dehydration (usually isotonic) and an inbalance in electrolytes. These abnormalities can be potentially life threatening, especially in infants, unless appropriately corrected. The most common etiologies for AING are rotaviruses and Norwalk viruses (see chart). Other viruses associated with AING are coronavirus-like particles, enteroviruses, adenoviruses, calciviruses, and possibly astroviruses.

ROTAVIRUS

Clinical Manifestations

Diarrhea is the major symptom. It can be severe, is usually watery and lasts about one week. Vomiting is sometimes present but usually is of shorter duration than the diarrhea. Fever may be present. Respiratory symptoms are commonly seen. If it is not prevented or reversed, severe dehydration may occur with associated lethargy, irritability and weakness.

Etiology and Epidemology

Rotavirus is a 70 nm diameter RNA virus with the appearance of a wheel rim. Rotavirus is primarily a pathogen of infants and young children. It is much less common in adults. In temperate climates, rotavirus infection accounts for about 50% of the children less than 2 years old who are hospitalized for diarrhea, and that usually occurs during the cooler months. In the tropics the infection occurs year round. In many third world countries it is responsible for much morbidity and mortality in infants.

The incubation period is believed to be one to three days, and the virus is spread via the fecal-oral route. The virus can continue to be shed in stool after symptoms have disappeared. Spread within institutions has been reported. While most children over 2 years of age and adults have antibody to rotavirus, the role of systemic antibody is protection from rotavirus is not clear. There are more than one serotype of rotavirus and sequential infection has been reported. Neonatal rotavirus infection does not confer immunity but may result in milder reinfections.

Diagnosis

While it is possible to culture rotavirus, it is very difficult and not practical in clinical settings. Rotavirus is best identified either by election microscopy (EM), or by serological technique. In many centers, EM may not be readily available. Serologic methods are used to identify rotavirus antigen. Enzyme linked immunosorbent assay, radioimmunoassay, counterimmunoelectrophoresis, as well as other methods have been used. *REMEMBER:* The definitive diagnosis of rotavirus gastroenteritis may be difficult, as a recent study has suggested that many asymptomatic infants may have rotavirus in the stool.

Treatment

No antiviral therapy currently exists that will treat rotavirus. Therapy is supportive. Correction of electrolyte inbalance and rehydration are the cornerstones of therapy. In mild to moderate cases where vomiting is infrequent or non-existant, oral rehydration may be appropriate. If the patient is unable to retain oral fluids or if the dehydration is more serious, intravenous rehydration may be indicated. *REMEMBER:* Correction of fluid and electrolyte abnormalities may produce undesirable consequences such as convulsions, especially when fluids are given too rapidly or incorrectly. An oral vaccine against rotavirus is under investigation.

Sequelae and Complications

Fatalities associated with rotavirus infection in the U.S.A. are rare and usually associated with severe dehydration or electrolyte abnormalities. Lactose malabsorption and intolerance after rotaviral diarrhea are common. Most cases of rotavirus infection are self-limited and resolve completely.

NORWALK AGENT

Clinical Manifestations

The illness usually begins suddenly. Symptoms include diarrhea, vomiting, nausea and abdominal cramps. In addition, fever (usually low-grade), anorexia, myalgias, malaise and headache can be seen. The symptoms usually abate within 24 to 48 hours. Hospitalization is rarely needed. Complications are rarely seen. Gastric emptying time may be prolonged and xylose and fat malabsorption may occur. Transient lymphopenia has been reported.

Etiology and Epidemology

The illness is frequently epidemic and is seen primarily in cooler months. Norwalk Agent gastroenteritis is rarely seen in infancy. It is an illness of school age children, teens and adults. Transmission is by the fecal-oral route. Food-borne infections have been reported as have infection associated with lake swimming. Its incubation period is 1 to 2 days. The virus is shed in stool for at least three days after the onset of illness, and may also be found in vomitus.

Immunity does not follow the expected pattern. Subjects exposed to the virus who become ill are more likely to become ill again on re-exposure despite the presence of antibody. Subjects exposed to virus who did not become ill do not become ill on re-exposure despite the lack of antibody. The presence of antibody against Norwalk Agent may, therefore, increase the risk for developing illness.

Diagnosis

Laboratory diagnosis is made by immunoelectron microscopy or immune adherence hemagglutination assay. Neither of these are yet commercially available, therefore, the diagnosis is usually made on clinical and epidemiologic grounds.

Treatment

There is no specific therapy for gastroenteritis due to Norwalk Agent. Most cases are mild and can be managed with oral fluid rehydration and symptomatic therapy.

Sequelae and Complications

Complete recovery is the rule. Malabsorption problems secondary to Norwalk Agent infection are transient. As this infection is infrequent in infants, severe life-threatening dehydration or electrolyte inbalance is rare.

OTHER AING

Other viral etiologies of gastroenteritis include coronavirus-like particles, astrovirus, adenovirus and the enteroviruses. In addition, calcivirus has been associated with mild gastroenteritis in children. Symptoms resemble those of the other AING. In neonates, gastroenteritis due to coronavirus-like particles have been associated with watery bloody stools and gastric distension. Therapy is supportive, and sequelae or complications are rare.

	Organism	Disease	Epidemiology
Rotarvirus	RNA; 70 nm diameter; double-shelled structure; wheelrim appearance.	Sporadic; usually infants/young children 1 week duration; diarrhea-watery may be associated with respiratory symptoms; fever, vomiting; disease in adults is rare.	major pathogen in infant gastroenteritis; occurs in cooler months in temperate climates; fecal-oral spread; 1-3 day incubation period; most children over 2 years old have antibody to rotavirus; immunity is probably type specific; found throughout the world; viral shedding may continue for more than 1 week.

Diagnosis

Enzyme-linked immuno-sorbent assay; electron microscopy; counter immuneoelectro-phoresis;

	Organism	Disease	Epidemiology
Norwalk Virus	27 nm diameter; parvovirus-like.	epidemic; usually mild; explosive onset; vomiting, diarrhea, nausea, abdominal cramp; myalgias; self-limited (24-28 hours); lymphopenia	$\frac{1}{3}$ AING is due to Norwalk viruses; rapid spread with a primary attack rate of up to 50%; rarely seen in infants; not seasonal; worldwide distribution; fecal-oral transmission; respiratory symptoms rare; $\frac{2}{3}$ of adults have antibody.

Diagnosis

Primarily clinical/epidemiological; immunoelectron microscopy-not readily available; radio-immune assay.

KEY POINTS

1. Rotavirus is primarily an illness of infants and young children. It is diagnosed by electron microscopy or antigen detection of a stool specimen.
2. Norwalk viruses are primarily pathogens of older children, adolescents and adults. The illness usually begins abruptly and lasts 24 to 48 hours, Laboratory confirmation is difficult.
3. Adenovirus, coronaviruses, astroviruses, enteroviruses, and calciviruses have also been associated with acute gastroenteritis.

REFERENCES

1. Bishop, RF, Barnes GL, Cipriani E, et al: Clinical immunity after neonatal rotavirus infection. N. Engl J. Med 1983; 309:72–76.
2. Blacklow NR, Cukor G: Viral gastroenteritis. N Eng J. Med 1981; 304:397–406.
3. Brandt CD, Kim HW, Rodriguez WJ, et al: Adenoviruses and pediatric gastroenteritis. J. Infect. Dis 1985; 151:437–443.
4. Friedman AD: Acute infectious nonbacterial gastroenteritis. Asepsis 1983; 5(4):4–6.
5. Fulginiti V: "New" pediatric infectious disease. Resid Staff Physic 1983; 22:36–39.
6. Gerna G, Passarani N, Battaglia M, et al: Human enteric coronaviruses: Antigenic relatedness to human coronavirus OC43 and possible etiologic role in viral gastroenteritis. J Infect Dis 1985; 151:796–803.
7. Griffin MR, Surowiec JJ, McCloskey DI, et al: Foodborne Norwalk Virus. Am J Epidemiol 1982; 115:178–184.
8. Kuritsky JN, Osterholm MT, Korlach JA, et al: A statewide assessment of the role of Norwalk virus in outbreaks of foodborne gastroenteritis. J. Infect Dis 1985; 151:568.
9. San Joaquin VH, Marks MI: New agents in diarrhea. Pediatr Infect Dis 1982; 1:53–65.
10. Santosham M, Daum RS, Dillman L, et al: Oral rehydration therapy of infantile diarrhea. N Engl J Med 1982; 306:1070–1076.
11. Steinhoff MC: Viruses and diarrhea - a review. Am J Dis Child 1978; 132:302–307.

SALMONELLAE

Clinical Manifestations

Salmonellae produce gastroenteritis by stimulating secretions of fluid by the intestinal mucosa and by local inflammation. Bacterial penetration of intestinal epithelium and multiplication in the lamina propria produces the inflammation. The small intestine is predominantly involved. Classic symptoms initially are nausea, vomiting and colicky abdominal pain. Diarrhea shortly ensues. Stools are often foul-smelling. Chills and fever can occur. Symptoms are usually self-limited and last about 5 days. In immunocompromised patients and infants, the illness is more likely to be prolonged and may spread to other sites. *REMEMBER:* Salmonella gastroenteritis usually does not produce bloody or mucousy stool. It rarely produces an atonic anal sphincter (as is sometimes seen in shigella) and toxicity is uncommon.

Etiology and Epidemiology

Many different serotypes of salmonella are responsible for infection in humans. In the U.S., the most common serotype is *S. typhimurium.* Typhoid fever is usually caused by *S. typhi.* While the incidence of typhoid fever has decreased in this country during the twentieth century, the incidence of other forms of salmonella infection has been on the increase. Infants appear to be much more susceptible to salmonella infection than older children or adults. It tends to be a disease of lower socio-economic groups. Patients with sickle cell anemia are at greater risk for serious and life-threatening salmonella infection. The infection is more common in late summer and fall than in winter.

While humans tend to be the primary reservoir for typhoid fever, we appear to be incidental victims for most other types of salmonella infection. The reservoir for most nontyphoid salmonella infections appears to be domestic animals. Food serves as an effective vector and growth medium for the bacteria. Humans are able to tolerate low doses of salmonella but develop symptoms when the inoculi are in high doses.

Among the many sources of human infection are chicken, eggs, dried milk, turtles, pet food, chocolate, and various meat products. Nosocomial spread and intrafamilial spread are not uncommon.

Diagnosis

It is difficult to diagnose salmonella gastroenteritis on clinical grounds. Diagnosis depends on bacteriologic identification. The bacterium is a Gram-negative aerobe. Properties such as inability to ferment lactose (most salmonella), and produce hydrogen sulfide (most salmonella), as well as the bacterium's motility, help identify the organism. Intestinal biopsy is rarely indicated in salmonella gastroenteritis. When done, superficial ulcers and hemorrhages may be seen along with enteritis or gastritis. Mucous membranes and lymphoid follicles may be swollen. Serologic techniques are available to diagnose salmonella infection but are rarely needed or useful for the diagnosis of gastroenteritis.

Treatment

Controversy surrounds the use of antibiotics for routine salmonella gastroenteritis. Many reports cited have been retrospective, uncontrolled or anecdotal. It is generally agreed however, that in routine gastroenteritis due to salmonella in immuno-competent patients, antibiotic therapy is not indicated. The young infant, the patient without an intact immune system, and the patient with ulcerative colitis may be exceptions in whom antibiotic therapy may be indicated until symptoms disappear. Ampicillin, amoxicillin, chloramphenicol, and trimethoprin-sulfamethoxazole are the more commonly used antibiotics. Resistance transfer factor (R-factor) are operative in the transfer of antimicrobial resistance to salmonella and may play a role in the increased antibiotic resistance seen in salmonella in the U.S. In most cases, only supportive care is indicated.

Sequelae and Complications

Chronic or protracted salmonella infection may occur without symptoms, with relapsing symptoms or with mild persistant symptoms. Salmonella infection has been seen without obvious gastroenteritis symptoms but with failure to thrive. Most extra-intestinal salmonella infections are secondary to either a symptomatic or asymptomatic gastrointestinal infection. Most organ systems have been involved in salmonella infection.

Salmonella osteomyelitis occurs, especially in children with sickle cell anemia. The lower extremities are most commonly involved. About a third occur in the femur. Arthritis appears to be less common than osteomyelitis and does not seem to be more common in patients with sickle cell anemia. The hip and knee joints are most commonly involved. Meningitis due to salmonella is primarily a disease of infants. It may have a prolonged course, require a long course of therapy, and is associated with a high mortality. Salmonella brain abscesses have been reported. Salmonella endocarditis and mycotic aneurysms have also been reported. Genitourinary and pulmonary infections with salmonella are uncommon but do occur. While the gallbladder is often involved asymptomatically in typhoid fever, acute cholecystitis has been reported due to salmonella.

KEY POINTS

1. Salmonella is a common cause of gastroenteritis in children.
2. It is usually self-limited and requires no antibiotic therapy, but with certain patients such as those who have sickle cell disease, those who are immunocompromised and infants, bacteremia and dissemination of the infection may occur.
3. Domestic animals are a major reservoir of infection.

REFERENCES

1. Drachman RH: Acute infectious gastroenteritis. Symposium on Infectious Disease in Pediatric Clinics of North America. 1974, 21(3):711-733.
2. Gill ON, Bartlett CLR, Sockett PN, et al: Outbreak of Salmonella napoli infection caused by contaminated chocolate bars. The Lancet. 1983; i:574-577.
3. Kazemi M, Gumpert TG, Mark MI: A controlled trial comparing sulfamethoxazole-trimethoprim, ampicillin, and no therapy in the treatment of salmonella gastroenteritis in children. J Pediat 1973. 83:646-650.
4. Nelson JD: Salmonella infection, in Infections in Children. Wedgewood RJ, Davis SD, Ray CG, Kelley VC, (eds); pp. 780-811, Harper & Row, Philadelphia, 1982.

5. Nelson SJ, Granoff D: Salmonella gastroenteritis in the first three months of life. Clinical Pediatrics 1982, 21:709-712.
6. O'Brien TF, Hopkins JD, Gilleece ES, et al: Molecular Epidemiology of antibiotic resistance in salmonella for animals and human beings in the U.S. New Eng J Med, 1982. 307:1-6.

SHIGELLA

Clinical Manifestations

Shigella presents in a wide variety of ways. Patients may be asymptomatic, may have mild watery diarrhea, colitis, dysentary or appear toxic. Because shigella infections present in different ways, it is difficult to describe a "typical" case. The incubation period is usually a week or less. Acutely, symptoms include fever, malaise and crampy abdominal pain. These are usually followed by diarrhea and occasionally with tenesmus, and blood and mucous in the stool. These symptoms describe the typical dysentary seen with shigella infection. Physical examination often reveals a tender abdomen, hyperactive bowel sounds, and signs of dehydration. Sigmoidoscopy, if done, may reveal hyperemia, multiple bleeding sites, thick purulent mucous secretions and pseudomembranes. More common than the dysenteric form of the infection is the watery diarrhea which is indistinguishable from other causes of diarrhea. *REMEMBER:* Anywhere from 10% to 45% of cases of shigella in children may present with seizures as the initial symptoms.

Etiology and Epidemiology

Shigella is spread by the anal-oral route. The incidence increases with overcrowded living conditions. Only a very small number of organisms are needed to cause disease. It has been suggested that as few as ten organisms may be sufficient to cause disease in healthy adults. Acidic conditions will inhibit shigella. Antacids may promote shigella infection.

The bacterium is hardy and can survive for extended periods in shrimp, oysters, milk, flour, and eggs. Humans are the major host. Unlike salmonellae, shigella is uncommon during the first year of life. The peak incidence in children is between the ages of 1 and 4 years.

Asymptomatic excretion of the organism occurs, especially in untreated patients. The major species responsible for disease in the U.S. is *S. sonnei.*

Diagnosis

In patients with the dysentery form of the illness, the diagnosis can frequently be suspected on clinical grounds. The presence of blood and mucopurulent material in the stool is supportive evidence. Sheets of polymorphonuclear leukocytes in the stool is also a helpful finding.

The total peripheral white blood cell (WBC) count is not usually of assistance in making the diagnosis. About 10% of patients with shigella infection have WBC counts less than 5,000; about 10% have WBC counts greater than 25,000, and the remaining 80% fall in between. However, the WBC differential count can be very useful. Large numbers of immature neutrophils is a classic finding. *REMEMBER:* When the number of bands exceeds the number of segmented neutrophils, think shigella. Definitive diagnosis is made by rectal swab culture. Shigella is an aerobic, Gram-negative rod that is non-motile and non-capsulated.

Treatment

Antibiotic therapy is effective in shortening the duration of symptoms and decreasing the duration of shedding of the bacteria in the stool. Because shigella may contain plasmids that carry drug-resistant mechanisms (R-factor), antibiotic sensitivity testing of clinical isolates is important for appropriate management of patients. Ampicillin is often effective. In areas where ampicillin-resistant shigella are seen, trimethoprim-sulfamethoxazole is a good alternative. REMEMBER: Most shigellae are resistant to clinically achievable levels of amoxicillin even though they may be ampicillin sensitive. Although most infected children should be treated even if they have only mild symptoms or are asymptomatic; asymptomatic or recovering adults who are not at risk to transmit the infection need not be treated. Appropriate supportive therapy is an essential adjunct to antibiotic therapy. Electrolyte abnormalities should be corrected and the patient should be rehydrated.

Sequelae and Complications

Most cases of shigellosis resolve spontaneously or with the assistance of appropriate antibiotics. However, a variety of complications have been reported. The accompanying chart summarizes some of these complications. Chronic carriers exist, usually in the malnourished, but are not common, and may respond poorly to antibiotics. Use of lactulose will decrease intestinal pH and inhibit shigella in these patients.

Complications of Shigellosis

Complications	Description
Arthritis	Acute, self-limited, follows G.I. symptoms; more common in adult's large joints, predominantly.
Bacteremia	Shigellemia is rare but does occur. Secondary bacteremia with other enteric pathogens more common than Shigellemia.
Ekirc	Fever, diarrhea, vomiting, convulsions leading to death secondary to shigella induced hypocalcemia reported in Japanese children who may be calcium deficient prior to infection.
Hemolytic-Uremic Syndrome	Most commonly associated with **S. dysenteriae** type 1.
Liver disease	Mild elevation of SGOT has been reported.
Meningitis	Extremely rare. Usually occurs in neonates.
Obstruction	Intussusception has been associated with Shigellosis.
Perforation	Has been reported rarely.
Reiter Syndrome	Urethritis, conjunctivitis, arthritis; HLA- B-27 may be predisposing factor.
Respiratory Complications	cough, coryza, chest pain may occur in 25% of patients. Pneumonia, if it occurs, is rare.
Seizures	**Common, may be considered a symptom** rather than complication.
Urinary tract infections	Usually S. Flexneri. May occur in absence of enteritis.
Vaginitis	Often chronic with a serosanquinous vaginal discharge.

KEY POINTS

1. Shigella has a variety of clinical presentations including a dysentary form which frequently is manifest by fever, cramps, bloody mucousy diarrhea, and malaise.
2. Treatment is of value in shortening the duration of symptoms and duration of bacterial shedding.
3. Seizures may be the presenting manifestation of shigellosis.
4. A high percentage of immature neutrophils is frequently seen in shigellosis.
5. Although there is a wide spectrum of complications from shigella infection, most occur infrequently.

REFERENCES

1. Ashkenazi S, Dinari G, Weitz R, et al: Convulsions in Shigellosis: Evaluation of possible risk factors. Am J Dis Child 1983; 137: 985–987.
2. Barrett-Connor E, Connor JD: Extraintestinal manifestations of Shigellosis. AM J Gastroenterol. 1970; 53:234–45.
3. Dupont HL, Hornick RB, Dawkins AT, et al: The response of man to virulent shigella flexneri 2 a. J. Infect. Dis. 1969; 119:296–299.
4. Haltalin KC, Nelson JD: Coliform septicemia complicating shigellosis in children. JAMA 1965; 192:441–443.
5. Nelson J, Kusmiesz H, Jackson L et al: Trimethoprim-sulfamethoxazole therapy for shigellosis. JAMA 1976; 235:1239–43.

CAMPYLOBACTER

Clinical Manifestations

Diarrhea is the most common complaint in patients with campylobacter gastroenteritis. Although an acute onset of symptoms is common, patients may also present with a longer course of persistant or recurrent symptoms over weeks to months. Patients not presenting with diarrhea may have fever and abdominal pain or asymptomatic rectal bleeding as a presentation. In addition to diarrhea, patients also commonly were febrile (usually mildly), and had abdominal pain (especially younger babies). Dehydration is not commonly seen. Stools were usually abnormal and were watery, often with mucus and blood.

The classic clinical course begins after a 2 day - 10 day period. Mild abdominal discomfort progresses to more severe pain and the onset of acute diarrhea. Vomiting and dehydration are not commonly seen. The disease is usually self-limiting and resolves in 3-5 days. Fever, although uncommon in young infants, may be seen in older children. In severe cases, the symptoms can mimic appendicitis or ulcerative colitis. In neonates it has been associated with asymptomatic bloody diarrhea.

Etiology and Epidemiology

Most human enteritis due to campylobacter is due to *C. fetus s.s. jejuni.* Stool should be cultured on antibiotic containing media (selective media). Campylobacter enteritis has been reported from many parts of the world, including both temperate and tropical regions. All age groups appear to be susceptible to infection, although the incidence may be highest in young children. The national incidence of campylobacter varies, but most countries studied report that campylobacter is responsible for 5-10% of diarrhea seen. Certain countries, like Canada, have reported a much higher incidence. The infection can occur throughout the year, but in the U.S. appears to be more common during the summer months.

Sources of campylobacter infection include chickens, dogs, unpasteurized milk, cats, untreated water, and sick animals. Person-to-person spread has been reported including vertical spread from mother to neonate. Transmission is by the fecal-oral route with contaminated foods or by contact with contaminated fecal material.

Diagnosis

Clinical symptoms, the characteristics of the stool and the season are all helpful in suggesting the diagnosis of campylobacter enteritis. Laboratory diagnosis is made by stool culture. The organism grows best in 42°C in a micro-aerophilic environment. Skirrow's medium is often used. *REMEMBER:* Gram stain may be helpful in making a rapid presumptive diagnosis. The presence of "seagull"-shaped or curved Gram negative rods suggest the diagnosis in patients with appropriate symptoms and stool characteristics.

Treatment

Most cases of campylobacter enteritis are mild and self-limited with symptoms resolving in several days. Despite this, organisms may persist in stool for weeks which may result in spread of the disease to family members and other close contacts. In addition, some cases of campylobacter enteritis are more serious and have a prolonged course. *In vitro* campylobacter has been shown to be sensitive to erythromycin, tetracycline, furazolidone, chloramphenicol and the aminoglycosides. Evidence from several studies show that erythromycin therapy reduces the duration of bacterial shedding but does not appear to significantly alter the clinical course; although an uncontrolled study suggested that if given early in the course of the disease, erythromycin may be clinically effective. Appropriate supportive care should be included in the treatment of patients with campylobacter enteritis.

Sequelae and Complications

Most cases of campylobacter enteritis are self-limited and relatively benign. Occasionally severe dehydration may occur and must be managed appropriately. Erythema nodosum, seizures, and Guillain-Barre syndrome have been reported in association with campylobacter enteritis. In addition, bacteremia may frequently occur in association with campylobacter enteritis. Endocarditis and meningitis have also been reported. Fatal cases have been reported predominantly in immunocompromised and neonatal patients.

KEY POINTS

1. Campylobacter enteritis is usually a self-limited illness with symptoms of diarrhea, fever, and abdominal pain.
2. The diagnosis is suggested by the presence of "seagull"-shaped Gram negative rods in a smear from a stool specimen.
3. Erythromycin therapy probably decreases the duration of bacterial shedding and may have an effect on the clinical course of the infection.

REFERENCES

1. Anders B, Lauer BA, Paisley JW et al: Double-blind placebo controlled trial of erythromycin for treatment of Campylobacter enteritis. Lancet 1982; 1:131–132.
2. Blaser, MJ, Reller LB: Campylobacter enteritis. N Engl J Med. 1981; 305:1443–1452.
3. Blaser MJ, Weiss SH, Barrett TJ: Campylobacter enteritis associated with a healthy cat. JAMA 1982; 247:816–817.
4. Buck GE, Kelly MT, Pichanick AM, et al: Campylobacter jejuni in newborns: A cause of asymptomatic bloody diarrhea. Am J Dis Child 1982; 136:744.
5. Ho DD, Ault MJ, Ault MA et al: Campylobacter enteritis - early diagnosis with Gram's stain. Arch Intern Med 1982; 142:1858–1860.
6. Karmali MA, Fleming PC: Campylobacter enteritis in children. J Pediatr 1979; 94:527-533.
7. Karmali MA, Norrish B, Lior H, et al: Campylobacter entero-colitis in a neonatal nursery. J Infect Dis 1984; 149:874–877.
8. Naqvi SH, Dunkle LM, Clapper MA: Age-specific presentation of campylobacter enteritis in children. Clinical Pediatrics. 1983; 22:98–100.
9. Pai CH, Cillis F, Tuomanen E et al: Erythromycin in the treatment of Campylobacter enteritis in children. Am J Dis Child 1983; 137:286-288.
10. San Joaquin VH, Welch DF: Campylobacter enteritis - A 3 year experience. Clinical Pediatrics 1984; 23:311–316.
11. Schwartz RH, Bryan C, Rodriguez WJ, et al: Experience with the microbiologic diagnosis of Campylobacter enteritis in an office practice, Ped Infect Dis 1983; 2:298–301.

YERSINIA

Clinical Presentation

The most common symptoms of gastroenteritis due to *Yersinia enterocolitica* (YE) are diarrhea, abdominal pain, vomiting and fever. Outbreaks have been reported in which the symptoms mimic appendicitis. Symptoms, especially the diarrhea, may last one to three weeks; but excretion of the organism may continue for weeks, even after symptoms have disappeared.

Etiology and Epidemiology

Yersinia enterocolitica gastroenteritis is more frequently diagnosed in Europe, Japan, and Canada than in most areas of the United States. Person-to-person spread; dog-to-human spread; swine, cattle, and cat-to-human spread; spread from water supplies; and contaminated foods like chocolate milk, have all been reported. In children, most cases of infection occur around two years of age.

Diagnosis

Diagnosis is best made by bacterial culture. YE can grow at 4° C and 25°C, and this characteristic aids in identifying the organism. The organism is motile at 25°C but not at 37°C.

Treatment

Most *Yersinia enterocolitica* are susceptible *in vitro* to trimethoprim-sulfamethoxazole and aminoglycosides. Therapy does not appear to be indicated in mild self-limited infections. In invasive disease, or in immunocompromised patients, use of antibiotics is indicated.

Sequelae and Complications

While YE gastroenteritis is usually a self-limited infection, occasionally diarrhea can become protracted and may mimic inflammatory bowel disease. Erythema nodosum, erythema multiforme and maculopapular rashes have been reported in association with YE infection. Arthritis, mostly in older patients can occur, usually after the gastrointestinal symptoms. Leukocytes can be found in the joint fluid in these patients. Septicemia, although rare, has been reported, usually in immunocompromised patients. Rare complications include thyroiditis, osteomyelitis, meningitis, carditis, hepatitis and hemolytic anemia.

KEY POINTS

1. *Y. Enterocolitica* is a relatively infrequently identified cause of gastroenteritis in the United States.
2. Diagnosis is made by culture, and in serious cases antibiotics may be of value.

REFERENCES

1. Kohl S: Yersinia enterocolitica infections in children. Ped Clinics N Am 1979; 26:433–440.
2. Marks MI, Pai CH, Lafleur L et al: Yersinia enterocolitica gastroenteritis: A prospective study of clinical, bacteriologic and epidemiologic features. J Pediatr 1980; 96:26–31.
3. San Joaquan VH, Marks MI: New Agents in diarrhea. Ped Inf Dis 1982; 1:53–65.

GIARDIASIS

Clinical Manifestations

Clinical diagnosis of giardia infection can be difficult because of the wide spectrum of symptoms. Infected hosts may be asymptomatic, may have mild non-specific symptoms or may have acute gastrointestinal disease. Commonly found symptoms include diarrhea, abdominal cramps, flatulence, distension, nausea, foul smelling greasy stools, and weight loss. Blood or pus in the stools is not usually seen. Constipation has been reported in younger children. Diarrhea is the most common symptom and can be acute or chronic. The incubation period is believed to be approximately 15 days and the infection lasts an average of 44 days. Most infected people are asymptomatic. Giardiasis may present as a chronic malabsorption syndrome, sometimes resembling sprue.

Etiology and Epidemiology

There are two stages in the life cycle of *Giardia lamblia;* a trophic and a cystic stage. Infection is usually achieved by ingestion of the cyst. Excystation begins in the stomach and continues through the duodenum. Trophozoites survive best at pH of 6.4 to 7.4. They colonize the distal duodenum and proximal jejuneum where they adhere to microvillus surfaces where they absorb nutrients. When trophozoites are swept down the intestines they again encyst.

Giardia infection is more common in children than adults and is more common in lower socioeconomic groups than in upper socioeconomic groups. Spread is frequently the result of contaminated water and food, or person-to-person contamination. Increased susceptibility may result from decreased gastric acidity and malnutrition. Giardiasis is associated with immunoglobulin deficiencies, especially IgA.

Prevalence rates usually reported are less than 10% of the general population. In developing nations, however, 15–30% of children under two years of age are infected. In the U.S., day-care facilities are commonly associated with spread of giardia among children. Spread from pet dogs to children has been reported. In the U.S., giardia is the most common intestinal parasite. There is a high incidence among homosexual men. The parasite has been implicated in disease worldwide. It is common in the tropics, but has also been reported from the Arctic.

Diagnosis

Diagnosis depends on a high index of suspicion and appropriate laboratory studies. When there is unexplained gastrointestinal symptoms, failure-to-thrive or weight-loss giardiasis should be a consideration. Stool examination for ova and parasites will frequently make the diagnosis. Trophozoites are passed in stool infrequently, and cysts are fairly hardy so that it is not essential for stools to be examined while fresh. Children may have very erratic patterns of cyst excretion and many days to weeks may lapse between cyst excretion. When possible, multiple stool specimens taken over several weeks is desirable, as it will increase the yield.

If stools for ova and parasite are negative and symptoms persist, aspiration of the duodenum and jejuneum is usually effective in making the diagnosis. The aspiration can be accomplished using a nasogastric tube. An alternative is the string method, available commercially as Entero-test capsule. In the rare case that it is not diagnosed by these methods, jejunal biopsy may be necessary. Counterimmunoelectrophoresis has also been used in the diagnosis of giardiasis.

Treatment

Patients usually respond rapidly to appropriate therapy. Furazolidone comes as a liquid or tablet preparation. It is palatable and side effects are infrequent. The most common side effect is gastrointestinal upset. *REMEMBER:* Drinking alcohol while taking furazolidone or for several days after will result in a disulfiram (Antabuse) reaction. This same reaction can also be seen in these patients after eating tyramine containing foods like chicken livers, unpasteurized cheese, and yeast extract. Treatment is 9 mg/kg/day divided into three doses orally for ten days.

An alternative therapy is quinacrine hydrochloride. This is usually not used in children as it is available only as 100 mg tablets which makes dosing in infants and young children very difficult. The dose is 6 mg/kg/day divided into three doses orally for 10 days. The tablet does not taste good, and also has a disulfiram effect. Gastrointestinal upset is common in children on this drug.

Metronidazole is not approved for the treatment of giardiasis in children and therefore should be reserved for children who can not tolerate the other treatments or who are treatment failures. Other drugs available outside the U.S. for treatment of giardiasis include nitrimidazole and omidazole. They resemble metronidazole and may be effective with high dose, short-course therapy.

It is recommended that symptomatic and non-symptomatic infected children be treated. All young pediatric contacts of index cases should also be treated. Asymptomatic infected high risk adults, such as homosexual men, and food handlers, should also be treated. As with many other causes of gastroenteritis, the incidence of infection can be reduced by good public health and sanitary techniques. Travelers to endemic areas and campers need to be cautious when using water. *REMEMBER:* Chlorination does not kill giardia cysts.

Sequelae and Complications

Rarely extra gastrointestinal symptoms have been associated with giardia infections. Neurologic symptoms of headache, dizziness and paresthesias have been reported. Malabsorption occurs with giardiasis. The degree of malabsorption varies depending on severity of the illness. Giardiasis has been reported to cause decreased absorption of oral antibiotics given for various bacterial infection. Anti-giardia therapy can result in improved response to oral antibiotic therapy. Giardiasis in malnourished children can create a vicious cycle of enhanced parasitic effects, decreasing immune function, and increased malnutrition secondary to the giardiasis. Ultimately, superinfection can lead to death.

KEY POINTS

1. Giardiasis is a fairly common cause of gastrointestinal infection in children. Symptoms vary greatly, but all children diagnosed to be infected with *G. lamblia* should be treated.
2. Diagnosis is made by examination of stool for ova and parasites or by examination of duodenal or jejunal contents.

REFERENCES

1. Black RE, Dykes AC, Sinclair SP, et al: Giardiasis in day care centers: Evidence of person-to-person transmission. Pediatric 1977. 60:486–491.
2. Burke JA: Giardiasis in childhood. Am J Dis Child 1975; 129:1304–1310.
3. Craft JC: Giardia and giardiasis in childhood. Ped Infect Dis 1982; 1:196–211.
4. Craft JC, Murphy TV, Nelson JD: Furazolidone and quinacrine: Comparative study of therapy for giardiasis in children. Am J Dis Child 1981, 135:164–166.
5. Meyer EA, Jarroll EL: Giardiasis. Am J Epidemiol 1980; 111:1–12.
6. Pickering LK, Woodward WE, DuPont HL et al: Occurrence of *Giardia lamblia* in children in day care centers. Pediatrics 1984; 104:522–526.
7. Schmerin MJ, Jones TC, Klein H: Giardiasis: Association with homosexuality. Ann Intern Med 1978; 88:801–803.
8. Solomons NW: Giardiasis: Nutritional implications. Rev Infect Dis. 1982; 4:859–869.

Miscellaneous Causes of Gastroenteritis

Organism	Symptoms	Epidemiology	Diagnosis	Treatment	Complications/ Sequelae
Entamoeba histolytica (Amebiasis)	-Mild to severe diarrhea, may be bloody and painful. -Invasive disease (dysentery) is associated with pain, blood & mucousy diarrhea. -May be asymptomatic.	-Fecal-oral spread. -World wide distribution. -Acquired from ingestion of cysts. -Man is reservior. -Can be transmitted by food or liquids.	1-Trophozoites/ cysts in stool specimen. 2-Trophozoites/ cysts from aspirate of rectum. 3-Serology available	1-Asymptomatic: Diloxanide furoate or diiodohydroxyqiun or Metronidazole 2-Intestinal disease; metronidazole or diiodohydroxyquin with tetracycline or with paromamycin.	1-Liver abscess-tender large liver, often associated with fever-may occur without gastrointestinal symptoms. 2-Can invade liver, lung heart and central nervous system. 3-Appendicitis.
Aeromonas hydrophilia	-Watery diarrhea with vomiting and fever; self-limited. or -Bloody/mucousy diarrhea. or -Prolonged diarrhea.	-World-wide distribution. -Found in both immune competent and immunocompromised patients. -Enterotoxin producing.	1-Gram-negative rods, motile single flagellum. 2-May be missed in routine stool culture unless oxidase testing is done (oxidase positive.	-Usually self-limited. -Organism is susceptible to: chloramphenicol, aminoglycosides, trimethoprimsulfamethoxazole, tetracycline.	Immune compromised patients and neonates are the primary victims of extragastrointestinal infection. Sites involved include: blood, skin urinary tract, wound, meninges, bone, and joints.

Miscellaneous Causes of Gastroenteritis

Organism	Symptoms	Epidemiology	Diagnosis	Treatment	Complications/ Sequelae
Plesiomonas shigelloides	-Acute onset mild/ moderate diarrhea. -Pain, fever, lassitude headache. -Occasionally vomiting. -Spontaneous resolution in about 1 week.	-Found in water/soil -Found in variety of animals including pets.	-Gram negative rod, motile with flagella.	1-Usually self-limited 2-Trimethoprim- sulfamethoxazole is effective as are the aminoglycosides.	1-Meningitis 2-Sepsis
Cryptosporidium (Cryptosporidiosis)	-In immunocompromised patients-- severe irreversible diarrhea. -In immunocompetent patients--self limited, occasionally severe.	-Primarily a disease of animals. -Originally seen in humans with AIDS. -Now seen in immunocompetent human hosts. -Several reports of illness among children attending daycare centers.	-Stool Examination	No currently available FDA approved therapy.	-High mortality among AIDS patients.

Miscellaneous Causes of Gastroenteritis

Organism	Symptoms	Epidemiology	Diagnosis	Treatment	Complications/ Sequelae
Vibrio cholerae (Cholera)	-Watery diarrhea usually without blood but with flecks of mucus. -Vomiting may precede diarrhea. -Severe dehydration may occur.	-Man is host. -Contaminated water and food often mode of transmission. -Seen primarily in Asia, Africa & parts of Europe. -Incubation usually 3-5 days.	-Gram-negative comma shaped motile rods can be seen on dark field microscopy of stool. -Can be cultured on selective media. -Serum antibodies can be measured.	1-Trimethoprim-sulfamethoxazole 2-Tetracycline	-Most complications associated with hypo-volemia secondary to dehydration, severe acidosis, electro-lyte disturbances.
E. coli	Enterotoxigenic watery diarrhea, fever, cramps 3-7 days. **Invasive** pus, mucus, blood, in stool **Enteropathogenic** watery diarrhea	-Traveler's diarrhea. -Not commonly seen in industrial nations. -Lasts about 1 week-rarely seen in North America. -Seen in summer.	Not routinely available Sereny test Serotyping	No evidence that treatment changes course of disease	-Severe dehydration -Dysentery-like syndrome

79

REFERENCES

1. Alpert G, Bell LM, Kirkpatrick CE, et al: Cryptosporidiosis in a day-care center. N Engl J Med 1984; 311:860–1.
2. Burke V, Gracey M, Robinson J, et al: The microbiology of childhood gastroenteritis: Aeromonas species and other infective agents. J Infect Dis 1983; 148:68–74.
3. CDC: Cryptosporidiosis among children attending day-care centers. MMWR 1984; 33:599–601.
4. Diamond LS: Amebiasis: Nutritional implications. Rev. Infect Dis 1982; 4:843–850.
5. Freij BJ: Aeromonas: biology of the organism and disease in children. Ped Infect Dis 1984; 3:164–175.
6. Gracey M, Burke V, Robinson J: Aeromonas - associated gastroenteritis. Lancet 1982; 2:1304–1306.
7. Krogstad DJ, Spencer HC, Healy GR: Current Concepts in Parasitology: Amebiasis. New Engl J Med 1978; 298:262–265.
8. McNeeley D, Ivy P, Craft JC et al: Plesiomonas: biology of the organism and diseases in children. Ped Infect Dis 1984; 3:176–181.
9. Merritt RJ, Caughlin E, Thomase DW et al: Spectrum of Amebiasis in children. Am J Dis Child 1982; 136:785–789.
10. Pastore G, Rizzo G, Fera G, et al: Trimethoprim-sulfamethoxazole in the treatment of cholera. Comparison with tetracycline and choloramphenicol. Chemotherapy 1977; 23:121–128.
11. Pollitzer R: Cholera. Geneva, World Health Organization, 1959.
12. San Joaquin VH, Mark MI: New Agents in diarrhea. Pediatr Infect Dis 1982; 1:53–65.

REVIEW QUESTIONS

1.) True or False
1. Norwalk viruses cause a severe gastroenteritis commonly seen in neonates.
2. Norwalk virus gastroenteritis is usually an epidemic illness.
3. Rotaviruses cause gastroenteritis in neonates.
4. One episode of rotavirus gastroenteritis causes life-time immunity.
5. If viewed under an electron microscope, rotaviruses appear to have a wheel-rim appearance.
6. Coronavirus-like particles can cause a gastroenteritis in neonates.

2.) Match the infection with the description.

A. Shigella
B. Salmonella
C. Campylobacter
D. Yersinia
E. Giardia
F. Amebia
G. Crytosporidium
H. *E. coli*

1. Acquired from ingestion of cysts; May cause liver abscesses, bloody mucousy diarrhea.
2. Usually self-limited; animals are a major reservoir—including chickens and turtles.
3. Blood and mucous in the stool; tenesmus may present with seizures; large numbers of immature neutrophils in peripheral white cell count.
4. Self-limited in immune competent, may be fatal in immune compromised; parasite; no approved therapy currently available.
5. Travelers' diarrhea, usually self-limited, watery diarrhea.
6. "Seagull"-shaped Gram negative rod, self-limited usually.
7. May mimic inflamatory bowel disease, associated with arthritis, can grow at 4°C and 25°C.
8. Diagnosis is made by identifying cysts in stool, small bowel aspiration, or the string method.

5

HEPATITIS

Clinical Manifestations

Hepatitis B presents with a variety of symptoms. Common signs and symptoms include anorexia, fever, headache, nausea, vomiting, lassitude, weakness, abdominal discomfort and pain. In children, anicteric hepatitis is more common than icteric hepatitis and tends to be a milder disease. The liver may be tender. Tapping on the lower right thorax laterally will often produce pain (Murphy's sign). Occasionally the spleen is enlarged. Less commonly, hepatitis may present as a serum-sickness-like syndrome. These children will have arthralgias or arthritis, resembling rheumatoid arthritis. They will have a negative test for rheumatoid factor. Joint symptoms are often associated with urticaria. In addition, papular acrodermatitis of childhood has been associated with hepatitis B infection.

Many patients have subclinical cases of hepatitis. These patients have no symptoms of disease and can only be diagnosed by laboratory studies.

Etiology and Epidemiology

Hepatitis B surface antigen (HB_sAg) is found in the outer shell (lipid-containing envelope) of the virion. HB_cAg is found in the inner core of the virion. The core contains viral DNA, polymerase, and kinase that phosphorylates the viral genome-specified major polypeptide of the core. Hepatitis e antigen (HB_eAg) appears to also be associated with the core.

The incubation period is approximately 90 days (40-180 days). A few weeks after exposure, HB_sAg and HB_eAg may appear. In most patients as antigen levels peak, clinical symptoms appear. Shortly before, or at the time of the first clinical symptoms, antibody to core antigen (Anti-HBc) appears. As Anti-HBc rises, HB_sAg usually falls. Anti-HBc will decrease significantly during the first years following infection. There is considerable variation in the serologic time course.

The carrier state of Hepatitis B is defined as persistence of HBsAg. While in the U.S. the carrier rate is about 0.1%, in other parts of the world, such as much of Asia, the rate is as high as 15%.

HBsAg has been detected in saliva, serum, blood, vaginal secretions, and breast milk; and is often found in association with other sexually transmitted diseases. Vertical transmission from mother to neonate can occur, especially at the time of birth. Early identification of pregnant women who are Hepatitis B carriers is important so that measures can be instituted to protect the infant. Infants infected with Hepatitis B frequently go on to become chronic carriers. In general, if the mother has acute hepatitis during the first trimester, the risk of the baby developing infection is about 10%. This risk increases the later in the pregnancy that the acute maternal infection occurs, up to about a 50% risk in the third trimester. Factors associated with higher rates of hepatitis B virus transmission to neonates include:

1. HBeAg without anti-HBe in maternal serum.
2. Asian racial origin.
3. High titer of HBsAg in the mother.
4. Presence of HBsAg in older siblings.

REMEMBER: Women who should have prenatal screening for HBsAg are those with histories of liver disease, who work or are treated in hemodialysis units, who work or reside in institutions for the mentally retarded, who were rejected as blood donors, who received multiple blood transfusions, who have frequent occupational exposure to blood, who are a household contact of a Hepatitis B carrier or hemodialysis patient, who have had multiple episodes of sexually transmitted diseases, or who use illicit drugs percutaneously. In addition, women of Asian, Pacific Island, or Alaskan Eskimo descent, or women born in Haiti or sub-Sahara Africa may be at increased risk.

Diagnosis

Many cases of hepatitis B go undiagnosed because the patients are asymptomatic. Patients who have symptoms suggestive of hepatitis should have liver function tests to confirm hepatic involvement. Elevated transaminases are usually seen in these patients. Acute active infection can best be confirmed by the presence of HBsAg with or without anti-HBc. In the early convalescence phase, anti-HBc may be seen alone. In patients with recent past infection both anti-HBs and anti-HBc may be present. When the infection was in the remote past, often only anti-HBs is present. To some extent HBeAg appears to correlate with degree of infectivity. In general, patients with anti-HBe have a lower titer of hepatitis B virus than do those with HBeAg.

Treatment and Prevention

At this time, the treatment of Hepatitis B is supportive. Most patients will develop antibody to HBsAg and recover completely from the illness. Research continues on antiviral and interferon therapy for this infection.

Because there is no specific treatment, and because patients occasionally go on to develop chronic or persistent infection, prevention is important. Both passive and active prevention is available. Two forms of passive protection are available. Regular immune globulin (I.G.) from non-preselected donors has a titer of anti HBs of about 1:100. Hepatitis B immune globulin (HBIG) is prepared from patients pre-selected for high antiHBs titer resulting in a titer of about 1:100,000. For post-exposure prophylaxis HBIG should be used, if available, for intense or intimate exposure; (e.g. hepatitis B contaminated needle stick, or sexual contact) or to infants born to mothers who had acute hepatitis during pregnancy or are known carriers.

The hepatitis B vaccine provides the means of active protection. Injection of HBsAg results in the production of antibody to HBs which is protective. Three shots over six months provide protection in over 95% of patients.

Current recommendations for newborns born to HBsAg positive mothers are to give the neonate 0.5 cc HBIG I.M. immediately after birth followed by the first dose of vaccine in the first week of life. The second vaccine dose is given one month later. Prior to the third dose at six months, the baby should be tested for HBsAg. If the baby is positive, the vaccine was a failure and the third does not need be given. Similar recommendations have been made for percutaneous exposure, homosexually active males, and for regular sexual exposure with a chronic carrier. Outside the neonatal period the dose of HBIG is 0.06 cc/Kg (5ml maximum) I.M. and 1 cc vaccine I.M. (Children under 10 years of age should receive 0.5. cc of vaccine.)

Sequelae and Complications

Most patients with hepatitis B have an uneventful recovery. Fulminent hepatitis leading to death is a rare outcome. About 10% of those infected may go on to become chronic carriers. About one-fourth of these develop chronic active hepatitis, some of whom may develop cirrhosis, cancer of the liver, or may die from their disease. Most of the carriers have chronic persistent hepatitis. This is not progressive.

Circulating immune complexes of HBsAg and antiHBs may result in associated findings of serum sickness-like illness, polyarteritis nodosa, and membranous glomerulonephritis. Aplastic anemia and infantile papular acrodermatitis have also been associated with hepatitis B.

KEY POINTS

(1) Time Course of typical hepatitis B infection:

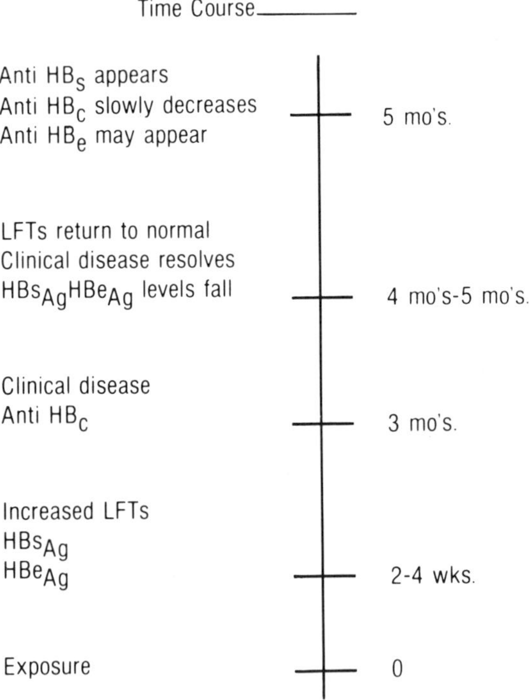

(2) Diagnosis:

HB$_s$Ag (with/without anti HB) suggests active infection.

Anti HB$_c$ alone suggests early recovery stage.

Anti HB$_c$ and anti HB$_s$ suggests recent past infection.

Anti HB$_s$ alone suggests remote past infection.

(3) High risk groups:

History of liver disease,

multiple blood transfusions or occupational exposure to blood products,

household contact or sexual contact with hepatitis B carrier,

hemodialysis worker or patient,

institution for mental retarded—worker or patient,

history of other sexually transmitted diseases,

percutaneous drug use,

Asian, Pacific Islands, Alaskan, or Eskimo descedent,

Hatian, sub-Sahara African,

infants born to mothers in these risk groups.

REFERENCES

1. Ahtone J, Maynard JE: Laboratory diagnosis of Hepatitis B. JAMA 1983; 249:2067–2069.
2. ACIP: Post-exposure Prophylaxis of Hepatitis B, MMWR 1984 33:285–290.
3. Bernier RH, Sampliner R, Gerety R, et al: Hepatitis B Infection in households of chronic carriers of Hepatitis B surface antigen. American Journal of Epidemiology, 1982; 116:199–211.
4. Callis LM, Clanxet J, Fortuny G, et al: Hepatitis B virus infection and vaccination in children undergoing hemodialysis. Acta Pediatr Scand 1985; 74:213–218.
5. King JW: A clinical approach to hepatitis B. Archives of Internal Medicine 1982. 142:925–928.
6. Lo KJ, Tong MJ, Chien MC, et al: The natural course of hepatitis B surface antigen-positive chronic active hepatitis in Taiwan. J Infect Dis 1982; 146:205–210.
7. Salvioli GP, Faldella G, Alessandroni R et al: Prevention of perinatal transmission of chronic hepatitis B surface antigen (HBsAg) carrier state. Pediatrics 1984; 73:408–9.

8. Surgenor DM, Chalmers TC, Conrad ME, et al: Clinical trials of Hepatitis B immune globulin. NEJM, 1975; 293:1–16.

9. Villarejos VM, Visona KA, Gutierrez A et al: Role of saliva, urine, and feces in the transmission of type B hepatitis. NEJM 1974, 291:1375–1380.

10. Werner BG, Grady GF: Accidental Hepatitis B Surface Antigen Positive Inoculations-Use of e antigen to estimate infectivity. Ann Int Med 1982; 97:367–369.

HEPATITIS A

Clinical Manifestations

Symptoms of hepatitis A are similar to those of hepatitis B, except that the incubation period is shorter (15-50 days). Neither the carrier state nor chronic hepatitis A have been definitively demonstrated.

Approximately two weeks after exposure, hepatitis A antigen (HAAg) can be demonstrated in stool. Two weeks later, serum transaminases rise. HAAg in stool peaks, and transaminases peak about the time clinical symptoms appear. With the appearance of jaundice, the excretion of HAAg rapidly falls off. While symptoms are still present, antibody to HAAg becomes detectable. IgM appears first and falls off 2-3 months after the onset of symptoms. IgG appears after clinical illness and persists.

Etiology and Epidemiology

Spread of hepatitis A is primarily by the fecal-oral route and is common in crowded, unsanitary conditions. Spread is common within households. It has been reported in daycare center outbreaks, and has been reported to be sexually transmitted in homosexual men. Various foods (raw clams, meat, milk, orange juice) and water contamination have also been implicated in spread of the disease. The spread of hepatitis A by transfusion of blood products rarely if ever occurs.

Diagnosis

Symptoms, signs, history, and time lapsed since exposure, are helpful in making the diagnosis. The presence of elevated transaminases helps confirm the diagnosis of hepatitis. Detection of antibody of HAAg helps identify the specific agent as hepatitis A virus. Hepatitis B, nonA-nonB hepatitis, CMV, toxoplasmosis and EBV should be included in the differential.

Treatment and Prevention

There is no specific therapy for hepatitis A. Treatment is supportive. Prevention is best done with observing good rules of hygiene and maintaining sanitary conditions. Post-exposure prophylaxis is done using conventional immune serum globulin (ISG) This should be given as soon after exposure as possible, preferably within 1-2 weeks of exposure. If given as recommended, it is 80-90% effective. ISG should also be given to travelers to countries with epidemic hepatitis. In school or institutional outbreaks, use of ISG may be indicated. 0.02 ml/KG of ISG should be administered. Those who require long-term prophylaxis, such as travelers to endemic areas of the world, should receive 0.06 ml/KG. This can be repeated every 4-6 months as indicated.

Sequelae and Complications

Complications and sequelae of hepatitis A are extremely rare. Full recovery is the rule.

KEY POINTS

(1) Time Course of typical hepatitis A.

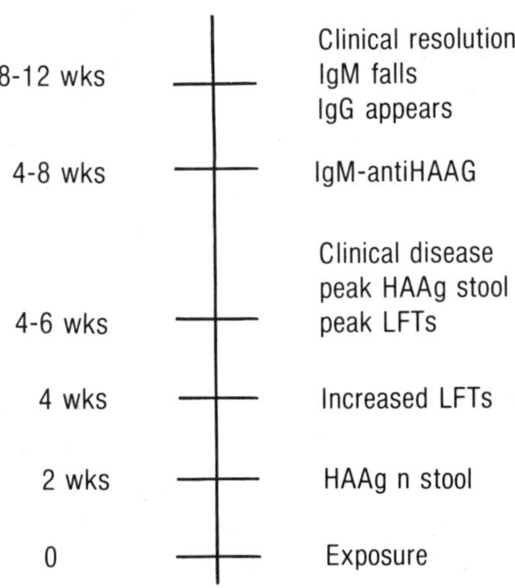

(2) Hepatitis A is primarily spread by the fecal-oral route.
(3) Prevention is by using immune serum globulin.

REFERENCES

1. Aach RD. Viral Hepatitis: In *Textbook of Pediatrics Infectious Diseases* (Feigin & Cherry eds) WB Saunders, 1981; 1:513–532.
2. Corey L. Holmes KK: Sexual transmission of Hepatitis A in homosexual men. NEJM 1980; 302:435–438.
3. Drenstag JL, Feinstone SM, Kapikian AZ, et al: Fecal shedding of hepatitis A antigen. Lancet, 1975, 1:765.
4. Vernon AA. Schable C, Francis D: A large outbreak of hepatitis A in a day-care center. Am J of Epidemiology, 1982; 115:325–331.
5. Villarejos VM, Serra CJ, Anderson-Visona K, et al: Hepatitis A virus infection in households. Am J of Epidemiology 1982; 114:577–586.

CAUSES OF MISCELLANEOUS HEPATITIS

NON-A, NON-B HEPATITIS

Non-A, Non-B hepatitis (NANB) is responsible for about 90% of the post-transfusion hepatitis in the United States. It is responsible for about 25% of the cases of sporadic hepatitis among hospitalized patients and may be responsible for over 40% of the sporadic cases of hepatitis in the community. It is likely that more than one etiologic agent is responsible for NANB hepatitis.

Symptoms resemble those of the other causes of hepatitis. The incubation period is an average of 7-8 weeks, with a range of two to 26 weeks. Although usually a milder disease than hepatitis A or B, fulminant cases have been reported. NANB hepatitis has been reported in newborn infants born to mothers with NANB hepatitis.

Diagnosis is based on exclusion of other causes of hepatitis and an appropriate clinical history. At best, most diagnosis of NANB hepatitis are provisional.

There is no specific therapy of NANB hepatitis. Supportive therapy is indicated. ISG may offer some protection or at least modify symptoms. The idea of giving ISG post-transfusion to prevent NANB hepatitis is arguable. Further study is needed.

Both chronic NANB hepatitis and NANB carrier state have been reported. Carriers may be totally asymptomatic and have normal liver function tests and still transmit the infection via blood.

DELTA AGENT HEPATITIS

Delta agent infection appears to occur in patients who are hepatitis B carriers. It appears that delta agent requires certain helper functions of hepatitis B virus for replication. The result is an acute hepatitis. Many of these patients go on to develop chronic hepatitis. Drug addicts who are hepatitis B carriers have a high incidence of delta infection.

The clinical presentation is similar to that of other infectious hepatitis and can not be distinguished on clinical grounds. Delta agent infection may occur anytime during the carrier state. Although recovery from infection is the rule, fulminant hepatitis has been reported.

(Hepatitis due to CMV and toxoplasmosis are discussed in the chapter on congenital infections. Hepatitis due to Epstein-Barr Virus is discussed in the section on EBV infections.)

KEY POINTS

1. Non-A, Non-B hepatitis is the major cause of post-transfusion hepatitis in the U.S.
2. Delta agent hepatitis occurs in patients who are hepatitis B carriers. The clinical disease is similar to that of hepatitis B.

REFERENCES

1. Alter MJ, Gerety RJ, Smallwood LA, et al: Sporadic Non-A, Non-B Hepatitis: Frequency and epidemiology in an Urban U.S. Poluation. J. Infect. Dis., 1982, 145:886–893.
2. Hansson BG, Moestrup T, Widell A, et al: Infection with delta agent in Sweden: Introduction to a new hepatitis agent. J. Infect Dis., 1982, 146: 472–478.
3. Moestrup T, Hansson BG, Widell A. et al: Clinical Aspects of delta agent. Brit. Med J 1983; 286:8–90.
4. Robinson WS: The enigma of non-A non-B hepatitis. J. Infect Dis., 1982; 145:387–395.
5. Sampliner RE: Chronic Non-A, Non B Liver disease. Arch Int Med 1981; 141:1581.
6. Tabor E, Seeff LB, Gerety RJ: Chronic non-A non-B hepatitis carrier state. NEJM 1980; 303:140–143.
7. Tong MJ, Thrusby M, Rakela J, et al: Studies of the maternal-infant transmission of the viruses which cause acute hepatitis. Gastroenterology 1981; 80:999–1004.

REVIEW QUESTIONS

1.) The incubation period for hepatitis B is approximately __________.

2.) Prior to the presence of symptoms, what laboratory tests will provide evidence of hepatitis B infection (3)?

3.) Hepatitis B carrier state is diagnosed by the persistence of __________.

4.) Prevention of hepatitis B is possible by using __________ or __________.

5.) The incubation period for hepatitis A is __________.

6.) The primary means of spread of hepatitis A is __________.

7.) Prevention of hepatitis A is possible using __________.

8.) Most post-transfusion hepatitis in the U.S. is probably __________ hepatitis.

9.) A prerequisite for delta hepatitis is a __________ infection.

6

MENINGITIS

Clinical Manifestations

A high index of suspicion, early diagnosis, and institution of appropriate treatment early in the illness is essential to achieve a satisfactory outcome in children with meningitis. The axiom that thinking about doing a lumbar puncture is sufficient reason to do it is valid. If all the spinal taps you do are positive then you probably are not doing enough of them and may have missed the diagnosis of meningitis on occasion.

Classic symptoms of meningitis include a stiff neck, headache, vomiting, nausea, and irritability. In addition, fever, anorexia, change in state of consciousness, a bulging fontanelle, seizures, photophobia, backache and cranial nerve involvement may be found. The actual symptoms in any given patient may be minimal, have some of the above, or may be classic with many or most of the symptoms listed. *REMEMBER:* Most infants do not exhibit classic symptoms.

Evidence of meningeal irritation may be difficult to see in infants and non-specific symptoms of irritability and poor feeding may be the only clues. Lack of a bulging fontanelle does not rule out meningitis. When signs like the Kernig (flexed thighs on abdomen, try to extend at knees) and Brudzinski (neck flexing gives knee and hip flexion) are present, it supports the diagnosis of meningitis. Increased intracranial pressure is usually present but papilledema is rarely observed. Inappropriate antidiuretic hormone syndrome often occurs. Failure to recognize this problem can result in increased intracranial pressure. Seizures prior to admission occur in 20–30% of children with meningitis.

Not all children with meningimus have meningitis or central nervous system infection. Some of the other causes include: pneumonia, cervical adenitis, discitis, cat scratch disease, appendicitis, juvenile rheumatoid arthritis, black-widow spider and scorpion bites, shigellosis, and retropharyngeal abscesses, among many others.

Etiology and Epidemiology

Outside of the neonatal age group, most bacterial meningitis is due to infection with *Hemophilus influenzae* type b, *Streptococcal pneumoniae* or *Niesseria meningitidis*. Most of these are due to *H. influenzae*. Those children less than one year of age appear to be at greatest risk. High risk also appears to be associated with being black, a Navajo Indian, or an Eskimo. The incidence is slightly higher in males than females. The incidence of *H. influenzae* meningitis has been increasing over the last few decades. Defects in leukocyte function, deficiency of certain complement components, low levels of immunoglobulins, T and B lymphocyte defects, splenectomy, sickle cell anemia and other hemaglobinopathies, immunosuppression and malnutrition are some of the conditions which predispose to meningitis.

There have been reports of meningitis developing in bacteremic patients after a lumbar puncture. Should neurological symptoms or meningeal signs develop despite an initial negative L.P., do not hesitate to repeat the L.P.

Diagnosis

The diagnosis of meningitis must be made as rapidly and accurately as possible. Optimal therapy depends on identifying and characterizing the specific pathogen responsible and then choosing the most appropriate treatment.

The workup for meningitis should include a lumbar puncture. Fluid should be obtained for cell count and differential, glucose, protein, Gram stain and culture. An additional tube of CSF fluid should be held in case additional studies are needed. A CBC, blood culture, urinalysis and urine culture, serum electrolytes, BUN and glucose may provide additional valuable information. When inappropriate ADH syndrome is suspected, serum and urine osmolality can be useful.

REMEMBER: In patients not previously treated with antibiotics prior to the time that a culture is taken, the culture remains the most valuable tool in the diagnosis of meningitis. It is a prudent policy not to narrow your antibiotic coverage based on Gram stain or other non-culture technique.

Once cultures are positive, sensitivities can be determined and antibiotics can then be adjusted safely.

Many non-specific assays have been devised to try and help us distinguish bacterial from non-bacterial disease. None are completely reliable and the decision to stop antibiotics based on these tests would be unwise at this time.

Other more specific rapid diagnostic tests are available which tell us the specific organism believed to be responsible for infection. Counterimmuno-electrophoresis (CIE), latex agglutination, and bacterial coagglutination are currently commonly used. These tests identify bacterial antigen and are more rapid than culture technique. They are particularly valuable in patients who have antibiotic therapy before the cultures were obtained. This prior antibiotic therapy may result in false negative cultures but should not affect these antigen detection systems.

The value of these techniques is limited because of false negative results often due to insufficient concentration of antigen in the CSF, and because of certain cross-over reactions which may result in identifying the wrong organism. In addition, identifying the organism by these techniques does not enable antibiotic sensitivities of the organism to be determined. RE-MEMBER: While most *H. influenzae* that are ampicillin resistant are resistant based on the production of beta-lactamase, there are other mechanisms of resistance also. Therefore, one should not use ampicillin alone for treatment of *H. influenzae* even if the organism is beta-lactamase negative (i.e., does not produce beta-lactamase) unless the sensitivity is confirmed by antibiotic sensitivity testing.

Treatment

Optimal therapy is determined by culture and antibiotic sensitivity results. In children and infants outside the neonatal period the three most common pathogens are *H. influenzae, St. pneumoniae,* and *N. meningitidis.* Initial therapy should, therefore, include antibiotics appropriate to cover these organisms. Ampicillin plus chloramphenicol is the usual combination. Chloramphenicol resistant *H. influenzae* remains fairly rare. Penicillin may be used as an alternate to ampicillin in combination with chloramphenicol.

Several of the cephalosporins have been shown to be effective in meningitis and if chloramphenicol can not be used, cefotaxime, ceflriaxone or cefuroxime are alternatives. Aplastic anemia is a rare but potentially life-threatening complication of chloramphenicol administration.

REMEMBER: Oral administration of chloramphenicol results in blood levels at least equal to that obtained by intravenous administration. Patients being treated with I.V. chloramphenicol who are showing clinical improvement, can usually be switched to oral medicine around day 5 of therapy. Obtaining chloramphenicol levels is recommended especially in infants and in patients receiving phenobarbital or dilantin. Both of these drugs alter chloramphenicol pharmokinetics.

Appropriate therapy should be continued for seven to ten days. Therapy should probably also be continued for at least 5 days after the patient is afebrile. Patients who show a good response during the first 24 hours of therapy and continued improvement thereafter probably do not need a repeat lumbar puncture on therapy. Lack of clinical response or clinical deterioration necessitates a repeat lumbar puncture. **REMEMBER:** Patients with *H. influenzae* may take longer to defervece than patients with other bacterial causes of meningitis. As long as there is overall clinical improvement, fever for about one week is within acceptable limits for resolving *H. influenzae* meningitis. The appearance of new symptoms, or the recurrence of fever after a period of being afebrile should create concern.

Repeat lumbar punctures, immediately after therapy has been stopped, do not appear to be of value in predicting relapse. In patients who follow a routine hospital course without complications and are asymptomatic at the end of therapy, repeat LPs are usually not indicated.

Appropriate supportive care is essential in the total care of the patient with meningitis. Inappropriate ADH syndrome should be managed with fluid restriction. Seizures should be controlled with anticonvulsants. The appearance of subdural effusions or intracranial abscesses may necessitate surgical intervention.

An essential component of treatment of meningitis is the prevention of its spread. Rifampin prophylaxis is recommended for household and nursery school contacts. Medical personnel with intimate contact with the patient (mouth-to-mouth resuscitation) can also receive prophylaxis.

Antibiotic prophylaxis should begin as soon as possible. For meningococcal infection rifampin should be given 20 mg/kd/day divided q12h x 2 days. If the organism is sensitive to sulfonamides, these may be used. The value of prophylaxis for *H. influenzae* remains controversial. Current recommendations are for the use of rifampin 20 mg/kg/day in one daily dose x4 days in households where there is at least one child (besides the index case) less than 4 years old. In those households, the entire family should receive prophylactic antibiotic. The index case should also receive rifampin as the antibiotics commonly used in treatment of *H. influenzae* infections do not routinely eliminate the nasopharyngeal carriage in the patient.

Sequelae and Complications

Antibiotic therapy has significantly reduced mortality in bacterial meningitis. Nevertheless, morbidity from the disease remains high, and significant sequelae may occur in up to half of children with meningitis. The list of possible consequences of meningitis include: hearing loss, seizure disorders, cranial nerve involvement, low IQ's, visual problems, obstructive hydrocephaly, paralysis, subdural effusions, and brain abscesses. Some, but not all, of the deficits are temporary.

A good neurological exam including auditory testing (brainstem auditory evoked potentials and/or hearing testing) should be done before discharge and then at follow-up visits.

Many signs and symptoms have been correlated with a poor prognosis. Among these are focal deficit prior to therapy, seizures prior to admission, low CSF glucose, low serum sodium, and high concentration of bacteria in the CSF.

KEY POINTS

BASIC WORKUP FOR MENINGITIS

DIAGNOSIS (should be modified as appropriate for each patient).
L.P. - culture, Gram stain or Acridine Orange Stain
   (Acridine Orange may be more sensitive, especially in patients already on antibiotics)
   glucose, protein, cell count and differential
Antigen detection (CIE or Latex Agglutination or Coagglutination)
Blood - culture, CBC, electrolytes, BUN, glucose, Osmolality
Urine - culture, antigen detection, urinalysis, osmolality
MANAGEMENT
Antibiotics - broad spectrum pending culture results and sensitivities.
Fluids - moderate restriction, monitor for evidence of IADHS.
Daily examination - monitor neurological symptoms, signs, head circumferences. Monitor for evidence of other sites of infection.
In patients with lack of improvement–
Look for additional sites of infection.

Look for evidence of subdural effusion.
Look for evidence of abscess.
Look for evidence of failure of therapy.
Workup should include: Physical exam; urinalysis; chest x-ray; transillumination of head, CT scan, or ultrasound of head; repeat LP.

REFERENCES

1. Feigin RD: Central Nervous System infections in *Textbook of* Pediatrics Infectious Diseases 1981. Feigin RD, Cherry JD (ed.) Saunders; pp 293–308.
2. Friedman AD, Ray CG: Rapid Diagnosis of Infections. Pediatric Infectious Diseases 1982; 1:366–373.
3. McCracken GH. New Concepts in the management of infants and children with meningitis. Pediatric Infectious Diseases 1983; 2:55-555 (suppl).
4. Philip AG, Baker CJ: Cerebral fluid C-reative protein in neonatal meningitis. J Pediatr 1983; 102:715–717.
5. Sarff LD, Platt LH, McCracken GH: Cerebrospinal fluid evaluation in meningitis. J Pediatr 1976; 88:473–477.
6. Schaad UB, Nelson JD, McCracken GH: Recrudescence and relapse in bacterial meningitis of childhood. Pediatrics 1981; 67:188–195.
7. Siegel JD: New Developments in Meningitis. Pediatric Infectious Diseases 1982; *1*:545–551 (suppl).
8. Smith AL: How to evaluate and treat meningitis. Resident and Staff Physician, Nov. 1977, 77–86.
9. Stein MT, Travner D: The child with a stiff neck. Clinical Pediatrics 1982; 21:559–563.
10. Teele DW, Dasefsky B, Rakusan T, Klein JO: Meningitis after lumbar puncture in children with bacteremia. NEJM 1981; 305:1079–1081.
11. Yogev R: Advances in diagnosis and treatment of childhood meningitis. Pediatric Infectious Diseases 1985; 4:321–325.

REVIEW QUESTIONS

1.) In children outside the neonatal period, the three most common bacterial causes of meningitis are (3) __________.
2.) Laboratory diagnosis of meningitis is usually made by L.P. Spinal fluid should be evaluated for (6) __________
3.) In children with meningitis monitoring, fluid intake and output and following urine and serum osmolality can help identify patients with the complication of __________
4.) True or False
   1. Infants with meningitis almost always will have a stiff neck.
   2. An infant with a flat or sunken fontanelle rarely will have meningitis.
   3. CIE is a fast diagnostic test that identifies bacterial antibody.
   4. *H. influenzae* that are not beta-lactamase producing are always ampicillin sensitive.
   5. Oral chloramphenicol achieves serum levels that are usually at least as good as levels achieved by intravenous administration.
   6. Seizures prior to the institution of therapy is a poor prognostic sign.

7

URINARY TRACT INFECTIONS

Clinical Manifestations

The symptoms of urinary tract infections (UTIs) in children are similar to those found in adults. The list of common symptoms include dysuria, frequency, urgency, abdominal pain, fever, and enuresis. Less frequently hematuria, abdominal tenderness, vaginal discharge, and anorexia occur.

Clinical diagnosis of UTIs in infants is more difficult than in older children. Infants infrequently present with symptoms common to older children. Nonspecific symptoms are common in the infant. Feeding problems, failure to thrive, diarrhea, vomiting, and fever are often presenting manifestations of UTIs in infants. Irritability, abnormal urine appearance, odor, jaundice, and central nervous system symptoms also are found. *REMEMBER:* In infants with feeding problems or poor weight gain it is essential to consider the diagnosis of UTI.

Signs of UTI found on physical exam are few. Upper urinary tract infection may be associated with costovertebral angle (CVA) tenderness; while lower tract infection is associated with suprapubic tenderness. *REMEMBER:* The combination of fever, chills, and CVA tenderness are classic for upper urinary tract infection (pyelonephritis).

Etiology and Epidemiology

Escherichea coli is the etiologic agent in most UTIs. The reservoir for most of these bacteria is the gastrointestinal tract. Retrograde spread of enteric bacteria up the urethra is responsible for many UTIs, especially in girls. In younger infants and neonates, infection of the urinary tract is often secondary to bacteremia or sepsis.

The incidence of UTIs is greater in females than males in all age groups except during the neonatal period when the incidence in male infants is about four times that found in female infants. Infections of the urinary tract are common in children. Only infections of the respiratory tract are more common. The incidence of bacteruria in school age girls is 5-10%.

Diagnosis

Urinalysis - (U/A) The urinalysis can provide a good deal of information which is of value in diagnosing infections and noninfectious diseases.

Color - Brown urine suggests the presence of bilirubin, red suggests hemoglobin or red blood cells, and dark brown suggests myoglobin or old blood. Beets can turn acidic urine red and aklaline urine yellow. Pyridium, povan, rifampin and red candies may all turn urine red or reddish orange.

Clarity - A hazy or cloudy urine suggests infection or kidney disease.

Specific Gravity - This can serve as an index of hydration, or kidney function or of central nervous system disease.

pH - An index of systemic pH may be abnormal in UTIs and in tubular disease.

Reducing substances - Clinitest measures glucose, fructose, galactose and lactose but may be falsely positive in patients receiving chloramphenicol, chloral hydrate, or ascorbic acid.

Ketones - The presence of ketones in the urine suggests starvation or diabetes.

Proteinuria and Hematuria - These are frequently present in patients with renal disease.

Urinary Sediment - The sediment is particularly valuable in patients where a UTI is suspected. Red cells or casts can be seen in tuberculosis, subacute bacterial endocarditis, cystitis, malaria, and acute apendicitis. Non-infectious causes include glomerulonephritis, neoplasm, trauma, systemic lupus erythematosis, polyarteritis nodosa, blood dyscrasias and certain drugs like anti-coagulants, asprin, phenobarbitol, and sulfonamides. *REMEMBER:* Red cell casts mean renal parenchymal disease and requires further evaluation.

White cells usually mean infection. Greater than 50 white blood cells (WBCs) per high power field or clumping of WBCs is strongly suggestive of UTIs but most infections are less obvious. *REMEMBER:* Lack of WBCs in the urine does not mean there is not infection. Chronic UTIs especially may be present without WBCs in the urinary sediment. Look for bacteria in urine.

Hyaline and epithelial casts may suggest renal disease, as do fatty casts. Culture - The "gold standard" for the diagnosis of UTIs is based on work done over 20 years ago, in which the presence of 100,000 bacteria per milliliter from midstream urine in adult females correlated well with the presence of UTIs. Since then this study has served as the basis for diagnosing UTIs not only in adult females, but also in adult males and children, and for diagnosing both upper and lower tract infection.

Recent evidence suggests rigidly following these criteria may miss a significant number of UTIs. Routine clean voided urine specimens can be obtained fairly easily in toilet trained children when the genital region is appropriately cleaned. In smaller children and infants reliable samples are best obtained by suprapubic aspiration or catheterization of the urethra. When done properly in young infants and neonates, the suprapubic tap is safe and reliable. If the suprapubic tap grows any number of organisms, the probability of this reflecting true infection is very high, especially if they are Gram negative bacilli. Catheterized specimens may have bacteria without true infection. Less than 1000 colonies/ml makes it very unlikely that a true UTI is present. *REMEMBER:* Clean catch urines are best obtained at first morning void after thoroughly cleaning the genital area with soap, water, and antiseptic solution. Midstream urine should be obtained.

Treatment

Therapy should cover the spectrum of organisms most commonly associated with UTIs. *Escherichia coli* is responsible for the vast majority of these infections. Other bacteria found include klebsiella, enterobacter, proteus, and less frequently, pseudomonas and staphylococcus. Priority is given to covering the enteric bacteria when choosing an antibiotic.

Acute UTIs can be effectively treated with either amoxicillin or a sulfonamide for 7-10 days. Upper tract infection should be treated for longer, at least two weeks. Repeat cultures at 48-72 hours after treatment has begun should be sterile. If they are not, an alternative antibiotic should be selected which does not also demonstrate *in vivo* resistance. *REMEMBER:* Antibiotics that concentrate in the urine and that show good antimicrobial activity at the pH of the patient's urine, will be most successful in sterilizing that patient's urine. Pseudomonas lower tract UTIs can be successfully treated with erythromycin if the urine is alkaline. Thus, a regimen of oral bicarbonate and erythromycin can successfully treat lower tract infection without the need for parenteral therapy. Other examples are the penicillins and nitrofurantoins which are much more active in acidic urine.

Shorter term therapy for uncomplicated lower tract UTIs has been shown to be effective in adults and may be effective in children also. Among the antibiotics studied for short course therapy are amoxcillin, ampicillin, trimethoprim-sulfamethoxazole, cefadroxil and amikacin. Regimens of single dose therapy or one to three days of therapy probably result in increased compliance but may be poorly effective in unsuspected upper tract infection. The issue of possibly higher recurrence rates after short course therapy has not yet been satisfactorily resolved.

Sequelae and Complications

Recurrences of UTIs are not uncommon. Rates of recurrences vary from 25 to 40%. The greater the number of previous infections the greater the chances of relapse. Conversely, the longer the infection free period after a UTI, the less likely is a recurrence. The frequency of relapse can be decreased by using suppressive antibiotic therapy. Nitrofurantoin or trimethoprim-sulfamethoxazole is frequently used. REMEMBER: Nitrofurantoin is associated with liver toxicity and pulmonary damage. Trimethoprim-sulfamethoxazole has been associated with neutropenia and rash. Stevens-Johnson syndrome has been reported. The risk of repeated UTIs must be weighed against the risk of drug side effects in each patient.

Careful follow-up of patients with UTIs is needed to monitor for the development of vesico-urethral reflux (VUR) which may result in renal scarring. VUR may occur in up to 50% of girls with a history of many UTIs. Intravenous pyelograms and voiding cystourethrograms after the first UTI provides baseline data for further follow-up. *REMEMBER:* VUR tends to improve with time in many (not all) patients. Renal scarring is more likely in pre-school age children than in older children.

KEY POINTS

1 *Diagnosis*
Obtain urine for analysis, culture, and sensitivity.
Infants and neonates - suprapubic

Older infants and children - midstream, first void clean catch (await culture results before beginning treatment in case culture is contaminated and repeat cultures are necessary).

If child is clinically ill and therapy cannot be withheld, then suprapubic or cath. specimen should be obtained and treatment begun immediately.

2 *Management*

Antibiotics - initial therapy appropriate for common organisms, e.g., amoxicillin, then change antibiotic based on sensitivity, if necessary.

Repeat culture on therapy to ensure effectiveness of therapy.

3 *Follow-up*

Post-therapy urine culture - 7 days post therapy workup for anatomical abnormalities IVP, VCU.

Periodic followup urines - at least every month x 3 followed every 3 months and then every 6 months. Follow-up for 2 years post-UTI.

REFERENCES

1. Lohr JA, Kesler RW, Hayden GF, et al.: Three-day therapy of lower urinary tract infections with nitrofurantoin macrocrystals: A randomized clinical trial. J of Pediatr 1981; 99:980-983.
2. Margileth AM, Pedreira FA, Hirshman GH, et al.: Urinary tract bacterial infections. Office diagnosis and management in Pediatric Clinics of North America 1976; 23:721-733.
3. Marks MI: Genitourinary infections in *Textbook of Pediatric Infectious Disease.* Feigin and Cherry (eds). Saunders Co., Philadelphia, 1981, pp. 348-366.
4. McCracken GH: Recurrent urinary tract infections in children. Pediatric Infectious Disease 1984; 3(3 suppl); 528-30.
5. Mou TW: Effect of urinary pH on the antimicrobial activity of antibiotics and chemotherapeutic agents. J. Urol. 1982; 87:978-987.
6. Ogra PL. Faden HS: Urinary tract infections in childhood: An update. J of Pediatr. 1985; 106:1023-1029.
7. Shapiro ED: Short course antimicrobial treatment of urinary tract infections in children: A critical analysis. Pediatric Infectious Disease 1982; 1:294-297.
8. Stamm WE, Counts GW, Running KR, et al.: Diagnosis of coliform infection in acute dysuric women. NEJM 1982; 307:463-467.
9. Zinner SH, Sabath LD, Casey JI, et al: Erythromycin and alkalinization of the urine in the treatment of urinary tract infections due to Gram-negative bacilli. Lancet 1971; 1:1267-1268.

REVIEW QUESTIONS

1.) The classic presentation of pyelonephritis include__________.(3)
2.) UTIs in neonates and infants may present with non-specific manifesta-tions such as __________. (5)
3.) The bacteria most commonly associated with UTIs is__________.
4.) White blood cell casts suggest__________.
5.) Rifampin may discolor urine and turn it what color?
6.) The presence of__________(number) bacteria/ml on a midstream clean catch voided urine suggest the presence of a UTI.
7.) Penicillins are more effective antibiotics in urine if the pH is __________. (acidic or alkaline)

8

SEXUALLY TRANSMITTED DISEASES

GONOCOCCAL URETHRITIS

Clinical Manifestations

Gonococcal urethritis usually presents as a sudden onset of dysuria, frequency, and urethral discharge in males. The discharge is usually purulent. Less common symptoms include scrotal swelling in the males, and evidence of proctitis in the homosexual male. The symptoms may be more severe in the morning. REMEMBER: Although uncommon (less than 20%), some infected males will be asymptomatic.

Symptoms in the infected female include a vaginal discharge and evidence of cystitis such as frequency and dysuria. Vulvar pain may be present. Asymptomatic cases in females are common and the incidence may be as high as 60%.

Etiology and Epidemiology

Neisseria gonorrhea is an intracellular Gram-negative diplococcus. There are roughly 1 million reported cases of gonorrhea in the U.S. each year. The actual number of cases is believed to be at least twice as many, or over 2 million cases of gonorrhea each year. Both the 15-19 year old group and the 20-24 year old group have particularly high incidence rates. The incubation period is usually 2-7 days. Young children with evidence of *Neisseria gonorrheae* infection should be investigated for sexual abuse.

Diagnosis

The clinical presentation along with associated physical findings such as meatal erythema in males, pain on rectal examination in homosexual males, and cervical friability or erythema in the female patient, may be helpful.

Laboratory studies are necessary to determine the specific etiologic agent causing the symptoms. Gram stain may be very useful, especially in the male patient. The presence of Gram negative intracellular diplococci on the smear of urthral exudate is usually considered diagnostic. REMEMBER: It is important that the bacteria are intracellular to make the diagnosis. Extracellular organisms are insufficient proof of gonorrhea. There may not be (in fact, usually are not) organisms in every leukocyte; therefore, detailed scrutiny of the slide is important. In females, the Gram stain is less valuable and is often not considered sufficient to either make or rule-out the diagnosis.

Confirmation of the diagnosis is made by culture. It is important to inoculate the specimen immediately after it is obtained and that the medium, usually Thayer-Martin, be at room temperature and not used directly from the refrigerator. Growth of the organism is best achieved in an enhanced CO_2 atmosphere. To make the diagnosis, the presence of oxidase positive Gram negative diplococci must be demonstrated. Positive cultures should be tested for penicillin sensitivity. Follow-up cultures after therapy are a good idea.

Recently, antigen detection systems have become available as aides in the diagnosis of gonorrhea. Their exact role in the cost-effective and efficient diagnosis of gonorrhea remains to be clarified.

Treatment

Standard therapy for gonorrhea in adolescents and adults is 4.8 million units aqueous procaine penicillin G divided into two simultaneous intramuscular injections and 1 gram probenacid given orally. Alternatives include the use of ampicillin (3.5 grams orally) or amoxicillin (3.0 grams orally) with 1 gram of probenacid orally. Tetracycline, 10 grams over 5 days as a qid regimen is also acceptable therapy. *REMEMBER:* Concurrent infection with chlamydia or ureaplasma is not uncommon, and may result in an apparent therapeutic failure of penicillin. If the etiology is pencillinase-producing *Neisseria gonorrheae* spectinomycin, cefoxitin or a third generation cephalosporin are among the alternatives available.

Sequelae and Complications

Simple urethritis/vaginitis may progress to other sites and cause epididymitis, prostatitis, cervicitis, endometritis and salpingitis. Other complications and syndromes associated with *N. gonorrheae* infection include: perihepatitis, pharyngitis, tenosynovitis, arthritis, endocarditis, dermatitis, proctitis, meningitis, septicemia, and conjunctivitis.

NON-GONOCOCCAL URETHRITIS (NGU)

Clinical Manifestations

It is difficult on clinical grounds to distinguish gonorrhea from non-gonococcal urethritis. Urethral discharge, if present, may vary from slightly mucoid to purulent. Dysuria may be present. Asymptomatic cases occur. The term "non-gonococcal urethritis" usually refers to infection in the male. Similar infection in the female patient is usually referred to as "urethral syndrome" and is associated with dysuria and pyuria without isolation of a significant number of organisms of usual urinary pathogens.

Etiology and Epidemiology

It is estimated that about half of NGU is due to *Chlamydia trachomatis,* about 30% is due to *Ureaplasma urealyticum,* and the remaining cases by a variety of organisms including *Trichomonas vaginalis, Candida albicans,* and *Herpes simplex.* The age distribution of NGU appears to parallel gonorrhea. The incubation period may exceed 10 days. Recurrences are common, and coinfection, often with *N. gonorrheae* is not uncommon. Young children with genital chlamydial infection should be investigated for possible sexual abuse.

Diagnosis

A presumptive diagnosis can be made in a patient with an appropriate clinical presentation, a negative Gram stain for *N. gonorrheae,* and a negative culture for *N. gonorrheae.* Confirmation is possible in laboratories where chlamydia or ureaplasma are grown. Antigen detection methods are commercially available to detect chlamydia in genital infections.

Treatment

Most chlamydial and ureaplasma genital infections can be treated with tetracycline or doxycycline for at least 7 days. As some ureaplasma are unresponsive to tetracycline, it is reasonable to use erythromycin if tetracycline therapy fails. Relapses are common. Co-infection with *N. gonorrheae* can occur and should be ruled out.

Sequelae and Complications

C. trachomatis can cause, in addition to urethritis, epididymitis prostatitis, cervicitis, proctitis, Reiter's syndrome, endometritis, salpingitis, perihepatitis and otitis. In infants, chlamydia causes conjunctivitis and pneumonia.

U. urealyticum has also been associated with salpingitis, chorioamnionitis, in addition to urethritis, and in infants is associated with pneumonia.

SYPHILIS

Clinical Manifestations

Primary syphilis is characterized by a painless chancre. The lesion is a papule that is eroded, with a raised border that is indurated. Not all chancres are typical. Syphilitic chancres are not limited to the genital area. Oral and anal lesions are not uncommon, especially among homosexual males. Lymphadenopathy may accompany lesions. The symptoms are usually self-limited even if not treated.

Secondary syphilis presents with a variety of cutaneous manifestations. In untreated patients, secondary syphilis may appear within six months of initial infection. Lesions may be macular, papular, or pustular but are not usually vesicular or bullous. Lesions also may appear on moist mucous membranes. These lesions often contain many spirochetes and are very contagious. The lesions of secondary syphilis usually disappear over months. Systemic symptoms of generalized lymphadenopathy, fever, malaise, sore throat, and headache may also be present.

Etiology and Epidemiology

Syphilis is caused by *Treponema pallidum,* a motile spirochete. About 30,000 cases of syphilis (primary and secondary) are reported each year. Twice that number may actually occur.

Diagnosis

A typical clinical presentation with typical lesions is helpful in making the diagnosis. Laboratory confirmation is necessary. Dark field preparation from lesions may show the spirochette. Serologic tests are frequently used. VDRL (Veneral Disease Research Laboratory) and RPR (rapid plasma reagin) tests are available to make a presumptive diagnosis of syphilis. These are not specific for *T. pallidum* antigen but instead measure antibody to phospholipids. A positive VDRL or RPR should be confirmed with a *T. pallidum* specific antigen test like the FTA (fluorescent treponemal antibody-absorption) test. REMEMBER: A variety of illnesses including other infections, malignancy and immune disorders may give false positive nonspecific (VDRL or RPR) test results.

Treatment

In patients with acquired syphilis of less than one year since initial infection, benzathine penicillin G (50,000 U/kg IM in one dose, not to exceed 2.4 million units) or aqueous procaine penicillin G, (50,000 U/kg IM daily for 8 days with the daily dose not exceeding 600,000 U) are recommended. If the patient is penicillin allergic, erythromycin or tetracycline (in older children) is recommended for 15 days. If neurosyphilis is present, benzathine penicillin should not be used.

If the infection has existed for greater than 1 year, benzathine penicillin should be given weekly for 3 weeks, or procaine penicillin for 15 days. Penicillin allergic patients should receive erythromycin or tetracycline for at least 30 days. Adequate therapy can be documented by a seroreversal of the VDRL or a fall in the titer within one year of therapy.

Sequelae and Complications

Complications include late syphilis and congenital syphilis.

TRICHOMONIASIS

Symptoms

Trichomoniasis is often asymptomatic, especially in men. Symptoms, when present, often include erythema and edema of the external genitalia. Frothy grayish discharge may be present. Vaginitis may be associated with cervicitis and punctate hemorrhages. Symptomatic males may present with urethritis.

Etiology and Epidemiology

T. vaginalis is a protozoa. Transmission is both sexually and through non-sexual contact. Reported prevalence rates vary from as low as 5% of gynecologic patients to as high as 75% of promiscuous populations. Trichomoniasis is uncommon in prepubescent females.

Diagnosis

Trichomonas vaginalis, a motile protozoan, can be seen by micoscopic examination of wet mount preparation. The prep should be taken of vaginal discharge. The specimen is mixed in a saline drop on a slide. One looks for the characteristic wobbling swimming motion of the organism. Culture methods are available. An alternative to a wet mount is a papanicolaou smear.

Treatment

T. vaginalis infections can be treated with a single oral 2 gram dose of metronidazole. It is usually recommended that sexual partners be treated, even if asymptomatic.

Sequelae and Complications

Complications and sequelae are infrequent. *T. vaginalis* may be associated with prostatitis and salpingitis. In addition, neonatal conjunctivitis has been reported.

GENITAL WARTS

Clinical Manifestations

Genital warts, *Condyloma acuminata,* are flesh colored growths usually appearing in the genital-perineal region. Lesions may occur near the glans penis, urethra, perianal region, vagina, cervix or vulva. The growths are described as sessile or papillary.

Etiology and Epidemiology

Condyloma acuminata are caused by human papillomavirus, which is a small DNA virus of the papovavirus group. Its spread is usually from sexual contact and its age distribution parallels that of gonorrhea. Although uncommon, infants can be infected with genital warts that have been transmitted by the mother. Human papillomavirus types 6 and 11 are associated with both genital warts and laryngeal warts. Types 16 and 18 are associated with both genital warts and genital cancer.

Diagnosis

Genital warts are usually diagnosed by clinical appearance. If there is a question regarding the diagnosis, histology can be done.

Treatment

There are several modalities for therapy. Podophylin can be applied on a weekly basis. Alternative treatment include cryotherapy, curretage, or electrocautery. Genital warts have been shown to respond to interferon given intramuscularly. Many warts will regress spontaneously.

Sequelae and Complications

Complications are rare. Malignant transformation has been reported infrequently. Acquisition by infants may result in laryngeal or bronchial papillomata which may cause respiratory distress.

SCABIES

Clinical Manifestations

A major symptom of scabies is itching. Lesions can frequently be found on soft skin folds, such as on the penis, scrotum, finger webs, wrist, elbows, nipples, buttocks, soles and umbilicus. Lesions are usually red papules. Characteristic burrows containing the mite can often be seen. The mites cause an allergic response frequently resulting in papular urticaria. Infants and children may have vesicles, few or no burrows, and atypical distribution of lesions.

Etiology and Epidemiology

Scabies is caused by *Sarcoptes scabei,* a small mite. Transmission is primarily person-to-person through close contact. Fomites are usually important sources only if they are heavily infected. It is believed that 2 to 4 percent of patients seen by dermatologists have scabies.

Diagnosis

The diagnosis is best made from microscopic examination of skin scrapings, looking for the mite or her eggs. Unexcoriated burrows or papules which are new and not secondarily infected are good sites for scrapings.

The procedure can easily be done by placing some mineral oil onto a scalpel blade, scraping the site and then adding the scrapings to additional mineral oil on a glass slide. It is examined under the microscope after placing a coverslip.

Treatment

Several scabicides are available as a lotion or cream, including lindane or gamma benzene hexachloride. It is absorbed through the skin and can be toxic. Symptoms include convulsions, nausea, vomiting and respiratory failure. Applying the lotion or cream and leaving it on for only 12 hours instead of 24 hours can reduce the risk of toxicity. It should be thoroughly washed off after the treatment period. A second application may be needed one week later since the treatment may not be ovicidal. Because itching is the result of the allergic response, it may persist for a few weeks despite adequate therapy.

Alternative therapy includes crotamiton cream applied a second time, 24 hours after the first application, and sulphur applied three consecutive nights. Both of these therapies should be followed by thorough bathing 24 hours after the last application. Outside the U.S., thiabendazole cream or benzyl benzoate are used successfully. An emulsion concentrate of benzyl benzoate, DDT, benzocaine and polysorbate, diluted with water has been recommended by the World Health Organization. Contaminated clothing and bedding should be thoroughly washed.

Sequelae and Complications

Secondary infection commonly occurs as a result of scratching papules and burrows. Impetigo, furunculosis or cellulitis may result. Pustular eczema may also occur. Nodular scabies involves the entire dermis and may extend into subcutaneous tissue. The reddish-brown nodules may persist despite adequate therapy. Norwegian scabies is manifested by thick crusted keratotic lesions of the palm and soles, often resembling psoriasis. It is usually the result of a large infestation of mites and is highly contagious.

LICE

Clinical Manifestations

Lice cause erythematous papules that itch. Nits will frequently be present at the base of hair in the pubis, anal, thigh and abdominal regions. Adult lice may also adhere to the hairs.

Etiology and Epidemiology

Pediculosis pubis is caused by *Phthirus pubis,* the pubic louse. It is a small (1-4 mm) oval grayish insect. The louse is usually transferred by bodily contact often during sexual activity. It is usually not contracted from bedding or clothing.

Diagnosis

Diagnosis is made by clinical observation of the louse. Alternatively microscopic identification of the nits at the base of the hair will also make the diagnosis.

Treatment

Treatment is with pyrethrin-based lotion or with gamma-benzene hexachloride. Eggs are not killed by these products so treatment should be repeated one week later. Disinfection of bedding and clothing is usually not needed for pubic lice.

Sequelae and Complications

Rarely, secondary infection causes impetigo, furunculosis or pustular eczema.

HERPES SIMPLEX VIRUS (HSV)

Clinical Manifestations

The spectrum of symptoms varies from mild to severe. Many patients experience soreness, itching, and dysuria, and the majority have tender inguinal or femoral lymphadenopathy. Systemic symptoms such as headache, and fever may also occur.

With their initial herpes infection, women frequently get a heavy vaginal discharge and erosive cervicitis. Men may have urethritis with dysuria and little or no discharge. Skin lesions, while not universal, are frequently seen. Lesions characteristically start out as vesicular or vesiculopustular lesions. The lesions are commonly found on the vulva or the shaft of the penis. During the first week, the lesions usually progress to ulcers. Discomfort usually is increased during this stage of the illness. Healing usually begins during the second week and all lesions are usually healed about three weeks after the onset of symptoms. Recurrent outbreaks tend to be milder than the initial infection.

Etiology and Epidemiology

Approximately 10% of the adult population in the U.S. has symptomatic genital herpes. HSV type I is primarily associated with cold sores and fever blisters. HSV type 2 is primarily associated with genital herpes. However, primarily because of orogenital contact, HSV-1 has been found in about 20% of genital herpes, and HSV-2 has been associated with orofacial infection.

Diagnosis

A history of recent sexual contact and the presence of typical lesions are helpful in making the diagnosis of genital herpes. *REMEMBER:* Other infections can cause a genital ulcer. *Treponema pallidum, Hemophilus ducreyi* and rarely, *Chlamydia trachomatis* have all been associated with genital ulcers. Syphilitic ulcers tend to be painless. Herpes and chancroid (*H. ducreyi*) lesions are usually painful if touched. *REMEMBER:* Herpes lyphadenopathy is usually slightly tender and firm, and usually non-fixed.

Syphilitic nodes are non-tender and firm. Chancroid and lymphogranuloma venereum (*C. trachomatis*) usually produce lymphadenopathy that is suppurative, if present at all. Diagnostic confirmation is best achieved by isolation of the virus in tissue culture. Cultures are usually positive in 48-72 hours. If viral cultures are not readily available, a scraping from a lesion can be stained by Giemsa or Papanicolaou stain for multinucleated giant cells or inclusion bodies within cells. Alternatively, immunofluorescent staining for herpes antigen can help detect the presence of Herpes simplex virus.

Treatment

Acyclovir has been shown to be effective in primary initial genital herpes. The drug is currently available as topical, oral and IV forms. In immunocompromised patients, the course of recurrent HSV infections may also be shortened with therapy.

Patients should take basic hygienic precautions to avoid autoinoculation to other parts of their body, to avoid sexual contact while lesions are present, and to avoid secondary bacterial infection by keeping lesions dry and clean. Emotional support is important, especially in patients with frequent recurrences.

Sequelae and Complications

A majority of patients with an initial HSV-type 2 infection will have recurrences. These recurrences can be either reactivation of latent virus that is in the sensory nerve root ganglia or, as there are several different strains of HSV-type 2, may be the result of exogenous reinfection. Prodromes prior to recurrences are common. Prodromal symptoms are usually itching or tingling. New lesions often appear 24-48 hours after the prodrome. Recurrences are usually milder than the initial infection. As many as 10% of recurrences are asymptomatic. Some recurrences seem to be associated with stress or hormonal changes.

Serious complications of genital herpes infections include meningitis and cervical cancer. The relationship between HSV-2 infection and cervical cancer is a statistical association. Immunocompromised patients and neonates can develop life-threatening systemic infection with HSV-type 2.

CHANCROID

Clinical Manifestations

The characteristic lesions are one or more soft chancres. The chancre is an ulcer that is tender, ragged, non-indurated, and often is covered with a gray-yellow necrotic exudate. Inguinal adenopathy may be present and is usually unilateral. Women may be asymptomatic.

Etiology and Epidemiology

Chancroid is caused by *Hemophilus ducreyi,* a non-motile Gram negative coccobacillus. The infection frequently occurs in association with other genital infections, especially herpes and syphilis. The infection is much more common in third world nations than in the developed nations. Infection does not produce immunity and reinfections occur. Asymptomatic females may serve as a significant reservoir of infection.

Diagnosis

Symptoms and the appearance of the lesions may suggest chancroid, but diagnosis depends on demonstration of *H. ducreyi* from the lesions. This may be difficult as cultures or smears of scrapings from the lesion may be useful in less than 30% of cases. Consequently diagnosis often depends on the appearance of the lesion and ruling-out other likely etiologies, especially syphilis.

Treatment

Sulfonamides are the drugs of choice. Two weeks of sulfisoxazole (1 gram po.qid) will usually result in a cure. Tetracycline and kanamycin are alternative treatments but are often less effective. Recent data suggests that erythromycin or trimethoprim-sulfamethoxazole may be suitable alternatives depending on the specific sensitivities of the *H. ducreyi* involved.

Sequelae and Complications

Deep scars secondary to the ulcers, a deformed penis, phimosis, paraphimosis, fistulas and secondary infections have all been reported.

Other sexually transmitted diseases such as CMV, hepatitis B and AIDS are discussed in other sections of this book.

KEY POINTS

1. Patients with a documented sexually transmitted disease may frequently have several different organisms causing infection. Apparent treatment failures may be related to this multiplicity of etiologies.
2. *N. gonorrhea* infection is frequently found in association with syphilis, chlamydia, or ureaplasma.
3. Primary herpes and *H. ducreyi* lesions are usually painful. Primary syphilitic chancre is usually painless.
4. Primary HSV-infections may respond to acyclovir therapy.
5. Penicillin is the treatment of choice for *N. gonorrhea,* and *T. pallidum* infections.
6. Tetracyclines usually provide adequate therapy for *C. trachomatis and U. urealyticum.*
7. *T. vaginalis* is treated with metronidazole.
8. Podophylin is frequently used to treat condyloma.

REFERENCES

1. Anonymous: Sexually Transmitted Disease Summary. CDC Publication 00-3380 Technical Information Service, Atlanta, Georgia.
2. Bell TA: Major sexually transmitted diseases of children and adolescents. Pediatr Infect Dis. 1983; 2:153–161.
3. Bowie WR: Etiology and treatment of nongonococcal urethritis. Sex Transm Dis 1978; 5:27–33.
4. Chacko MR, Louchik JC: Chlamydia trachomatis: Infection in sexually active adolescents: Prevalence and risk factors. Pediatr 1984; 73:-836–840.
5. Felman YM, Hoke AW: Wellcome Atlas of Sexually transmitted diseases. Burroughs Wellcome Co. USA, 1985; pp 18-34.
6. Lee TJ, Sparling PF: Syphilis: An algorithm JAMA 1979; 242:1187–1189.
7. Lykke-Olesen L, Pedersen TG, Larsen L et al: Epidemic of chancroid in Greenland, 1977. Lancet 1979; 1:654–655.

8. Murphy MD: Office laboratory diagnosis of sexually transmitted disease. Pediatr Infect Dis. 1983; 2:146–152.

9. Nilsen AE, Aasen T, Halsos AM, et al: Efficacy of oral acyclovir in the treatment of initial and recurrent genital herpes. Lancet 1982; 2:571–573.

10. Rein, MF: Therapeutic decisions in the treatment of sexually transmitted diseases. An Overview. Sex Trans Dis 1981; 8(s):93–99.

11. Rosenfeld WD, Litman N: Urogenital tract infections in male adolescent. Pediatrics in Review. 1983; 4:257–265.

12. Schachter J: Chlamydial infections. N Engl J Med 1978; 298:428–435, 490–495, 540–549

13. Stamm WE, Running K, McKeuitt M, et al: Treatment of the acute urethral syndrome. N Engl J Med 1982; 307:463–68.

14. Stewart DB: The gynecologic lesions of lymphogranuloma verereum and granuloma inguinale. Med Clin North Am 1964; 43:773–786.

REVIEW QUESTIONS

1.) Match infection with appropriate therapy: (each drug may be used more than once).

1. Chlamydia	A. Metronidazole
2. *N. gonorrhea*	B. Tetracycline
3. Herpes	C. Podophylin
4. *H. ducreyi*	D. Sulfasoxazole
5. *T. pallidum*	E. Acyclovir
6. *U. urealyticum*	F. Penicillin
7. *T. vaginalis*	G. Gamma-benzene hexachloride
8. Condylomata	
9. *Phthirus pubis*	
10. *Sarcoptes scabei*	

2.) Match the diagnostic test with the diagnosis:

A. rapid plasma reagin	1. Herpes
B. motile protozoa on wet mount	2. Gonorrhea
C. skin scraping from burrows	3. Syphilis
D. microscopic examination of nits at the base of hair	4. Lice
E. Giemsa stained lesion scraping showing multinucleated giant cells	5. Scabies
F. intracellular Gram negative diplococci.	6. Trichomoniasis

3.) True or False
   1. Penicillin is appropriate therapy of combined *N. gonorrhea* and *C. trachomatis* infections.
   2. *C. trachomatis* and *U. urealyticum* account for the majority of cases of non-gonococcal urethritis.
   3. A positive VDRL makes a definitive diagnosis of syphilis.
   4. Papillomaviruses cause condyloma acuminata.
   5. HSV-1 and HSV-2 may both cause genital herpes.
   6. Syphilitic nodes are usually non-tender and firm.
   7. Syphilitic ulcers are usually painless.

9

BONE, JOINT, SOFT TISSUE AND SKIN INFECTIONS

OSTEOMYELITIS

Clinical Manifestations

Symptoms of osteomyelitis depend on the location of the infection. Infections of the long bones are most common, and the lower extremities are more frequently involved than the upper extremities. As a result, a limp is a common finding in osteomyelitis. There is usually point tenderness over the site of infection. Pain is usually present. It is the focality of the symptoms that suggests the diagnosis and the location. In some children there is a mild prodrome of low-grade fever and malaise which is associated with the bacteremia that occurs prior to the localized symptoms.

In neonates, the symptoms of osteomyelitis are more subtle. The baby may be irritable and fussy. An elevated temperature may be present, but is an infrequent finding. The affected limb may be swollen and tender and attempts at passive movement will usually elicit crying or evidence of irritability. The neonate will not voluntarily move the involved limb or will move it infrequently. Systemic symptoms are not frequently seen. Multiple sites may be involved and joint involvement is not infrequent.

Etiology and Epidemiology

The most common organism causing osteomyelitis is *Staphylococcus aureus.* Other organisms causing osteomyelitis included Group A streptococci, *Haemophilus influenzae, Strep. pneumoniae, Pseudomonas aurigenosa,* salmonellae, and other gram negative enterobacteriaceae. Anaerobes, candida, mycobacteria, among others, are infrequent causes. In neonates, Group B streptococci and coliforms are also etiologic agents of osteomyelitis.

The most common sites for infections are the femur and the tibia. Less commonly, the other long bones are involved. Other bones are involved relatively infrequently. Group B streptococcus, a common etiology in neonates, frequently occurs in the proximal humerus. Osteomyelitis is more common in males than females, and is more common in children than middle age adults.

Diagnosis

Patients with a history or physical finding compatible with osteomyelitis should be further evaluated. Radiographs of the suspected sites of infection may be very useful. Early in the disease only small local deep soft tissue swelling on a region of the metaphysis may be evident. Within the first week of symptoms, the x-ray usually further reveals swelling of adjacent muscles, and the obliteration of interposed translucent fat planes because of the presence of edema. Usually by day 10 to 21 after symptoms have appeared, the x-ray will show evidence of bony destruction and periosteal new bone formation.

Radiologic changes in the neonate may differ from that in the older child. Most commonly seen is deep soft tissue swelling. Evidence for multiple bone involvement is also seen. Joints may also be involved. Localized rare faction and subperiosteal new bone formation is also seen. Widened joint spaces, periosteal elevation and lytic lesions are seen on x-ray less frequently.

Radionuclide scanning is an alternative to x-ray. Scanning is more sensitive and can, therefore, frequently demonstrate evidence of osteomyelitis before conventional x-rays can. Skilled interpretation of the scans is important to reduce the risk of false positive scans.

Once the site of osteomyelitis is found, aspiration or drainage procedures should be done to identify the etiologic agent. Blood cultures should also be obtained, but are frequently negative.

Treatment

Once the organisms have been identified and sensitivity testing is done, an appropriate antibiotic can be chosen. Empiric therapy should provide adequate coverage for at least staphylococci, H. influenzae, and group A streptococci, pending gram stain, culture, and sensitivity results. In neonates, group B streptococci and enteric organisms should also be covered. Osteomyelitis involving the foot, especially the calcaneous, requires pseudomonas coverage also. Concern for salmonella should result in appropriate coverage in patients with splenic dysfunction, like patients with sickle cell disease. Therapy is then adjusted based on laboratory results.

Treatment is usually initially given intravenously. Failure of treatment appears to be duration related, and antibiotics should be continued for at least 4 to 6 weeks. In staphylococcal osteomyelitis, oral therapy may be used after signs and symptoms of osteomyelitis are gone. Doses should be adjusted based on serum bactericidal levels. Oral antistaphyloccal penicillin, antistaphylococcal cephalosporins and clindamycin have all been used successfully in oral therapy. Compliance with oral therapy is essential for cure. Surgical debridement and drainage are also useful. It has been reported that pseudomonas osteomyelitis of the foot can be treated adequately with good debridement and two to three weeks of appropriate intravenous antibiotics.

Sequelae and Complications

Neonates may develop bone destruction or deformity after osteomyelitis. Spread of the infection to other sites such as the meninges is infrequent, but does occur. The development of recurrent or chronic osteomyelitis is frequently the result of inappropriate or insufficient treatment of the initial osteomyelitis.

ARTHRITIS

Clinical Manifestations

Systemic symptoms include fever and occasionally malaise. The affected joint is usually swollen, warm, red and tender. Palpation of the joint produces evidence of effusion. There is limitation of motion of the involved joint. Movement of the joint will frequently elicit pain. In neonates, septic arthritis commonly occurs in hip joints; flexion of the hip with swelling of the thighs or buttocks are frequently seen.

Etiology and Epidemiology

Staphylococci, streptococci, pneumonococci and *H. influenzae* make up the vast majority of cases of septic arthritis. Age related incidence rates suggest that staphylococci, streptococci and gram negative bacteria make up the majority of cases in infants less than three months of age. In children between 3 months and 4 years, *H. influenzae* and streptococci become increasingly more common and over 4 years of age most cases are due to staphylococci. In adolescents and in neonates, *Neisseria gonorrhea* is occasionally seen. Viruses can occasionally cause arthritis. Many have been implicated including rubella, mumps, varicella zoster and Epstein-Barr viruses.

Septic arthritis is more common in males than females. Over 75% of children with *H. influenzae* arthritis report a history of otitis media or other respiratory infection during the 2 weeks preceding the arthritis. Patients with staphylococcal arthritis frequently report a recent history of skin or soft tissue infection. *REMEMBER:* Neonatal septic arthritis of the hip can follow a femoral venipuncture, therefore, this procedure should be avoided when possible.

Diagnosis

Radiographs show evidence of capsular swelling. Joints should be aspirated for Gram stain, and culture. Blood should also be cultured. Joint fluid should also be examined for its ability to clot. Septic fluid from joints will clot rapidly. The white cell count of the fluid is usually much higher (average greater than 70,000 cells/ml) than in non-septic arthritis and the cells are usually overwhelmingly polymorphonuclear leukocytes. The glucose is about 30% of the blood glucose.

Treatment

Initial therapy in children should be effective against staphylococci and *H. influenzae*. Frequently, an anti-staphylococal penicillin and chloramphenicol are used. Once the organism is identified, the therapy can be appropriately altered. Therapy is usually continued for 3 to 4 weeks. Oral therapy has been used successfully following an initial course of intravenous antibiotics and careful monitoring of bactericidal levels. Desirable peak serum bactericidal titers are at least 1:8.

Surgical drainage is an important component of therapy. Drainage should be carried out as soon as possible. Repeated aspirations of the affected joint are sometimes necessary.

Sequelae and Complications

Spontaneous ankylosis and pathologic dislocations have been reported, especially in patients in whom therapy is delayed. *H. influenzae* arthritis appears in general to have a better prognosis than does staphyloccal arthritis.

DISCITIS

Clinical Manifestations

Backache, a limp, localized tenderness to spinal percussion and, in younger children, refusal to walk are common symptoms. Duration of symptoms prior to diagnosis averages about 10 weeks. An upper respiratory infection frequently precedes symptoms. The sedimentation rate is usually elevated, but less than 50.

Etiology and Epidemiology

The most common organism recovered from biopsy specimens is *Staphlyococcus aureus*. Many specimens do not grow any organisms. The disease is most common under five years of age. There is no sex preference. The lumbar region is most commonly involved.

Diagnosis

In patients with the above symptoms, radiographs of affected areas of the spine will show disc space narrowing usually between L4 and L5 or L3 and L4. Obtaining a specimen from the affected area will help in determining the organisms. This disease must be distinguished from vertebral osteomyelitis. In vertebral osteomyelitis, pain is a major symptom. There is frequently fever and elevated white blood cell count and the x-ray shows bony destruction.

Treatment

Antistaphylococcal therapy is usually given. Treatment is continued for 4 to 6 months and may be given orally.

Sequelae and Complications

Young children do well. They usually reconstitute the disc space and have no complications. Older patients may develop spinal fusion.

SKIN AND SOFT TISSUE INFECTIONS

IMPETIGO

Impetigo is a superficial skin infection usually due to group A streptococci or less frequently to *Staphlyococcus aureus*. Mixed infections also occur. Lesions frequently begin as vesicles then later become crusted. The crust is typically yellow-gold and thick. Localized adenopathy may occur but systemic symptoms are infrequent. The lesions are not painful but are pruritic. They are very contagious and spread among siblings and friends is common.

Diagnosis is usually made based on the typical appearance of the lesions, but if the diagnosis is in question, Gram stain and culture of the vesicle will usually demonstrate the presence of either streptococci or staphylococci. The group A streptococci responsible for impetigo are in general different serotypes than those causing pharyngitis.

A good clinical response is usually achieved with penicillin or erythromycin therapy. Intramuscular benzathine penicillin as a single dose, or 10 days of oral penicillin, or erythromycin is effective. If bullae are present, the etiology is likely to be *Staphylococcus aureus* and treatment with a penicillinase-resistant penicillin or erythromycin should adequately treat the infection.

Post-streptococcal acute glomerulonephritis (PSAGN) is the major complication of impetigo. This complication of impetigo is most commonly seen in preschool children, usually about 3 weeks after the skin infection. PSAGN can also occur after pharyngitis caused by certain strains of group A streptococcus.

STAPHYLOCOCCAL SCALDED SKIN SYNDROME (SSSS)

The skin lesions in SSSS are primarily the result of damage caused by the exfoliative exotoxin produced by the phage group II *S. aureus* responsible for the infection. *S. aureus* is not usually recovered from the skin lesions, but usually from other sites such as blood, abscess, etc.

The lesions are typically bullae. There is not usually an inflammatory reaction associated with the lesions. Fever and scarlatinaform rash are frequently seen. Bullae form and rupture. Exfoliation results in exposure of areas of bright red skin surfaces. Treatment is with penicillinase-resistant penicillins. Fluids must be closely monitored and appropriately replaced.

TOXIC SHOCK SYNDROME (TSS)

135

Toxic shock syndrome is an illness associated with fever, a scarlatinaform rash, hypotension, desquamation, and involvment of multiple organ systems. The syndrome is associated with *Staphylococcus aureus* infection. It is believed that symptoms are the result of exotoxin. The source of the *S. aureus* infection should be sought. When appropriate, surgical drainage should be done. Antistaphylococcal antibiotics should be used systemically.

CELLULITIS

Periorbital cellulitis is discussed in the ocular infections chapter. Cellulitis in children can occur on other areas of the face. It is also found frequently on extremities. *Staphylococcus aureus,* group A streptococcus, and *H. influenzae* are responsible for the majority of cases seen in pediatric patients. *H. influenzae* is found more frequently on the face than on the extremities.

Cellulitis is frequently associated with fever. The affected area of skin is usually warm, red and tender. Diagnosis of cellulitis is based on the clinical presentation. In order to optimize therapy, isolation of the infecting organism should be attempted whenever possible. Material for culture can sometimes be obtained by aspirating the leading edge of the cellulitis. Injection of a small amount of non-bactericidal saline into the leading edge prior to aspirating may aid in recovery of the organism. Blood should also be cultured, as it is positive in the majority of cases due to *H. influenzae.* In patients with streptococcal cellulitis (usually on the extremities or perianal region), often a red streak of lymphangitis will be present.

Initial therapy for cellulitis in small children should cover for *H. influenzae* as well as streptococci and *S. aureus.* In older children, coverage for *H. influenzae* becomes less important. Initial therapy can consist of an antistaphylococcal penicillin plus chloramphenicol or a broad-spectrum cephalosporin such as cefuroxime if the child is young. Older children can usually be treated with penicillin, or if staphylococci are suspect, anti-staphylococcal penicillin. Therapy is then modified based on culture results and clinical response. No significant clinical response is likely during the first 6 to 12 hours so it is frequently difficult to gauge clinical effectiveness the first day of therapy.

KEY POINTS

1. Focality of symptoms help make the diagnosis of osteomyelitis in children. Symptoms in the neonate may be more subtle.

2. Aspiration of the area of bone involved is essential for identification of the organism and selection of appropriate antibiotic coverage.
3. Pseudomonas is frequently present when the osteomyelitis is of the calcaneous bone.
4. Infected joints should be aspirated to identify the etiology of the arthritis.
5. Femoral venipuncture is a risk factor for the development of septic arthritis of the hip in infants.
6. Discitis should be suspected in children with a limp, backache, tenderness to spinal percussion or a refusal to walk.
7. Impetigo usually appears as yellow-gold, thick crusts which may start out as vesicles.
8. Scalded skin syndrome is due to an exfoliative exotoxin produced by *Staphylococcus aureus. S. aureus* is usually not recovered from the lesions.
9. Toxic shock syndrome is a multisystem illness associated with staphylococcal infection.
10. Cellulitis in children is frequently caused by either Staphylococci or *H. influenzae.* Antibiotics that are chosen initially should at least cover for these organisms.

REFERENCES

1. Carter S, Feldman WE: Etiology and treatment of facial cellulitis in pediatric patients. Pediatr Infect Dis 1983; 2:222–224.
2. Chusid MJ, Jacobs WM, Sty JR: Pseudomonas arthritis following puncture wounds of the foot. J. Pediatr 1979; 94:429–431.
3. Dunkle LM, Brock N: Long-term follow-up of ambulatory management of osteomyelitis. Clinical Pediatrics 1982; 21:650–655.
4. Fischer GW, Popch GA, Sullivan DE, et al: Diskitis: A prospective diagnostic analysis. Pediatrics 1978; 62:543–548.
5. Fox L, Sprunt K: Neonatal osteomyelitis. Pediatrics 1978; 62: 535–542.
6. Jacobs RF, Adelman L, Sack CM, et al: Management of *Pseudomonas* osteochondritis complicating puncture wounds of the foot. Pediatrics 1982; 69:432–435.
7. Nelson, JD, Bucholz RW, Kusmiesz H, et al: Benefits and risks of sequential parenteral-oral therapy for supportive bone and joint infections. J. Pediatric Orth 1982; 2:255–262.

8. Rudoy RC, Nakashima G: Diagnostic valve of needle aspiration in *Haemophilus influenzae* type b cellulitis. J. Pediatr 1981; 94:924–925.

9. Smith D: *Haemophilus influenzae* cellulitis. Am J Dis Child 1976; 130:1193–1194.

10. Uman SJ, Kunin CM: Needle aspiration in the diagnosis of soft tissue infections. Arch Intern Med 1975; 135:959–961.

11. Walduogel FA, Vassy H. Osteomyelitis: The past decade. N Engl J Med 1980; 303:360–370.

12. Weiss A, Friendly DM, Eglin K, et al: Bacterial periorbital and orbital cellulitis in childhood. Ophthalmology 1983; 90:195–203.

REVIEW QUESTIONS

1.) True or False
   1. Most common sites of osteomyelitis are the long bones.
   2. During the first few days of symptoms of osteomyelitis, a normal x-ray of the suspected area of infection rules out the diagnosis of osteomyelitis.
   3. The most common organism found in osteomyelitis is *Staphylococcus aureus.*
   4. Surgical drainage is an important component in the treatment of arthritis.
   5. Refusal to walk and localized spinal tenderness suggests the diagnosis of discitis.
   6. Vertebral osteomyelitis is usually painless.
   7. Staphylococci can be routinely cultured from the skin lesions found in scalded skin syndrome and toxic shock syndrome.
   8. The etiologic agent causing cellulitis can sometimes be isolated from the leading edge of the cellulitis.

10

BITES

Dogs and Cats

Clinical Manifestations

Signs of infection usually occur within 72 hours of the bite. When *Pasteurella multocida* is the primary pathogen, infection is usually evident within 24 hours and is often characterized by severe pain, redness and swelling. Fever and adenopathy are not constant findings. In contrast, staphylococci and streptococci cause infections that have a less rapid start and may be associated with some adenopathy and fever. Despite these differences it is difficult to determine the particular pathogen without obtaining cultures in individual cases.

Etiology and Epidemiology

Pets can be responsible for a wide variety of human infections. Bites from these animals are relatively common. It is thought that cat bites become infected more frequently than dog bites. The oral flora of the animal is usually responsible for the infection. Staphylococci, streptococci, and *P. multocida* are common pathogens in these infected bites. *P. multocida* infection appears to be more commonly seen following bites from cats than dogs.

Diagnosis and Treatment

Not all bites become infected. Early intervention after the bite is important in preventing infection. Steps that should be taken as soon after the bite as possible include: thorough cleansing of the wound; debridement; tetanus prophylaxis, if indicated; evaluation for the need for rabies prophylaxis; and in particular circumstances, antibiotic prophylaxis.

There is controversy regarding the use of antibiotics for prophylaxis of bites. Routine use of prophylactic antibiotics does not seem to be indicated; however, there may be certain circumstances when prophylaxis should be considered. Puncture wounds are frequently the result of cat bites. They may be quite deep and difficult to adequately clean. Prophylactic antibiotics may be of value in that circumstance. In addition, several investigators have recommended prophylactic antibiotics for deep wounds involving tendons, bone or facial wounds.

Antibiotic therapy depends on the particular pathogen. Empiric therapy usually covers staphylococci, streptococci, and *P. multocida*. Penicillin plus an anti-staphylococcal antibiotic has been recommended. Penicillinase resistant penicillins have poor antimicrobial activity against *P. multocida*. Alternative therapy, in penicillin allergic patients, would be erythromycin. Therapy can be adjusted based on culture results and sensitivities.

Sequelae and Complications

In patients who do not respond to appropriate antimicrobial therapy, a thorough evaluation should be done looking for other foci of infection. Osteomyelitis, arthritis, sepsis, meningitis, and endocarditis have all been reported. Less frequent consequences of bites include: cat scratch disease, tularemia, plague, tetanus, and rabies (see chart).

Snake Bites

Clinical Manifestations

The venom from pit vipers produces destruction of local tissue; alterations in blood coagulation and cells; cardiovascular changes; and changes in capillary permeability leading to blood loss, hemorrhage, edema, shock, renal failure and even death. In contrast, coral snakes may produce little local reaction, but within a few hours of being bitten, ptosis, blurred vision, and a curare-like syndrome may develop. Symptoms may include dyspnea, numbness, dysphagia, muscle spasm and coma.

Etiology and Epidemiology

Poisonous snakes in the United States include rattlesnakes, copperheads, water moccasins, and coral snakes. The first three are pit vipers.

Diagnosis

Snakes may be difficult to identify and, when available, an expert should be asked to identify the snake. When a herpetologist is not available, certain clues may help to identify poisonous snakes. Pit vipers have facial pits between the eye and nose on each side of the face. They also have eliptical eyes (as opposed to round, in many non-poisonous snakes), and fangs. Non-poisonous snakes have a double row of subcaudal plates behind the anal plate. Rattlesnakes have a single row of plates followed by a double row followed by the rattles at the end. Copperheads and water moccasins have the same plate configuration as rattlesnakes but without the rattles. Coral snakes have a characteristic color pattern of red, yellow (or white) and black bands. Non-poisonous snakes usually have red bands bordered by black bands.

Treatment

Once it has been established that a patient was bitten by a venomous snake, treatment should be instituted to 1) neutralize the venom and 2) support the patient until symptoms are gone. Antivenin should be given as soon as possible but only after testing for sensitivity to antivenin is done. Enough antivenin should be given to stop the progression of symptoms. Twenty ml to 150 ml of antivenin should be given, depending on the severity of symptoms. When needed, tetanus prophylaxis should be given. Cardiovascular, respiratory and neurological systems should be closely monitored and supportive care given as needed. REMEMBER: Never inject antivenin locally into fingers or toes.

Sequelae and Complications

Complications of snake bites depend on which snake is involved. Local tissue destruction sometimes leading to loss of a digit can occur. Extensive plastic surgery is sometimes required. Systemic effects lead to a variety of problems and can, if not adequately controlled, result in death.

The risk from snake bite can be reduced by patients knowing the characteristics of poisonous snakes, seeking medical help as soon after the bite as possible and taking basic preventive measures to reduce the risk of being bitten.

Scorpion Bites

Clinical Manifestations

Scorpion bites may cause a variety of symptoms. Tachycardia, hypertension, hyperglycemia, mydriasis, gastric distension, increased salivation, hyperesthesia, local pain at the envenomation site, and respiratory distress have all been reported. Neurologic manifestations include: seizures, hyperthermia, nystagmus, blurred vision and transient blindness. Death occurs but is rare.

Etiology and Epidemiology

Scorpion bites are not uncommon. Over 1,000 cases were reported to the Arizona Poison and Drug Information Center in 1982 alone. Most scorpion bites occur between April and November since most scorpions hibernate during the winter. While most victims are adults, most serious envenomations occur in children less than 2 years of age.

Diagnosis

Diagnosis is usually made by identification of a scorpion as the cause of the sting. A small erythematous area may appear at the envenomation site.

Treatment

Treatment of scorpion stings in adults and teenagers is usually limited to symptomatic relief including the localized application of ice to the sting site. Younger children often require more aggressive care. Therapy includes maintaining an open airway; control of seizures, agitation, and hyperactivity with Phenobarbitol; antivenin (only currently available in Arizona) for tachycardia, hyperthermia or hypertension; and propranolol for tachyarrhythmias. The use of antivenin and propranolol remains controversial. Well controlled studies are lacking. Other supportive measures should be instituted as needed.

Sequelae and Complications

Potential risks of antivenin use include anaphylaxis and serum sickness. Respiratory depression, shock and death are rare complications of envenomation and can usually be avoided with good intensive care support.

ZOONOSES

Organism	Source	Disease	Treatment	Comment
Pasturella multocida	Dogs and Cats	Cellulitis Osteomyelitis Endocarditis Meningitis Pneumonia	Penicillin	-Usually from animal bite -Non-bite droplet transmission occurs
Yersinia pestis	Rodents Fleas Pets	Bubonic Plague	Streptomycin Tetracycline Chloramphenicol	Usually west of 100th meridian.
Francisella tularensis	Rabbits, rodents, cats, contaminated meat/water, Anthropods.	Ulceroglandular Ocularglandular Pharyngeal Pneumonia Typhoidal	Streptomycin Tetracycline Chloramphenicol	Inhalation of droplets occurs, can result in disease.
Salmonella	Turtles, birds, and dogs.	Gastroenteritis most common.	Usually self-limited	About 2 million cases per year.
Leptospira	Dogs, Cattle	Biphasic illness. Also atypical form.	Penicillin of questionable value, since usually self-limited	About 100 cases per year.
Yersinia enterocolitica	Pets	Mesenteric lymphadenitis. Erythema multiforme.	Trimethoprim-sulfamethoxazole	Also person-to-person, contaminated food.
Chlamydia	Birds	Psittacosis	Tetracycline, Chloraphenicol.	Tetracycline prophylaxis of pet birds may help prevent infection.

Organism	Source	Disease	Treatment	Comment
Rabies Virus	U.S. wild animals. Mexican dogs. (Usually not rodents or lagomorphs)	Rabies	None (supportive)	Vaccine-safe efficacious Skunks, racoons, bats may have long periods without symptoms.
Lymphocytic choriomeningitis virus	House mouse, hamster	Lymphocytic-choriomeningitis	None (supportive)	Flu-like illness followed by CNS involvement.
Etiology of Cat scratch disease	Cats	Cat scratch disease	Supportive	Usually self-limited

Miscellaneous Zoonoses

Cryptococcus neoformans - Pigeons
Diphylidium caninum - (tapeworm) dogs
Dirofilaria immitis - Dogs-to-mosquito-to-man
Histoplasma capsulatum - pythons, sheep, ticks, aerosol, person-to-person rare.
Ringworm - cats
Toxocara - pets, causes visceral larvae.
Toxoplasma - cats

KEY POINT

1 Dog and cat bites require good wound cleansing and debridement, appropriate use of tetanus and rabies vaccine (see Chapter 18), and judicious use of antibiotics.
2 It is important to identify the type of snake responsible for a bite so that appropriate therapy can be instituted. Snakes with red bands bordered with black bands are usually *not* poisonous.
3 Scorpion bites in young children are potentially life threatening and require intensive monitoring and aggressive supportive care.

REFERENCES

1. Chun YT, Berkelhamer JE, Harold TE: Dog bites in children less than 4 years old. Pediatrics 1982; 69:119–121.
2. Goscienski PJ: Zoonoses. Pediatr Infect Dis 1983; 2:69–81.
3. Henderson BM, Dujon EB: Snake bites in children. Journal of Pediatric Surgery 1973; 8:729–733.
4. Jarvis WR, Banks S, Synder E, et al: Pasteurella multocida osteomyelitis following dog bite. Am J Dis Child 1981; 135: 625–627.
5. March SM: Infections due to dog and cat bites. Pediatr Infect Dis 1982; 1:351–356.
6. McCollough NC, Gennaro JF: Treatment of venomous snakebites in the United States. Clinical Toxicology 1970; 3:483–500.
7. Nelson JD: Diseases acquired from pets. Pediatr Infect Dis 1983; 2(suppl) 556–560.
8. Rachesky IJ, Banner W, Dansky J, et al: Treatment of *Centruroides exilicauda* envenomation. Am J Dis Child 1984; 138:1136–1139.
9. Wingert WA, Wainschel J: Diagnosis and Management of Envenomation by Poisonous Snakes. S. Medical Journal 1975; 68:1015–1026.

REVIEW QUESTIONS

1.) The most common Gram negative organism in cat bites is
__________.

2.) Antibiotic coverage is sometimes indicated in_________ bites because
the bite is often a deep puncture wound which may be difficult to clean.

3.) Pit vipers include ________(3).

4.) A curare-like syndrome may develop after a __________ snake bite.

5.) Alternating red, yellow (or white), and black bands are typical of
________snakes.

6.) Red bands bordered by black bands are typically found in ________
snakes.

7.) Scorpion bites are rare during ________(season).

8.) ________ is often carried by dogs, birds, and turtles and is responsible
for a usually self-limited gastroenteritis in humans.

11

NEONATAL SEPSIS

Clinical Manifestations

Signs and symptoms of neonatal sepsis are non-specific. Common findings include: temperature instability, poor feeding, irritability, lethargy, vomiting, diarrhea, abdominal distension, jaundice and respiratory distress. Additional findings may include apnea and cyanosis. Any one or combination of these clinical manifestations may be present. As the disease progresses, hypoxemia and shock may develop. Respiratory symptoms and chest radiographic findings may be indistinguishable from hyaline membrane disease. REMEMBER: It is essential to have a high index of suspicion of possible sepsis in the newborn. Subtle findings early in the course of the disease may be missed resulting in a delay in the institution of therapy.

Group B streptococcal disease in the newborn can present within the first few days of life and often during the first few hours. It is associated frequently with maternal complications of pregnancy. It is acute, rapidly progressive, and can be fatal. Initially, it may resemble respiratory distress syndrome but progression is rapid and death may occur in as little as 12 hours.

Late onset disease usually appears one to two weeks after delivery. Meningeal involvement is very common. The mortality rate is lower than with the early onset disease and the history of maternal complications of pregnancy is often lacking.

Etiology and Epidemiology

Certain babies are at a high risk for neonatal sepsis. Risk factors may be present in mother or neonate. Mothers with endometritis, urinary tract infections or bacteremia place their infants at increased risk of acquiring infection. Mothers who are colonized by certain pathogens (like group B streptococcus) or mothers without antibody to specific pathogens may also place their newborn babies at increased risk of infection. If there is a history of prolonged rupture of membranes, premature labor, or maternal fever, the infant should be monitored closely for possible infection. Other factors that have been associated with neonatal sepsis are prolonged labor, invasive monitoring of the fetus, and coitus near the time of birth.

Neonates with congenital anomalies who are asphyxiated, or who are premature, are at risk for infection. In addition, neonates receiving hyperalimentation are also at risk for sepsis.

Most neonatal sepsis in the U.S. is a result of infection with *Kl Escherichia coli* or group B streptococcus. In some other parts of the world streptococcus is a relatively rare cause of neonatal infection. In contrast, *Listeria monocytogenes* is more common in countries like Spain, and salmonella is seen relatively frequently in Latin America. Recent data from Canada suggests that *Streptococcus viridans* is being seen more frequently, at least in some regions, and may emerge as a major neonatal pathogen. Staphylococcus and enterics other than *E. coli* can also occasionally be responsible for neonatal infection. Coagulase negative staphylococcal neonatal sepsis is becoming increasingly frequent in some pediatric centers.

While greater than half of the babies born to mothers colonized with group B streptococcus of K1 *E. coli* will themselves be colonized by 72 hours of age, only 1–2% of these colonized infants will develop invasive disease. It does appear, however, the number of sites colonized and the quantity of bacteria recovered is related to the risk of disease. Risk increases if the amniotic fluid is infected, if the infant is a "premie" or if the membranes have been ruptured for at least 24 hours.

Diagnosis

Initially the most important component of diagnosis is a high index of suspicion. The earlier neonatal sepsis is suspected, the more rapidly a definitive diagnosis can be made. Non-microbiologic laboratory data may also be helpful. Neutropenia is a helpful clue, however other problems such as asphyxia, and maternal hypertension may also result in neutropenia. The immature to total neutrophil ratio appears to be more useful. A high immature to total neutrophil count is more likely in a septic neonate than in a neonate whose mother had hypertension, or than in a neonate with asphyxia. Further supportive evidence can be gotten by examining the neutrophils for degenerative changes such as toxic granulation and vacuolization.

Other studies such as erythrocyte sedimentation rate, C-reactive protein, buffy coat smear, Limulus lysate essay, and antigen detection methods such as countercurrent immunoelectrophoresis and latex agglutination may be of use in increasing your suspicion of infection.

The definitive diagnosis is made by microbiologic culture. Blood, CSF, and urine cultures are useful, although cultures of urine taken during the first 12 hours of life are rarely positive. Gastric aspirate cultures are not particularly useful in deciding whether or not a neonate is infected. *REMEMBER:* As many as 30% of infants with sepsis may have concommittant meningitis. The L.P. may be a rapid way to make a presumptive diagnosis. Gram stain or acridine orange stain may help identify the presence and type of bacteria. Some studies suggest acridine orange is superior to Gram stain in identifying bacteria in the CSF. Countercurrent immunoelectrophoresis and latex agglutination of CSF fluid may also help in presumptive diagnosis.

Infants who continue to look and act septic despite a negative workup for bacteria should get a more thorough workup. Herpes simplex infection can be acquired perinatally and infants infected with herpes may initially present like a septic neonate. The absence of cutaneous herpetic lesions does not rule out neonatal herpes. Rarely, *Mycoplasma hominis* has caused neonatal infection. Premature infants with central venous catheters, hyperalimentation, or prolonged antibiotic use are set-ups for candida infections such as sepsis or meningitis.

Treatment

Initially therapy should cover the more common pathogens. The use of ampicillin along with an aminoglycoside is common practice. Some authorities recommend the use of a third generation cephalosporin in place of the aminoglycoside if there is evidence for meningitis. Aminoglycosides, in general, penetrate poorly and unpredictably into the CSF while many of the third generation cephalosporins achieve CSF levels many times the M.I.C. (minimal inhibitory concentration). Once sensitivities of the organism are known, the antibiotic regimen can be appropriately adjusted. During the first week of life the recommended dose of ampicillin is 25 mg/kg q 12 h. After 1 week of age, 25 mg/kg q 8 h is given. Gentamicin is usually given as 2 mg/kg q 12h and is given 2 mg/kg q 8 h after 1 week of age.

Two of the third generation cephalosporins commonly used are cefotaxime (50 mg/kg/dose) given q 12 hours during the first week of life and q 8 hours thereafter, and moxalaclam (50 mg/kg/dose) given in the same regimen as cefotaxime.

In addition to antibiotic therapy, leukocyte transfusions appear to be of value in some septic newborns. Where leukapheresis is not available, double volume exchange transfusions may be effective. Preliminary data in adults suggest that early administration of nalaxone to patients with septic shock can reverse the effects of shock. Whether this will be confirmed in well controlled studies, and whether it will be effective in neonates is not yet clear.

Sequelae and Complications

Septic neonates may seed to virtually any site in the body. Meningitis can occur and may result in ventriculitis subdural empyema formation, or abscess formation. Otitis can frequently be seen. Seeding to bones, joints, soft tissue and the urinary tract can occur.

Mortality rates vary by hospital and by etiology. Rates of fatalities range from 20% to 75%. Many surviving infants may have permanent neurological sequelae as the result of CNS involvement.

KEY POINTS

1. Common bacterial etiologies for neonatal sepsis and meningitis include group B streptococcus and *E. coli.*
2. Septic appearing neonates with negative bacterial cultures should be evaluated for possible herpes infection.
3. Ampicillin plus an aminoglycoside is traditional initial therapy for neonatal sepsis. If Gram negative meningitis is suspected, a third generation cephalosporin may be considered in place of the aminoglycoside.
4. Outcome is related in part to early diagnosis and initiation of appropriate therapy. It is important to have a high degree of suspicion of sepsis in neonates.

REFERENCES

1. Baumgart S, Hall SE, Campos JM, et al: Sepsis with coagulase-negative staphylococci in critically ill newborns. Am J Dis Child 1983; 137:-461–463.

2. Boe O, Diderichsen J, Matre R: Isolation of *Mycoplasma hominis* from cerebrospinal fluid. Scand J Infect Dis 1973; 5:285–288.

3. Britton JR: The evaluation of possible sepsis in the newborn infant. Infectious Diseases Newsletter 1982; 1:97–99.

4. Cairo MS, Rucker R, Bennetts GA, et al: Improved survival of newborns receiving leukocyte transfusions for sepsis. Pediatrics 1984; 74:887–892.

5. Corrigan JJ: Thrombocytopenia: A laboratory sign of septicemia in infants and children. J Pediatr 1974; 85:219–221.

6. Engle WD, Rsosenfeld CR: Neutropenia in high-risk neonates. J Pediatr 1984; 105:982–986.

7. Gnehn H, Klein JO: Management of neonatal sepsis and meningitis. Pediatr Ann. 1983; 12:195–206.

8. Harris MC, Polin RA: Neonatal septicimeia. Pediatric Clinics of North America. 1983; 30: 243–257.

9. Johnson DE, Thompson TR, Green TP, et al: Systemic candidiasis in very low-birth weight infants (greater than 1,500 Grams). Pediatrics 1984; 73:138–143.

10. Kleiman MB, Reynolds JK, Watts NH: Superiority of acridine orange stain versus Gram stain in partially treated bacterial meningitis. J Pediatr, 1984; 104:401–403.

11. Liv CH, Lehan C, Speer M, et al: Degenerative changes in neutrophils: an indicator of bacterial infection. Pediatrics. 1984; 74: 823–827.

12. Pass MA, Gray BM, Khare S, et al: Prospective studies of group B streptococcal infections in infants. J Pediatr 1979; 95:437–43.

13. Schreiber JR, Maynard E, Lew MA: Candida antigen detection in two premature neonates with disseminated candidasis. Pediatrics 1984; 74:838–841.

14. Siegel JD: Neonatal Sepsis. Pediatr Infect Dis 1982; 1:339–344.

15. Siegel JD, McCracken GH: Sepsis neonatorum. N. Engl J Med. 1981; 304:642–647.

16. Spigelblatt L, Saintonge J, Chicoine R, et al: Changing pattern of neonatal streptococcal septicemia. Pediatr Infect Dis 1985; 4:56–58.

17. Wasserman RL: Unconventional therapies for neonatal sepsis. Pediatr Infect Dis 1983; 2:421–423.
18. Wientzen RL, McCracken GH: Pathogenesis and Management of neonatal sepsis and meningitis. Curr Prob Pediatr 1977; 8:22–35.

REVIEW QUESTIONS

1.) Early onset group B streptococcal infection in neonates usually presented as ____________.

2.) Urine cultures are ____________ (usually or rarely) positive during the first 12 hours of life in septic neonates.

3.) ____________ should be considered in bacterial culture negative septic neonates even if no skin lesions are present.

4.) Maternal risk factors associated with neonatal sepsis include ____________(5)

5.) Risk factors in neonates associated with sepsis include ____________(3)

12

PERINATAL INFECTIONS

Throughout gestation the fetus is at risk for infection from the mother. During delivery, as the neonate passes through the birth canal, again there is risk of infection, and then, once out in the world, the infant may come into contact with a wide variety of pathogens. This chapter will deal with some of the more common and more interesting causes of perinatal infection.

CYTOMEGALOVIRUS (CMV)

Clinical Manifestations

While CMV is believed to be the most common congenital infection, symptomatic disease is relatively uncommon. As many as 90% of neonates with CMV infection have no symptoms at birth. In those patients with symptoms, petechiae, hepatosplenomegaly, jaundice and microcephaly are common. More than half of symptomatic patients will have one or more of these clinical findings. Other fairly common findings include small for gestational age, prematurity, inguinal hernias and chorioretinitis.

Not all of the apparently asymptomatic neonates remain asymptomatic. Some will go on to develop psychomotor retardation, learning disabilities, dental defects or hearing loss. Hearing loss can be progressive with further loss of hearing even after the first year of life.

Acquisition of CMV natally may be asymptomatic. When symptoms are present, the patient often has a pneumonitis with a prolonged course, without fever.

Etiology and Epidemiology

CMV, one of the herpes viruses, is endemic throughout the world. Nearly 1% of all neonates are born with CMV infection but its incidence varies in different populations. There is a direct correlation between the rate of pre-existing antibody in the mothers and the rate of congenital infection in that same population. Maternal antibody neither protects against reactivation of infection during pregnancy, nor does it prevent spread of the infections to the fetus.

CMV is spread person-to-person and can be found in saliva, semen, urine, cervical and vaginal secretions, breast milk and blood. Infected babies can be contagious from months to years after birth.

While about 1% of neonates are born with CMV infection, acquisition can occur in the postnatal period, and at a lesser rate throughout childhood. Depending on the population involved in developed nations, anywhere from 40-80% of prepubertal children have evidence of CMV infection. In other areas of the world 90-100% of children are infected.

Primary infection in the pregnant mother leads to infection in the fetus in less than 50 percent of cases. Reactivation infection in the pregnant woman can also lead to fetal infection.

Perinatal infection may result from prenatal infection shortly before delivery, from infection during birth, or postnatally from infected individuals or from blood transfusions.

Diagnosis

Characteristic findings in congenital CMV infections are retinopathy that is described as depigmented punched-out perivascular areas with little or no exudate; perivascular cerebral calcifications; microcephaly; hepatosplenomegaly; hyperbilirubinemia; thrombocytopenia "celery stalking" (radiolucent longitudinal streaks); and inguinal hernias. CMV acquired natally may present with a protracted febrile pneumonitis. The diagnosis of CMV is best confirmed by isolation of the virus from the infected neonate. Specimens of urine and saliva can be successfully cultured from infected infants. If the specimen is maintained at 4°C, it can be transported without significant loss of titer. Frozen specimens, or those at room temperature may have a significant fall in titer. If the titer of virus in the specimen is high, the culture may demonstrate evidence of the virus in a few days.

Cultures should be held for 4-6 weeks, however, to insure that a low titer specimen is not mistakenly read as negative. Serologic tests for CMV are not as satisfactory as culture in diagnosing congenital or natally acquired CMV infection. The use of IgG antibodies for diagnosis requires simultaneous serologic testing of both mother and neonate, and if antibody is present, then serial samples from the infant should be obtained since maternal IgG antibody crosses the placenta and will initially be present in the neonate's serum.

Treatment

There is currently no available therapy for CMV. Trials of interferon therapy and various antiviral drugs have been disappointing. It is, therefore, important that pregnant women avoid contact with known CMV excretors. There are currently on-going trials of CMV vaccines to determine their safety and efficacy. Because reactivation of CMV infections in pregnant women can be associated with fetal acquisition of CMV infection, it is not yet clear the role the vaccine might play in preventing congenital CMV infection.

Sequelae and Complications

In serious congenital infection, patients may develop progressive central nervous system (CNS), hepatic, and pulmonary damage leading to severe permanent disabilities, or death. CMV infection is strongly associated with deafness and with mental retardation. Even infants who are apparently asymptomatic at birth, may develop a variety of developmental abnormalities; many of which become apparent during the first two years of life. Patients may also develop dental defects including discoloration of teeth with abnormal appearing enamel. The incidence of dental carries and tooth damage is very high in this group. Perinatal infection in premature infants is associated with hepatosplenomegaly, aseptic appearance, pneumonitis and thrombocytopenia. Atypical lymphocytosis and hemolytic anemia can also be seen. In these premature infants, mortality may be as high as 10%.

RUBELLA

Clinical Manifestations

Classic congenital rubella syndrome can be a devastating disease. Eye findings include cataracts, glaucoma, microphthalmia, and "salt and pepper" retinopathy. Central nervous system (CNS) damage results in microcephaly, mental retardation, and hearing loss. Liver involvement occurs. The infant may be jaundiced, have hepatosplenomegaly and evidence of cholestasis. Interstitial pneumonitis may be present. Cardiac defects include patent ductus arteriosis, pulmonary artery stenosis and myocarditis. Hemolysis may occur, thrombocytopenia may be present, and the baby may have a blueberry muffin appearance due to erythrogenic arrests in the skin.

The presence of purpura in these infants is associated with a high risk of death during the first year of life.

Babies with congenital rubella syndrome may demonstrate impaired production of antibodies to types 1 and 3 poliovirus, measles, and diphtheria after immunization. Long bone radiographs may demonstrate linear metaphyseal striations ("celery stalking"), usually most pronounced near the knees. This finding may resolve by six months of age. These babies will also demonstrate retardation of knee epiphyseal maturation as they grow and develop.

Asymptomatic cases occur, and apparently asymptomatic infants may develop symptoms during infancy.

Etiology and Epidemiology

Congenital rubella syndrome occurs in 0.05% of live births. Congenitally infected infants may continue to shed virus for months after birth and are a hazard to seronegative pregnant women. Reinfection can occur but because of a booster antibody response, viremia does not occur. Hence, there is no viral spread to the fetus in a pregnant woman who has antibody to rubella prior to her pregnancy. Vaccine programs are primarily designed to reduce the risk and incidence of congenital rubella.

Diagnosis

A presumptive diagnosis can be made if there is a maternal history compatible with rubella during pregnancy or if maternal seroconversion occurred during pregnancy. That history, along with stigmata of congenital rubella in the neonate is strongly suggestive of the diagnosis.

Confirmation can be done by isolation of the virus from throat, stool, urine or conjunctiva during the first month of life. Alternatively, serial serologic testing of mother and infant can also establish the diagnosis.

Treatment

There is currently not any therapy available for rubella. This makes prevention very important. The availability of rubella screening programs and rubella vaccine programs should ultimately make congenital rubella syndrome an exceedingly rare disease.

Sequelae and Complications

The mortality from congenital rubella is about 16%. It is believed that less than 20% of infected neonates will have no long-term sequelae. Deafness, congenital heart disease and psychomotor retardation are the most common long-term effects. Other defects include retinopathy, cataracts and glaucoma.

Late manifestations of the congenital rubella syndrome include diabetes mellitus (20% of patients) which usually presents in the second or third decade of life; chronic lymphocytic thyroiditis, thymic hypoplasia, pancreatic insufficiency and panencephelitis.

TOXOPLASMOSIS

Clinical Manifestations

Characteristic findings of toxoplasmosis include microphthalmia, uveitis, cataracts, disruption of the globe, and chorioretinitis often accompanied by an exudate giving the macular the appearance of a headlight of an oncoming car in the fog. Central nervous system (CNS) characteristics that are seen are intracerebral calcifications (as compared to periventricular calcifications in CMV), microcephaly, hydrocephaly and mental retardation.

Etiology and Epidemiology

Toxoplasmosis is a parasitic infection caused by *Toxoplasma gondii.* The prevalence rate of infection in humans varies with the geographic region and has been reported to occur in anywhere from 5% to 95% of adults. Transmission of toxoplasma is primarily the result of ingestion of poorly cooked meats or from exposure to cat feces. Flies and roaches may also play a role in the spread.

In the U.S., the prevalence rate of infection in young adults has been reported to be 20% or less. It is estimated that six of every 1000 pregnant women in the U.S. will acquire a primary toxoplasma infection during pregnancy. The incidence of congenital toxoplasmosis is about 0.1% of live births. The incidence of congenital toxoplasmosis is higher in parts of Europe, and South and Central America. *In utero* transmission rates are about 39% and only a primary maternal toxoplasma infection will lead to an infected fetus.

Diagnosis

An appropriate maternal history and evidence of classic symptoms in the neonate is helpful in suggesting the diagnosis. When the CNS is involved, a high cerebrospinal fluid (CSF) protein (disproportionately high as compared to the CSF leukocyte count) is helpful in making a presumptive diagnosis.

Laboratory confirmation is necessary to be sure of the diagnosis. Isolation of *T. gondii* can be done from specimens of placenta, CSF or blood.

Cultures may take up to six weeks to show proof of infection. Specimens are inoculated either into mice or tissue culture. Serologic methods are also available for diagnosis. Serial titers are necessary if IgG antibody is being measured. IgM determinations can also be done from neonatal serum to make the diagnosis.

Treatment

Current therapy regimens are not ideal. These regimens are not based on good controlled human studies. Reactivation of infection after therapy has been reported. Therapy usually consists of at least four weeks of treatment with both pyrimethamine and sulfadiazine. Despite inadequate human experimentation data, the risk of ongoing postnatal damage to the CNS probably justifies treatment. *REMEMBER:* Pyrimethamine is bone marrow toxic. Significant toxicity in newborns can usually be prevented by giving folinic acid (1 mg/kg q 24 hours beginning on day 5 of pyrimethamine therapy).

Recommended doses of pyrimethamine are 1 mg/kg/day divided into 2 daily doses. On day 1, a loading dose of 2 mg/kg/day should be used. If side effects or toxicities develop (bone marrow suppression, pancytopenia, or single cellular element depression) the dose should be reduced. Sulfadiazine can be given at 150 mg/kg/day divided into four doses.

If chorioretinitis is present, is has been recommended that prednisone therapy accompany the above treatment regimen and that it continue for at least four weeks. Serum antibodies usually persist despite adequate therapy.

Sequelae and Complications

Chorioretinitis may be present at birth or may develop later in infants with subclinical neonatal infection. Brain dysfunction may not become apparent during early infancy and varies from mild to severe. Other late sequelae include precocious puberty and deafness.

SYPHILIS

Clinical Manifestations

There are a variety of findings in congenital syphilis. Eye findings include eye chancres and chorioretinitis. Periostosis (paresis of Parrot) is painful. Osteochondritis can be seen on radiograph as transverse radiolucent and opaque bands. This usually heals during the first 6 months of life. Lymphadenopathy, hepatosplenomegaly, meningoencephalitis, papular skin rashes and eczematoid skin rashes are also seen. Sniffles (mucous membrane discharge that is positive for *Treponema pallidum*) abnormal CNS findings and self-limited hemolytic anemia are also present in the early stages of the illness. Later (after 2 years of age), Hutchinson's teeth (notched upper incisors), Mulberry molars (dome-shaped with abnormal cusps), Rhagades facies (linear atrophic scars radiating from the nose and mouth), eighth nerve deafness, neurosyphilis (tabes, paresis, mental retardation, seizures, spasticity, eye abnormalities, speech defects and hemiplegia), interstitial keratitis and joint deformities can occur.

Etiology and Epidemiology

Syphilis is caused by the spirochete *Treponema pallidum.* Mothers in the early stages of syphilis pose the greatest risk to the fetus. Congenital syphilis is relatively rare. In the past few years, only about 150 cases of congenital syphilis have been reported each year as compared with over 17,000 cases per year in the early 1940's. Spread of *T. pallidum* is the result of sexual contact (direct physical contact with an infectious lesion) or transplacental spread. Hematogenous spread of the organism is more common during the early stages of the disease thus reducing the chances of transplacental spread in pregnant women with late or latent infection.

Diagnosis

A maternal history of syphilis or appropriate symptoms in the neonate may suggest the diagnosis. Laboratory tests are necessary to confirm the diagnosis. There are two classes of serologic tests for syphilis. Reagin tests (non-treponemal) are the Venereal Diseases Research Laboratory slide test

(VDRL) and the rapid plasma reagin test (RPR). These tests detect antibody to cardiolipin-lecithin antigen (nonspecific). Falsely positive non-treponemal tests may result from various infectious diseases, malignancies; inflammatory and immunologic disease. False negative test results occur in late or tertiary-acquired syphilis. The fluorescent treponemal antibody absorption test (FTA-Abs) and the micro-hemagglutinin-Treponema pallidum test (MHA-Tp) are treponemal tests and measure antibody specifically directed against treponemal antigens. Reagin positive patients should have the diagnosis confirmed by a treponemal test.

In neonates, the infant will have a positive test for IgG antibodies if the mother's serologies are also positive, even if the infant is not infected. This is due to maternal IgG antibodies crossing the placenta, and applies to both reagin and treponemal-specific tests. Maternal antibody levels in infant serum should decrease over the first 1–3 months of life. Persistent or rising titer over several months in the infant is diagnostic of active infection. An adjunct to serologic diagnosis is the darkfield microscopic examination of exudate from skin lesions in the infected infant.

Treatment

Congenital syphilis is a preventable disease. VDRLs done routinely on pregnant women can enable adequate therapy of the mother and adequate treatment or prevention in the fetus. Infants born to mothers who had syphilis during pregnancy should be treated. In general, if the mother was not treated for her infection, was treated inadequately, or had non-penicillin therapy, the infant should be treated as soon after birth as possible. If the mother was adequately treated, the risk to the infant is slight, although these infants should be followed closely to insure that their reagin tests become negative.

In infants with suspected infection, the CSF must be examined. If the CNS is not involved, recommended therapy is one dose of benzathine penicillin G, 50,000 Units/kg, intramuscularly. If neurosyphilis is present or if it has not been ruled out, then aqueous crystalline penicillin G, 50,000 Units/kg/day divided into two daily doses should be given intramuscularly or intravenously for at least ten days (or single daily dose procaine penicillin may be used for at least ten days). *REMEMBER:* A Jarisch-Herxheimer reaction (febrile response to penicillin) is occasionally seen but is not usually of such severity to warrant discontinuation of therapy.

Post therapy follow-up includes periodic (usually every 3 months) quantitative reagin testing to document seroreversal which usually occurs within one year of therapy. In CNS syphilis, a repeat CSF examination one year after therapy should demonstrate a negative CSF-VDRL and a fall in CSF protein.

Sequelae and Complications

Congenital syphilis has a mortality of about 2%. Untreated, the disease can result in permanent damage. Blindness, deafness, mental retardation, seizures, "saddle nose" and "saber-shin" (tibial bowing) deformities can be seen.

HERPES SIMPLEX (HSV)

Clinical Manifestations

Herpes infection of the neonate can be asymptomatic. Symptomatic disease may present in any of several different forms. Disseminated disease may be present with or without CNS involvement. Disseminated disease usually presents during the first three weeks of life. Common symptoms include anorexia, vomiting, lethargy and fever. Other symptoms include jaundice, hepatomegaly, purpura, cyanosis, apnea, respiratory distress, rash and cardiovascular collapse. Irritability and seizures may suggest CNS involvement. Although not always present initially, skin lesions, oral ulcerations or keratitis will eventually occur in about 50% of disseminated disease. Liver and adrenal gland involvement is common. About 20% of infected infants will have abnormal chest x-rays. Bleeding diathesis may occur in up to 25% of neonates with disseminated herpes. Bleeding is frequently from the gastrointestinal tract.

CNS disease can occur without evidence of dissemination to other organ systems. Fifty percent of patients with CNS infection have no evidence of dissemination. Typically the CSF has a leukocytosis (50–200 cells) with both lymphocytes and polys, lymphs usually predominate. The CSF protein is usually elevated and often is greater than 1 gram. Hemorrhagic brain disease can occur, and red cells may be seen in the CSF.

Eye involvement of herpes infection in the neonate can take the form of keratoconjunctivitis, chorioretinitis or microphthalmia. When the infection is localized to the skin, vesicles are usually present. Lesions in the mouth occur in less than 10% of disseminated disease and can also occur as the only manifestation of infection.

Etiology and Epidemiology

Evidence exists for three modes of acquisition of herpes infection by the neonate. Infection can occur during the birth process. Infection can be acquired during passage through the birth canal or infection may ascend and cause infection if the membranes are ruptured. Postnatal infection is less common and is usually from a non-genital maternal source such as oral or skin lesions. Even less frequent and perhaps somewhat controversal is transplacental spread. Evidence of herpetic lesions at birth and associated congenital abnormalities such as chorioretinitis suggest the likelihood that herpes can be spread transplacentally. Supporting evidence includes reports of viremia with herpes, elevated IgG in cord blood, and an increased risk of abortion in pregnant women with genital herpes.

Neonatal herpes can be either herpes type 1 or 2. Approximately 80% of neonatal herpes is type 2. This corresponds with the 80% rate of genital herpes which is also type 2.

Neonatal HSV infection is more common in premature than full-term infants. The outcome of infection is similar however. The risk appears to be greatest when the pregnant women has a primary infection. The titer of virus in recurrent infection and the number of lesions are usually less than in primary infection. Antibodies do not protect against infection although it is possible that transplacental antibody may modify the disease. *REMEMBER:* As many as half of the infants who get HSV infection *never* have skin lesions. More than 70% of infants with skin lesions will develop disease at other sites. Fetal scalp monitors appear to be a risk factor for CNS dissemination. Most infants who develop herpetic lesions at the monitor site disseminate to the CNS.

The mortality rate from disseminated disease is above 50%. CNS disease alone results in death in up to 40% of infected infants. Morbidity is high.

Diagnosis

Diagnosis depends on maternal history and the symptoms and physical examination findings of the infant. Definitive diagnosis depends on demonstrating an active HSV infection.

If lesions are present, the base of the lesions are scraped. Scrapings can be stained by Czank stain or Pap stain. Smears are examined for intranuclear inclusions or multinucleated giant cells. These techniques are about 75% sensitive but can not distinguish between HSV and Herpes zoster infection.

Definitive diagnosis is best made by viral culture. Viral cultures are frequently positive within 48–72 hours. Immunofluorescent assays and electronmicroscopy can be of assistance in making a rapid diagnosis.

Serololgy is not particularly useful for neonatal diagnosis. IgM may not be detectable during the first week or two, therefore it is not usually useful to quickly diagnose herpes. IgG is not of value unless serial sera are obtained over several weeks.

In CNS disease, herpes is recovered from the CSF less than 50% of the time. Localization of CNS infection can be best made by computerized tomography CT or EEG. If a localized area of abnormality is found (often in the temporal lobe) a brain biopsy will provide a definitive diagnosis. Where brain biopsy is not feasible, a positive HSV culture from another body site in the presence of CNS symptoms, and an abnormal CT or EEG can also make the diagnosis.

Treatment

Adenine arabinoside (Vidarabine, Ara-A) therapy has resulted in decreased morbidity and mortality in neonatal HSV infection, especially in CNS infection. Early institution of therapy is essential. Prognosis appears to be better in neonates with skin lesions when treatment is instituted prior to dissemination. Acyclovir appears to be effective also. Acyclovir appears to be relatively safe and effective and requires a smaller fluid volume for infusion than does Viadarabine.

Sequelae and Complications

Mortality from CNS HSV infection ranges from 10% to 40%. Early institution of therapy has reduced mortality. Nevertheless, only half of the survivors are neurologically intact at one year of age. Mortality, even with therapy, is over 50% in neonates with disseminated disease. Less than 20% are normal at one year of age. Infants with skin lesions and disseminated disease who survive will have recurrences of the skin lesions during their first year of life. If recurrences occur after the first month of life they are not likely to progress or disseminate.

HEPATITIS B

Clinical Manifestations

Most neonates infected with hepatitis B virus are asymptomatic, some show mild elevations in serum transaminase levels, and some develop mild hepatitis. Severe fulminant hepatitis is rare in the neonatal period. Mild hepatitis B usually is anicteric and epidemic.

Pregnant women who contract hepatitis B infection during pregnancy or who are chronic carriers, may transmit the infection to their babies. In the U.S. and Western Europe, the carrier rate is less than 1% of the population. Less than 10% of the population have antibody. In contrast, carriage rates of up to 20% have been reported in parts of Asia and Africa, and greater than 50% have antibody.

Virus can be found in saliva, seman, blood, breast milk and other body secretions. Most infections in neonates appear to occur around the time of delivery. The later in pregnancy that acute maternal infection occurs, the more likely the neonate will become infected. Postnatal exposure is also a continued risk to the infant. It is not clear what role, if any, breast feeding has in the transmission of the virus, but it does not appear to be a major route of infection.

Diagnosis

Diagnosis is made by serology. If the mother had acute infection during pregnancy or if the mother is a hepatitis B carrier, the infant should have serology done as soon after birth as possible. Presence of hepatitis B antigen in the neonate makes the diagnosis.

Treatment

The goal is to prevent infection in the newborn. Identifying infected pregnant women or mothers is important so that infants can receive prophylactic therapy. Newborns born to hepatitis B surface antigen positive mothers should receive hepatitis B immune globulin, preferably within 24 hours of birth. This should be followed by hepatitis B vaccine if the infant is hepatitis B surface antigen negative. The vaccine should be administered within the first week of life and should be followed one month later by the second dose. Prior to the third dose, at 6 months, serology for hepatitis B surface antigen should be done. If surface antigen is present, than prophylaxis has failed and the third dose need not be given.

Sequelae and Complications

Infected infants may develop the carrier state. Chronic active hepatitis is uncommon in infants. Fatalities are rare. There appears to be an association of the carrier state and the development of liver cancer in adults. It is not known if infants who acquire hepatitis B in infancy are also at risk for liver cancer.

VARICELLA

Clinical Manifestations

Varicella zoster virus may infect the fetus and result in congenital defects, or may infect the baby in the perinatal period resulting in a more typical varicella picture. Congenital varicella appears to be rare. Defects include scarring, limb hypoplasia, encephalitis, paralysis, rudimentary digits, eye abnormalities and clubfeet. These infants are low birth weight and have increased susceptibility to infection.

The effects of perinatal infection depends on the timing of the maternal infection in relationship to the baby's delivery. If disease onset in the mother is less than five days prior to delivery or if the infant develops infection five to ten days after birth, the infection is serious and often fatal. If varicella occurs in the mother five days or more before delivery or in the infant less than five days after delivery, the infection is usually mild due to the development and transfer of maternal antibody. This mild form of the disease resembles the disease in older children.

Etiology and Epidemiology

By the age of 15 years, 90% of the population has had varicella. The incidence of maternal chickenpox is believed to be less than one case per 1000 pregnancies. The incubation period is 10 to 21 days. Prior to the appearance of the rash, viremia occurs which enables spread to the fetus.

Diagnosis

Diagnosis of congenital varicella is often difficult. Cultures may be negative and serology may also be negative. A maternal history of varicella during pregnancy and the typical defects in the neonate may be the only evidence of diagnosis.

Perinatal varicella can usually be diagnosed by maternal history of infection, of exposure near the time of delivery, and the typical clinical presentation in the neonate. Confusion with Herpes simplex viral infection sometimes occurs, and viral cultures are necessary to make a definitive diagnosis.

Treatment

The goal is prevention. Infants born to mothers who develop varicella within 5 days prior to delivery, or within 48 hours after delivery should receive varicella zoster immune globulin (V.Z.I.G.). V.Z.I.G. is also recommended for premature infants exposed postnatally, if the mother is seronegative for varicella, or has an uncertain varicella history. *REMEMBER:* Most infants greater than 28 weeks gestation will have transplacentally acquired maternal antibody and will be at least partially protected if the mother is immune.

Treatment data for varicella are mostly from studies in the immunocompromised child. Data suggest that vidarabine, acyclovir and interferon are all efficacious. Early institution of therapy appears to be essential to prevent dissemination. Therapy with vidarabine or acyclovir is usually administered for 5–7 days.

Sequelae and Complications

Damage from congenital varicella can be severe. Fatalities have occurred in many of the congenital varicella infections reported.

Perinatal varicella can also result in serious disease. Neonates are at risk for dissemination, and when disease onset in the mother is less than five days before delivery, or in the neonate 5–10 days after delivery, death can occur. In those risk groups the fatality rate has been reported as high as 30%.

ENTEROVIRUSES

Clinical Manifestations

Enteroviral infection in the neonate may present with a wide variety of symptoms. Common symptoms include hypothermia or hyperthermia, irritability, anorexia, vomiting and lethargy. Less commonly, diarrhea, abdominal distension, rash and central nervous system signs may be present. None of these clinical manifestations are unique to enteroviral infection. It is, therefore, difficult to distinguish enteroviral infection from herpes simplex infection or bacterial sepsis in the neonate.

Biphasic illness may occur. Mild symptoms lasting a few days are followed by an apparent recovery lasting usually less than 5 days. Severe manifestations follow including: meningitis, myocarditis and systemic manifestations, like disseminated intravascular coagulation.

Etiology and Epidemiology

Neonatal enteroviral infections are frequently seen during known community epidemics. This usually occurs in the summer or early fall months. Typically the mother will report having a viral-like illness near the time of delivery.

Diagnosis

Diagnosis is based on the characteristics previously described. The presence of an erythematous maculopapular rash or myocarditis should further increase suspicion of enteroviral infection. Treatable etiologies such as bacterial sepsis or meningitis, and herpes simplex infections should be ruled out. The direct method of confirming the diagnosis is viral culture. Samples of throat swabbing, stool and cerebrospinal fluid (CSF) are most useful.

Treatment

There is no antiviral therapy effective against enteroviruses currently available. Therapy consists of coverage for treatable etiologies until they have been ruled out, and supportive care.

Sequelae and Complications

Enteroviral infection in the neonate is not benign. Sequelae reported include ocular abnormalities, seizures, spasticity, decreased intelligence, decreased speech and language development.

Mortality was highest in low birth weight and low gestational age infants.

KEY POINTS

1. CMV is the most common congenital infection. It is responsible for classic congenital manifestations such as hepatosplenomegaly, jaundice, microcephaly, chorioretinitis and small for gestational age. CMV infection is also associated with psychomotor retardation, learning disabilities, dental defects and hearing loss.

2. Congenital rubella is preventable by appropriate antibody screening of women prior to pregnancy and immunization of those women who are seronegative. The congenital syndrome consists of involvement of the eyes, CNS, liver, heart, and spleen. In addition, some affected infants have immunological, hematological, skeletal and pulmonary manifestations.

3. Toxoplasmosis can be acquired by pregnant women from cat feces or poorly cooked infected meat. The parasite may then be passed on to the fetus resulting in a congenital toxoplasmosis infection. Early postnatal institution of therapy may halt progression of the infection.

4. Congenital syphilis can usually be prevented by routine serologic testing of pregnant women and treatment of those women with serologic evidence of infection. Untreated congenital infection may result in the development of Hutchinson's teeth, Mulberry molars, Rhagades facies, eighth nerve deafness, neurosyphilis, keratitis and joint deformities.

5. Untreated, *Herpes simplex* infection in the neonate can be devastating and often fatal. Symptoms frequently resemble those of bacterial sepsis or meningitis. Early institution of antiviral therapy has resulted in a decreased mortality.

6. Perinatally acquired hepatitis B infection frequently results in the carrier state in infants. Early identification of possible exposures and the institution of both passive and active antibody protection can significantly reduce the risk of the infant becoming infected.

7. Perinatal varicella is potentially fatal in infants who are premature, infants born to mothers who develop varicella within 5 days prior to delivery, or infants born to mothers who show symptoms of varicella within 48 hours of delivery. These infants should receive V.Z.I.G. to abort or modify their infection.

8. Perinatal enterovirus infection may present as sepsis or meningitis and frequently needs to be differentiated from herpes or bacterial infection.

REFERENCES

1. Alford CA, Pass RF: Epidemiology of Chronic Congenital and perinatal infections in man. In Clinics in Perinatology, (Plotkin SA, Starr SE, eds), 1981; WB Saunders Co. Philadelphia; 8(3):397-414.

2. Overall JC: Viral infections of the fetus and neonate in *Textbook of Pediatrics Infectious Diseases* (Fergin R, Cherry J, eds) 1981; W.B. Saunders Co., Philadelphia, pp 684-720.

3. Stagno S: Diagnosis of Viral Infections of the Newborn Infant. in. Clinics in Perinatology, (Plotkin SA, Staff SE, eds), 1981; W.B. Saunders Co., Philadelphia; 8(3):397–414.

4. Stango S, Pass RF, Dworsky ME, et al: Congenital and Perinatal Cytomegalovirus Infections: Clinical characteristics and pathogenic factors in CMV: *Pathogenesis and prevention of human infection* (Plotkin SA, Michelso S, Pagnno JS, Rapp F, eds), 1984; Alan R. Liss Inc., N.Y. pp 65–86.

5. Whitley RJ, Nahmias AJ, Visintine AM, et al: The natural history of herpes simplex virus infection of mother and newborn. Pediatrics 1980; 66:489–494.

REVIEW QUESTIONS

Match characteristics in column A with the infection in column B that is most closely associated with that characteristic. (Column B entries can be used more than once.)

A

1.) Frequently affects temporal lobe of brain
2.) Patents ductus arteriosus and pulmonary artery stenosis
3.) Periventricular calcification
4.) Treated with penicillin
5.) Recommended that pregnant women avoid cat feces
6.) Hyperimmune antibody and vaccine can prevent development of the carrier state
7.) Currently no specific treatment available, may mimic bacterial sepsis
8.) Hutchinson's teeth
9.) Inguinal hernias
10.) Rare congenital syndrome includes scarring, limb hypoplasia, encephalitis, paralysis, redimentary digits, eye abnormalities, and clubfeet

B

A. CMV
B. Herpes simplex
C. Rubella
D. Syphilis
E. Toxoplasmosis
F. Varicella
G. Enterovirus
H. Hepatitis B

13

INFECTIONS OF THE HEART

ENDOCARDITIS

Clinical Manifestations

The diagnosis of endocarditis in children often requires a high index of suspicion of the illness. Findings may be subtle, especially in patients with subacute bacterial endocarditis. Unexplained fever in patients at high risk for endocarditis necessitates a careful investigation for endocarditis. Patients at high risk include patients with congenital heart disease, rheumatic heart disease and postoperative cardiac patients.

Acute bacterial endocarditis (ABE) frequently is rapidly progressive. Hemorrhages, meningitis and infectious arthritis may be present. In addition, there may be evidence of embolic phenomena. When present, a change in a heart murmur is suggestive of endocarditis. Subacute bacterial endocarditis (SBE) is usually more subtle. Fever, if present, is often low-grade. Murmurs can frequently be heard. This disease usually begins relatively slowly. Physical findings that may be helpful include splenomegaly, Janeway spots (macules on the volar surface of hands and feet), Osler nodes (tender nodules) and Roth spots (hemorrhages with clear centers on the ocular fundus).

Etiology and Epidemiology

Endocarditis is frequently the result of introduction of the person's own flora into the bloodstream. Dental manipulation, rectal or colon manipulations, urinary tract manipulation, intravenous therapy and tonsillectomy are some of the ways that a transient bacteremia may be set up, leading to endocarditis. Intravenous drug abusers may also inject bacteria leading to endocarditis. Most endocarditis is due to Gram positive organisms, especially staphylococci and streptococci. Gram negative organisms include *Haemophilus, Actinobacillus, Cardiobacterium, Eikenella* and *Kingella.* After entering the blood, the organism will attach to damaged endocardium, or valves; and may adhere to microthrombi at the site of damage. Vegetations that are formed consist of bacteria, fibrin and necrotic debris. There are few white cells present in the vegetation. The most common congenital heart lesions associated with endocarditis are tetrology of Fallot, aortic valvular abnormalities and ventricular septal defects.

Diagnosis

Fever and murmur in a patient should suggest the possibility of endocarditis. Even in the absence of fever, the presence of other symptoms, particularly in a patient at risk, should result in a careful evaluation for endocarditis. Echocardiograms may be useful in identifying vegetations.

Blood cultures are essential for determining the etiology of the endocarditis. SBE is frequently caused by organisms that are usually thought of as being of low virulence, therefore, multiple blood cultures using strict sterile procedures can be helpful in finding the organism and avoiding contamination. Five or six separately drawn blood cultures should be obtained. Cultures must be maintained for several weeks to enable slow-growing organisms to grow. It is important to remember that unusual organisms may cause endocarditis. Clinically apparent endocarditis associated with negative blood cultures may be due to anaerobes, fungi and viruses, among others. An elevated WBC and erythrocyte sedimentation rate (ESR) are consistent with, but not diagnostic of, endocarditis. Mild hemolytic anemia and microscopic hematuria may also be present.

Treatment

The specific therapy depends on the organism isolated and the specific sensitivities of that organism. Synergy may be demonstrated with certain antibiotic combinations and this may result in an increased chance of cure. The dose of antibiotic may need to be adjusted based on the serum bacteriocidal levels obtained. Therapy should be instituted after adequate blood cultures are obtained. Effectiveness of therapy should be based on clinical improvement and follow-up blood cultures. Most patients with endocarditis are treated for four weeks or more. Patients with particularly resistant organisms or slow clinical improvement may need prolonged therapy.

Sequelae and Complications

Untreated, the disease is usually fatal. Septic embolization, especially to the brain may occur. Central nervous system changes should be a warning sign of possible embolization. Cardiac deterioration may occur as a result of progressive damage to valves or cardiac tissue. Surgical intervention may sometimes be required to replace incompetent or seriously damaged valves. Prognosis depends on several factors including the degree of damage prior to initiation of appropriate therapy, the location of the cardiac damage, and the sensitivity of the organism being treated.

Prevention of Bacterial Endocarditis

Endocarditis prophylaxis is recommended for patients with a variety of conditions including: prosthetic cardiac valves, most congenital cardiac malformations, systemic-pulmonary shunts (constructed), acquired valvular dysfunction (including rheumatic valvular disease), idiopathic hypertrophic subaortic stenosis, previous history of bacterial endocarditis and mitral valve prolapse with insufficiency (good data on the risk associated with mitral valve prolapse are lacking). Prophylaxis should be instituted for dental procedures that are likely to cause gingival bleeding (not including simple orthodontic appliance adjustment or loss of deciduous teeth), tonsillectomy, adenoidectomy, surgical procedures involving the respiratory tract, bronchoscopy, incision and drainage of infected tissue, and a variety of gastrointestinal and genitourinary procedures.

The American Heart Association recommends that "at-risk" patients undergoing dental or respiratory tract procedures should receive penicillin V 2 grams orally 1 hour prior to the procedure, and 1 gram orally 6 hours later. Patients weighing less than 27 kg should receive half the recommended dose. An alternative regimen is aqueous penicillin G intramuscularly or intravenously 50,000 Units/kg (maximum 2 million units) 1/2 to 1 hour before, and 25,000 Units/kg (maximum 1 million units) 6 hours later. In high risk patients (prosthetic valves or systemic-pulmonary shunts) parenteral therapy is preferred. Ampicillin, 50 mg/kg/dose (maximum 2 grams) plus gentamicin, 2 mg/kg/dose (1.5 mg/kg/dose in adults) given intravenously or intramuscularly 30 minutes before the procedure is then followed by oral penicillin V 6 hours later or the parenteral regimen may be repeated 8 hours later.

In penicillin allergic patients, erythromycin 20 mg/kg 1 hour before the procedure (maximum 1 gram) orally, and ½ that dose 6 hours later, can be used; or Vancomycin 20 mg/kg/dose (maximum 1 gram) should be given slowly over 1 hour prior to the procedure. A repeat dose of Vancomycin is not necessary.

Recommendations for gastrointestinal or genitourinary procedures include: ampicillin plus gentamicin given parenterally ½ hour to 1 hour before the procedure and then 8 hours later. The dose is as for dental procedures. Minor procedures can be prophylaxed with amoxicillin 50 mg/kg/dose orally, given 1 hour before and a ½ dose given 6 hours later. Penicillin allergic patients can receive vancomycin slowly intravenously as described above, with a repeat dose 8–12 hours later.

MYOCARDITIS

Clinical Manifestations

The spectrum of clinical manifestations of myocarditis is large. The illness may be asymptomatic. In extreme cases the illness is rapidly progressive and fatal. Symptoms are the result of myocardial dysfunction or dysrhythmias. Serious symptoms can be seen in neonates with myocarditis. Lethargy, failure-to-thrive, fever and anorexia are often seen in these newborns. In addition, many of these infants are cyanotic, have respiratory distress and have abnormal electrocardiograms.

Older children may have an indulent course. Low-grade fever and respiratory symptoms are often seen initially. Abdominal pain may be present. Manifestations of cardiac disease in these children include pallor, tachypnea, mottling, tachycardia, a gallup rhythm and hepatomegaly.

Etiology and Epidemiology

Myocarditis may be caused by a wide variety of organisms. Viral etiologies include Coxsackie B, Coxsackie A and echoviruses. Many other viruses have been implicated less frequently. A variety of bacteria, rickettsia, parasites and fungi have also been implicated as causes of myocarditis. Mycobacterial myocarditis occurs, but is rare. Non-infectious etiologies have also been reported. Myocarditis may also result from toxins produced in diphtheria and by scorpions.

Epidemics do occur, usually in neonates, and are frequently due to Coxsackie B. Maternal infection late in pregnancy may result in infection in the fetus or in the neonate. Postnatal spread is by fecal-oral route or by airborne route.

Diagnosis

Patients with the clinical presentation described above should be suspected of having myocarditis. Other clues include an exaggerated tachycardia, a gallop in the presence of an otherwise quiet precordium and an enlarged heart on x-ray, if cardiac failure has occured. The EKG usually shows diffuse low-voltage QRS complexes. Low amplitude T waves or inverted T waves may also be present. Q waves are usually small or absent in leads V5 and V6.

Specific etiologies can often be determined by obtaining appropriate cultures. Nasopharyngeal, blood and stool cultures may be valuable to diagnose viral infection. Isolation of the organism from the myocardium may also be desirable. Isolation of the virus from a non-cardiac source and a four-fold change in antibody titer to that virus will prove the etiology. Bacterial cultures can also be helpful.

Treatment

Treatment for most viral myocarditis is supportive care. Maintaining adequate respiratory and cardiac function is essential. Bed rest, oxygen and appropriate cardiac drugs are the mainstay of supportive care. If a bacterial etiology is found, appropriate antibiotics should be used.

Sequelae and Complications

The prognosis depends on the etiology. Coxsackie B myocarditis in infants may have mortality rates as high as 75%. In older children, the mortality rate appears to be less than 25%. Of those who recover, abnormal EKGs may persist. It is therefore important for those children who survive to have extended periodic follow-ups.

PERICARDITIS

Clinical Manifestations

Children who are septic and have cardiomegaly should be suspected of having pericarditis. They will usually have decreased heart sounds, a pericardial friction rub and precordial pain. *REMEMBER:* The most common triad of symptoms is tachycardia, fever and tachypnea. These along with abnormal cardiac findings on physical examination, EKG, or x-ray should strongly suggest the diagnosis. If the pericardial sac is full of fluid, cardiac tamponade may occur resulting in decreased venous return and decreased cardiac output. Pulsus peridoxus, an exaggerated fall in systolic blood pressure with inspiration, may be seen in patients with pericarditis.

Etiology and Epidemiology

Although purulent pericarditis occurs in all pediatric age groups, it is most common in children less than two years of age. Most cases of purulent pericarditis are secondary to another site of infection, especially the lungs. *Staphylococcus aureus* is most commonly isolated. *Haemophilus influenzae* type B is also frequently seen. Other bacteria, aerobic and anaerobic, are seen less frequently. Fungal pericarditis is uncommon but appears to be seen primarily in immunocompromised or immunosuppressed patients or patients on long-term antibiotic therapy.

Diagnosis

Patients with the symptoms described above should be evaluated for pericarditis. Chest x-rays may show a rapidly enlarging heart without increased pulmonary markings or a globular heart without increased pulmonary markings. Electrocardiogram may also be helpful. Low voltage QRS complexes result from periocardial effusion. Elevations of ST segments are frequently seen in some leads, and T wave inversion occurs. Definitive diagnosis is made by examining pericardial fluid. Appropriate cultures, slides and antigen detection tests should be obtained. Blood cultures frequently yield the causative organisms.

Treatment

Therapy must be directed to draining the pericardial sac, providing supportive care, and appropriate antimicrobial therapy. Definitive antimicrobial therapy depends on identifying the pathogen. Initial broad spectrum coverage should provide for anti-staphylococcus coverage as well as coverage for *H. influenzae,* meningococcus, pneumonococcus and streptococcus. Therapy is usually continued for three to four weeks. *REMEMBER:* Pericardial drainage significantly improves the survival rate in purulent pericarditis.

Sequelae and Complications

Mortality rates for purulent pericarditis have been reported to be as high as 70%. Those who survive usually have no significant sequelae.

ACUTE RHEUMATIC FEVER

Clinical Manifestations

The diagnosis of acute rheumatic fever (ARF) is based on the Jones Criteria, a set of major and minor manifestations of the disease. Major criteria include evidence of carditis, polyarthritis, chorea, erythema marginatum, and subcutaneous nodules. Minor criteria include: fever, arthralgias, previous ARF or rheumatic heart disease, increased erythrocyte sedimentation rate or positive C-reaction protein, leukocytosis and prolonged PR interval on EKG.

The typical course is for the patient to have a pharyngitis due to group A beta-hemolytic streptococci. If untreated, ARF may result. Fever, malaise and anorexia are common findings. Carditis and arthritis are the most common major criteria found. The arthritis is migratory and usually involves the larger joints. Carditis may declare itself with a murmur of mitral insufficiency and/or a murmur of aortic insufficiency. Radiologic evidence of cardiomegaly, an abnormal EKG or congestive heart failure may be present. Less frequently Sydenham chorea is seen. The onset of the chorea may be weeks to months after the streptococcal infection and may be the only manifestation of ARF. Erythema marginatum is a pinkish macular rash which fuses to form a serpiginous pattern that may come and go over several weeks. Subcutaneous nodules are infrequently seen.

Etiology and Epidemiology

ARF occurs most commonly in children 5 to 15 years old and thus parallels the incidence of group A beta-hemolytic streptococcal infections. The incidence is highest in the spring and winter months. While ARF is a consequence of streptococcal pharyngitis that goes untreated, it is not an inevitable consequence. Only about 3% of patients with untreated streptococcal pharyngitis go on to develop ARF.

Diagnosis

Diagnosis requires evidence of a recent streptococcal infection plus either two major Jones Critieria or one major and two minor Jones Criteria.

Evidence for streptococcal infection includes a positive throat culture, recent scarlet fever, increased ASO titer, or increase in other streptococcal antibodies. Chorea may occur as a sole criteria because its onset frequently is delayed several months.

Treatment

Salicylate therapy for one to two weeks will significantly improve symptoms. Penicillin therapy for streptococcal infection should be instituted followed by a prophylactic regimen of penicillin to prevent further occurrences. Cardiac symptoms must be managed appropriately, and in severe cases, cardiac surgery may be indicated.

Sequelae and Complications

Residual heart damage is common. Mitral insufficiency sometimes accompanied by aortic insufficiency is common. Ten year mortality rates of 80% have been reduced because of the use of antibiotic prophylaxis and corrective surgery. Patients should receive prophylactic antibiotics, preferably parenterally and should receive additional prophylaxis prior to certain dental and surgical procedures.

KEY POINTS

1. SBE may present with very non-specific and subtle manifestations. Fever, a new murmur or change in existing murmur, and splenomegaly should suggest the possibility of SBE.
2. Antibiotic prophylaxis is recommended for patients with a variety of conditions including: prosthetic valves, most congenital cardiac malformations, constricted systemic-pulmonary shunts, acquired valvular dysfunction, idiopathic hypertrophic subaortic stenosis, previous history of bacterial endocarditis and mitral valve prolapse with insufficiency.
3. Myocarditis is frequently due to enterovirus infection. In infants, the associated mortality may be high.
4. The most common triad of symptoms in patients with pericarditis are tachypnea, tachycardia and fever. Purulent pericarditis is frequently associated with decreased heart sounds, a pericardial friction rub and precordial pain.

5. Acute rheumatic fever is diagnosed based on finding two major criteria or 1 major and 2 minor criteria in association with evidence of streptococcal infection.

REFERENCES

1. Bentovich S, Rodriguez-Torres R, Lin J-S: Virologic studies in children with acute myocarditis. Am J Dis Child, 1968; 115:207–209.
2. Burch GE, Sun SC, Chu KC, et al: Interstitial and Coxackievirus B myocarditis in infants and children. JAMA, 1968; 203:1–8.
3. Cleary TG, Kohl S: Anti-infective therapy of infectious endocarditis. Ped Clin N Am, 1983; 30:349–364.
4. Coleman DL, Horwitz RI, Andriole VT: Associations between serum inhibitory and bactericidal concentrations and therapeutic outcome in bacterial endocarditis. Amer J Med, 1982; 73:260–267.
5. Dery P, Marks MI, Shapeara R: Clinical manifestations of coxsackievirus infections in children. Amer J Dis Child, 1974; 128:464–468.
6. Duff DF. Myocarditis. In Feigin RD and Cherry JD (eds), *Textbook of Pediatric Infectious Diseases,* 1981, Philadelphia, WB Saunders. pp 255–269.
7. Echeverria P, Smith EWP, Ingrams D, et al: Hemophilus Influenzae b pericarditis in children. Pediatrics, 1975; 56:808–818.
8. Harford CG: Bacterial Endocarditis. In Feigin RD, Cherry JD (eds): *Textbook of Pediatric Infectious Diseases,* Philadelphia, WB Saunders Co, 1981. pp 235–240.
9. Hermans PE: The Clinical Manifestations of infective endocarditis. Mayo Clin Proc, 1982; 57:15–21.
10. Johnson DH, Rosenthal A, Nadas AS: A forty-year reviewed bacterial endocarditis in infancy and childhood. Circulation, 1975; 51:581–588.
11. Lerner AM: Coxsackievirus myocardiopathy, J Infect. Dis., 1969; 120:496–499.
12. Sande MA, Scheld WM: Combination antibiotic therapy in bacterial endocarditis. Annals Int Med, 1980; 92:390–395.
13. Schwartz RH, Hepner SI, Ziai M: Incidence of Acute Rheumatic Fever: A suburban community hospital experience during the 1970's. Clin. Pediatr., 1983; 22:798–801.

14. Shulman ST, Amren DP, Bisno AL, et al: Prevention of bacterial endocarditis - a statement for health professionals by the Committee on Rheumatic Fever and Bacterial Endocarditis of the Council on Cardiovascular Diseases in the Young of the American Heart Association. AJDC, 1985; 139:232–235.
15. Shulman ST, Amren DP, Bisno AL, et al: Prevention of bacterial endocarditis. Am J Dis Child, 1985; 139:232–235.
16. Strauss AW, Santa Maria M, Goldring D: Constrictive pericarditis in Children. Am J Dis Child, 1975; 129:822–826.
17. Weinstein L, Schlesinger JJ: Pathoanatomic pathophysiologic and clinical correlations in endocarditis. N Engl J Med, 1974; 291:832–836.
18. Weir EK, Joffe HS: Purulent pericarditis in children: An analysis of 28 cases. Thorax, 1977; 32:438.

REVIEW QUESTIONS

Match description in Column A with appropriate item from Column B

A	B
A. Macules on the volar surface of hands and feet	1. Purulent pericarditis
B. Hemorrhages with clear centers on the ocular fundus	2. Roth spots
C. Criteria for antibiotic prophylaxis include:	3. Congenital cardiac malformations and prosthetic valves
D. Pericardial friction rub, cardiac tamponade, precordial pain	4. Rheumatic fever
E. Jones Criteria	5. Janeway spots
F. Carditis, polyarthritis, chorea, subcutaneous nodules, erythema marginatum	6. Major Jones Criteria

14

FEVER OF UNKNOWN ORIGIN

The term "fever of unknown origin" (FUO) is loosely used in pediatrics to simply describe a fever in a patient who has not yet had a diagnosis made. More precisely, an FUO in a pediatric patient is unexplained fever of at least two weeks duration. It has also been suggested that the diagnosis FUO might be reserved for those patients who still have no apparent diagnosis after a one week investigation. Regardless of the precise definition used, one needs to develop a logical method of evaluating FUOs.

Most pediatric FUO is the result of atypical presentations of common pediatric illnesses. Most are due to infectious diseases and collagen vascular disease. Malignancy in children infrequently presents as only fever. Always rule out the possibility of drug fever before beginning an exhaustive evaluation for fever. Fever must be documented preferably in the hospital to avoid factitious fever. In general, children with FUOs have a better prognosis than adults and frequently the fever will spontaneously resolve without an etiology being found.

A Word About Fever

How best to measure temperature and how much significance needs to be placed on the actual temperature measured are subjects that frequently preoccupy both pediatricians and parents of their patients. In general, rectal temperatures are most accurate and reproducible. *REMEMBER:* Temperatures in children are usually higher than adults. The average temperature (rectal) in children 1½ years old is 99.8°F (37.7°C). Temperatures decrease toward adult levels during adolescence. Temperatures peak between 5 p.m. and 7 p.m. and minimum temperatures occur between 2 a.m. and 6 a.m. An active, healthy child may have a rectal temperature of 100.4°F (38.0°C) in the early evening.

Fever can be classified based on the pattern it follows. Sustained fever persists throughout the day without much variation. Intermittent fevers return to normal at least once per day. Relapsing fevers are fevers alternating with variable periods of being afebrile. Septic fevers are characterized by wide variations in temperature. Double quotidian fevers return to normal twice a day. The chart gives examples of diagnoses associated with each of these patterns. Although these patterns are frequently seen with their associated diseases, the absence of the appropriate pattern does not rule out the diagnosis.

Making the Diagnosis

Identifying the etiology of FUOs requires a detailed history and careful physical examination. History obtained must include a thorough review of travel, medications, pica and animal exposure. In addition, a history of hereditary and familial illnesses is valuable. Special attention should be paid to physical signs such as red weeping eyes, often seen in periarteritis nodosa; and bulbar conjunctivitis, seen occasionally with leptospirosis. Other clues include: lack of sweating which is seen with moderate to severe dehydration, and anhydrotic ectodermal dysplasia; lack of tears, lack of sweat, and absent corneal reflex in association with a smooth tongue and fever suggest familial dysautonamia; and palpebral conjunctivitis seen in a variety of illnesses including Epstein-Barr virus infection, cat scratch disease, tuberculosis and lupus erythematosus. It is important to look for sinus tenderness, bone tenderness and muscle tenderness. Sinus tenderness, when present, is a useful sign suggesting sinusitis. Bone tenderness suggests osteomyelitis or invasive neoplastic disease. Muscle tenderness can be seen in association with trichinosis, viral infections, or collagen vascular diseases. *REMEMBER:* Subdiaphragmatic abscess may present with a sore trapezius muscle. Rectal examination may reveal tender pararectal lymph nodes or guiac positive stools. A careful dental examination is often valuable.

If the history and physical examination suggest a likely diagnosis, appropriate laboratory tests should be done to confirm it. If a diagnosis is not evident, an initial series of laboratory tests should be done. Each case must be individualized but initial screening tests frequently obtained include a complete blood count and differential white blood cell count, sedimentation rate, PPD, chest radiograph, liver enzymes, febrile agglutinins, anti-nuclear antibodies, serum protein electrophoresis and urinalysis. Additional studies can include VMA spot urine; blood, urine and stool cultures for bacteria; urine for cytomegalovirus; nasopharyngeal viral cultures; Epstein-Barr virus titers; and urine and serum for leptospirosis.

If the above workup does not provide an appropriate etiology for the FUO, a decision about when and if to pursue further workup must be made. A child with a FUO who is not particularly ill, nor is the fever significantly affecting the child's functioning, may not benefit from a further, more extensive and expensive workout. However, a child who is adversely affected by his illness needs a more extensive evaluation. This may include abdominal ultrasound or body computerized tomography, a bone scan, liver-spleen scan, intravenous pyelogram, a bone marrow aspiration and biopsy, and an upper and lower gastrointestinal radiographic contrast series. A child who is deteriorating or remains seriously ill may require a liver biopsy or laparotomy.

Differential Diagnosis

The list of possible causes of FUO in children is exhaustive. Nevertheless, some diagnoses are more common than others. Infections that present as FUOs include urinary tract infections, dental infections, Epstein-Barr virus, cytomegalic virus, viral hepatitis (A, B, nonA, nonB), tuberculosis, abscesses, osteomyelitis, sinusitis and salmonellosis. Other less frequent infections include leptospirosis, Q fever, brucellosis, toxoplasmosis, tularemia, syphilis, malaria and sarcoidosis. Noninfectious causes include collagen vascular disease, inflammatory bowel diseases, factitious fever and malignancies such as neuroblastoma, Hodgkin's disease and lymphoma.

(For details related to the diagnosis and treatment of the infections mentioned above, see appropriate sections in the book.)

Selected Noninfectious Etiologies of FUO

1. Juvenile Rheumatoid Arthritis (JRA) - Fever is part of the symptom complex of all three forms of JRA. In particular the systemic form of JRA is almost always associated with fever. Double quotidian fever and septic patterns of fever are frequently seen in systemic JRA. Arthritic symptoms may be delayed, even for years after the initial febrile symptoms. Children may appear toxic. Diagnosis is difficult as it is usually one of exclusion.

2. Regional Enteritis — Fever is a major sign of regional enteritis in children. Gastrointestinal symptoms may initially be lacking but a careful radiological examination of the gastrointestinal tract may suggest enteritis.

3. Drug Fever - Any drug can be implicated in causing FUOs. Topical preparations, especially those that are absorbed, may also be implicated. Fever may occur soon after the drug therapy is initiated or may be delayed a week or more. The usual patterns are either intermittent or continuous. The fall in fever back to normal may occur shortly after discontinuation of therapy, but if the drug has a long half-life in the body, fever may persist long after therapy is stopped.

4. Factitious Fever - Factitious fever is not real fever. The patient falsely reports elevated temperature for his own secondary gain. This type of "fever" can be diagnosed by hospitalization and having personnel take the temperature with a thermometer brought into the room at the time when the temperature will be measured, checking that it is down below normal before inserting and taking rectal rather than oral temperatures. This diagnosis can be suspected in patients who have normal temperatures when taken under supervision but elevated temperatures when no one is supervising the patient. A normal pulse in the presence of a reportedly high temperature should also raise the question of factitious fever. Lack of variation of the temperature and lack of diaphoresis with apparent rapid falls in temperature may also suggest this diagnosis.

Fever Pattern	Description	Examples	
Sustained	Fever remains elevated throughout the day.	Typhoid fever. Bacteremia.	Pneumococcal pneumonia. Rickettsial diseases.
Intermittant	Fever returns to normal at least once per day.	Malaria. (non-falciparum) Tuberculosis	Abscesses.
Relapsing	Fever alternating with variable periods without fever.	Malaria Meningococcemia Rat bite fever	Brucellosis
Septic	Wide variations in temperature.	Abscesses Tuberculosis	Malaria
Double Quotidiam	Temperature returns to normal twice a day.	Endocarditis (N. gonorrheae) Kala azar Tuberculosis (Miliary)	

KEY POINTS

1. Most FUO in pediatric patients is the result of unusual presentations of common pediatric illnesses. Most common etiologies are infectious or collagen vascular.
2. Before evaluating a patient for a FUO, document the presence of fever.
3. The evaluation for FUO should proceed in a logical sequence. Generalized broad screening tests should be followed with more specific focused studies once the general areas of abnormalities are pinpointed.
4. The first step in evaluating patients with FUOs who are currently taking medication is to stop the medicine if possible, and see if the fever resolves.

REFERENCES

1. Bernheim HA, Block LH, Atkins E: Fever pathogenesis, pathophysiology and purpose. Ann Intern Med, 1979; 91:261–270.
2. Dinarello CA, Wolff SM: Pathogenesis of fever in man. New Eng J Med, 1978; 298: 607–612.
3. Feigin RD: Fever of unknown origin in Feigin RD, Cherry J (eds), *Textbook of Pediatric Infectious Diseases.* Saunder Co., Philadelphia, 1982; pp. 787–795.
4. Kluger MJ: Fever. Pediatrics, 1980; 66:720–724.
5. Kresch MJ: Axillary temperature as a screening test for fever in children. J Pediatrics, 1984; 104:596–599.
6. Levinson SL, Barondess JA: Occult dental infection as a cause of fever of obscure origin. Am J Medicine, 1979; 66:463–467.
7. Musher DM: Fever of unknown origin: Diagnostic principles. Hospital Practice, 1982; 89–95.
8. Pizzo PA, Lovejoy FH, Smith DH: Prolonged fever in childhood: Review of 100 cases. Pediatrics, 1975; 55:468–473.

REVIEW QUESTIONS

1.) Match items in Column A with those in Column B

A | B

A. Sustained fever
B. Septic fever
C. Subdiaphramatic abscess
D. Peak temperatures
E. Minimum temperatures
F. Double quotidian fever

1. Sore trapezius muscle
2. 2 A.M. to 6 A.M.
3. Fever returns to normal twice a day
4. Wide variations in temperatures
5. Fever that persists throughout the day with little variation
6. 5 P.M. to 7 P.M.

2.) True or False
1. Malignancy accounts for most of the pediatric FUOs.
2. Regional enteritis may initially present with fever and without gastrointestinal symptoms.
3. Drug fever can occur with topical preparation use.
4. An active healthy child may have a temperature of 100.4°F in the early evening.

15

PARASITIC INFECTIONS

Parasitic infections have worldwide distribution. In the United States, parasitic infections are being increasingly recognized as causes of diseases. The influx of Asian and Central American refugees into the U.S. has resulted in additional increases in the frequency of a variety of illnesses; parasitic and non-parasitic. The importance of parasitic diseases in many underdeveloped and developing nations is greater than in most of the industrialized world. The incidence of some parasitic infections in third world nations extends into the hundreds of thousands.

This chapter will cover those parasitic infections important in North America as well as some of the more common parasites found in other areas of the world. Suspicion of a parasitic etiology of a disease often depends on a detailed, reliable travel history, especially outside the U.S., and a detailed history of unusual food and water sources. Increasingly, a reliable sexual history may also provide clues to parasitic infections.

The chart in this chapter contains a summary of some of the parasitic infections discussed in this chapter as well as brief description of a few additional parasitic infections.

ENTAMOEBA HISTOLYTICA

Clinical Manifestations

Most commonly, *E. histolytica* produces an asymptomatic infection. When symptoms are present they may present a variety of clinical pictures. Most commonly, if symptoms are present, they are mild. Abdominal distension, flatulence, constipation, or loose stools are seen. Perhaps the most typical symptom complex is acute diarrhea with cramping. Much less common is dysentery. Amoebic dysentery is associated with frequent fever, headache and chills. Bloody diarrhea with mucous and pain are typical of dysentery. Amoeba can spread via the bloodstream to the liver, lungs, pleura, heart, skin and brain. Spread of the amoebic infection to extraintestinal organs may occur at the same time as the dysentery. More commonly, however, extraintestinal infection occurs months to years after intestinal infection. Most patients with hepatic amoebic abscess, for example, have no intestinal symptoms nor any recent history of intestinal symptoms.

Etiology and Epidemiology

E. histolytica is a protozoa. It is the etiologic agent of amebiasis. These organisms are single cell animals that are capable of all necessary reproductive and metabolic processes. The organism appears in two stages, a trophozoite and a cyst stage. The cyst stage is protective against adverse environmental factors. *E. histolytica* do not require a vector for spread. The trophozoite stage, which normally resides in the colon of its host, is invasive.

It is estimated that 10% of the world's population is infected with *E. histolytica*. Over 30,000 deaths each year are attributable to amoebic infection. Prevalence rates in underdeveloped nations often approaches 50% of the population. These high rates seem to reflect the poor sanitation, crowding, socioeconomic status and cultural habits.

In the U.S., estimated prevalence is less than 5% but certain populations within the U.S. have a significantly higher rate. Up to 30% of the male homosexual population in the U.S. may be colonized with amoeba. Institutionalized mentally retarded people are reported to have a prevalence over

70%. Migrant workers and recent immigrants to the southwestern U.S. reportedly also have a high prevalence of infection.

Infection is usually a result of oral ingestion of the cyst. Spread is person-to-person, or from contaminated food or drink. The patient may be contagious intermittently if untreated.

Diagnosis

In patients with suspected amoebic infection, three stools should be submitted to the laboratory for evaluation. The diagnosis is made by identifying cysts or trophozoites in stool specimens. The success of laboratory diagnosis depends on the experience of the personnel examining the specimen, the type of staining done, whether the specimen is concentrated and whether amoebic cultures are done. *E. histolytica* will grow on egg enrichment media and this may be helpful in a specimen with few amoeba present. In invasive disease, serology may be helpful. Asymptomatic cyst passers usually have negative serology, whereas most patients with invasive disease will have a positive amoebic serology. Endoscopy can also be useful. Colitis due to *E. histolytica* appears as punctate hemorrhages or ulcers with exudative centers and hyperemic borders.

Patients with extraintestinal amoebic disease may not have gastrointestinal symptoms, and stool examination may not demonstrate amoeba. Amoebic serologies are usually positive but if it is early in the clinical course, the serology may be negative. Amoebic abscesses appear as cold central areas with a hot rim on gallium scan. Aspiration of abscess material will yield the typical brown "anchovy paste" fluid. The fluid is usually acidic and inflammatory cells are absent. The parasites are usually in the rim of the abscess; not in aspirated fluid. *REMEMBER:* Patients with amoebic liver abscess are usually not jaundiced, usually do have fever and abdominal pain and frequently have elevated alkaline phosphatase and transaminases.

Treatment

There are several different regimens available to treat amoebic infection. For asymptomatic carriers (cyst passers), diloxanide furoate, available from the CDC is recommended. The dose is 20 mg/kg/day divided in three doses, for ten days. Iodoquinol has also been recommended but in high doses is associated with optic neuritis. Paromomycin and tetracycline have also been used effectively. In endemic areas many physicians do not treat unless the patient is symptomatic since reinfection is likely.

Patients with mild to moderate symptoms usually are treated with metronidazole 35–50 mg/kg/day divided into 3 doses for 10 days plus diodohydroxyquin (Diodoquin) 30–40 mg/kg/day divided into 3 doses for 20 days. Diodoquin is chemically related to iodoquinol. More severe intestinal disease may also be treated with Diodoquin plus metronidazole or with the combination of dehydroemetine plus Diodoquin.

Liver abscesses should be treated with metronidazole plus Diodoquin. In very large or unresponsive abscesses, surgical drainage may be necessary.

Prevention of amoebic disease is related to upgrading sanitary conditions including proper cleaning of foods prior to consuming them, good personal hygiene, and adequate purification of drinking water (moderate amounts of chlorine or iodine will usually not kill amoeba). *REMEMBER:* Boiling water ensures the absence of amoeba. Avoiding sexual practices that permit fecal contact can also reduce the incidence of amoebic infection.

Sequelae and Complications

Prompt diagnosis and treatment can frequently prevent complications. Intestinal perforation and peritonitis as a result of toxic and necrotizing amoebic colitis can occur. Secondarily, sepsis may develop and can rapidly be fatal. Massive intestinal hemorrhage is another complication associated with fatal cases of amoebic diseases. Fistulas, colonic strictures and intussusception have been reported. Liver abscesses may rupture into the abdomen or into the pleural space. Cerebral abscesses have been reported, although very rarely in children.

GIARDIA LAMBLIA

Clinical Manifestations

Asymptomatic infection occurs. Clinical presentation of symptomatic disease varies. Mild diarrhea can occur. It is usually acute, may be self-limited and will mimic viral gastroenteritis. There is also a more chronic symptom complex of malabsorption, weight loss and diarrhea. These children may present as failures-to-thrive. Acute diseases due to giardia involve complaints of diarrhea, cramps, bloating, flatulence, nausea, anorexia and malaise. Fever, vomiting and tenesmus also are occasionally seen. Stools are often described as malodorous and greasy. Leukocytes are usually not found in the stools and pus and blood are also absent.

Etiology and Epidemiology

Giardia has a worldwide distribution. It is the most commonly identified intestinal parasite in the U.S. Prevalence rates in the U.S. vary from region to region but have been reported as high as 20%. It is also the most common etiology of waterborne outbreaks of diarrhea in the U.S.

The organism is a flagellated protozoan. There are two stages to its life cycle, a trophozoite stage and a cystic stage. In the intestine, the trophozoite forms a cyst. Once the cyst matures, division may take place resulting in two trophozoites.

Transmission of giardia is primarily person-to-person and by fecally contaminated water supplies. Infection appears to be relatively uncommon during the first year of life in the U.S. Endemic infection peaks during the second to seventh year of life. The incidence of non-epidemic giardia infection reflects, to some extent, levels of personal hygiene.

Infection with and transmission of giardia is particularly common in day care centers where the prevalence of stools with cysts has been as high as 50%; and homosexual men have an incidence of giardia as high as 20%. While day care center children are frequently symptomatic, the gay population has symptoms less frequently. Many patients, after a period of acute illness, will become asymptomatic but continue to shed cysts and are therefore still infectious.

Giardia infection can be found in association with hypogamma-globulinemia and the absence of plasma cells in the intestinal lamina propia. Malnourished children frequently have symptomatic giardiasis which in turn exacerbates their malnutrition creating a still more debilitated patient.

Diagnosis

A clinical presentation of diarrhea and malabsorption, especially when associated with significant weight loss, should prompt the consideration of a diagnosis of giardia infection. Stools should be examined for the presence of cysts or trophozoites. When proper techniques are used and an experienced examiner does the microscopic stool examination, the yield is usually over 50% for one stool examination and 90% for three stools.

When stool examination fails to reveal cysts or trophozoites, and a strong suspicion of giardia remains, sampling of duodenal contents is indicated. Procedures used include the string test (gelatin capsule containing a string is swallowed, allowed to dissolve in the stomach and the string is allowed to pass into the duodenum. The free end of the string is secured outside the mouth prior to ingesting the capsule. The string is then removed after at least 4 hours in the duodenum), duodenal aspiration, and duodenal biopsy. These techniques are believed to increase the yield over stool examination alone. *REMEMBER:* When obtaining stools for giardia, the organism is usually passed intermittently. Therefore, multiple specimens obtained on different days will help increase the yield.

Treatment

Although quinacrine hydrochloride is the drug of choice, it is frequently not well tolerated by children. When taken appropriately (6 mg/kg/day, up to 300 mg maximum, divided into three doses for 5 days) efficacy is 90%. Metronidazole is safe and effective for short course therapy in adults. It has not been extensively studied in children but is generally better tolerated than quinacrine. There are concerns about possible mutagenicity. It is given as 15 mg/kg/day, up to 750 mg maximum, in three doses for 5 to 10 days. Its cure rate is comparable to that of quinacrine. Furazolidone, given 5 mg/kg/day, divided into four doses, for 7 to 10 days, comes in a liquid preparation and, therefore, may be better suited for children than metronidazole. It may be somewhat less effective than either quinacrine or metronidazole. Relapses or treatment failures should be treated with a second course of therapy using the same drug or one of the alternative drugs. In low endemic areas, reinfection can frequently be prevented by investigation of family members and other likely sources of infection and treatment of all infected people. Good hygiene will also reduce the spread of giardia.

Sequelae and Complications

In untreated cases and cases that do not spontaneously resolve, malabsorption can result in significant weight loss and failure-to-thrive. Deficiency of vitamin A, vitamin B_{12}, and protein can be seen, especially in already malnourished children. Disaccharidase deficiency can occur, and a lactose intolerance syndrome can persist even for weeks after effective antigiardia therapy.

ASCARIS LUMBRACOIDES

Clinical Manifestations

Ascaris infection can be asymptomatic. If symptoms occur during the migratory phase (when the larvae pass to the lungs and then in to the gut), they usually include fever and symptoms of acute pneumonitis. Moderate eosinophilia may be present. Heavy intestinal infection with ascaris can be associated with intestinal obstruction. Less severe infections have been associated with maldigestion and poor absorption of protein. Steatorrhea may also be present. Ascaris appears to be more strongly associated with malnutrition in less developed areas of the world than in the U.S.

Etiology and Epidemiology

Ascaris lumbracoides is responsible for about 1 billion cases worldwide, making it the most prevalent helminth infection. The organism, which is predominantly found in tropical regions is also found in temperate climates. Ascaris adult worms inhabit the lumen of the small intestine and live up to 2 years. A female worm produces thousands of eggs each day that are passed in stool. Embryos form within these eggs and when ingested by humans, the embryos penetrate the small intestine wall, enter the blood stream, pass to the heart and on to the lungs; where they pass into aveoli, bronchi and the trachea. They are then swallowed and passed into the intestine where they develop into adult worms. The cycle then begins again.

Ascaris eggs deposited into soil take at least 2 weeks to become infectious. The time from ingestion of eggs to the development of an adult worm is about two months. The eggs are quite hardy, and can survive temperatures below 0°C and anaerobic environments. When soil conditions are favorable, the ova can survive for years. Sunlight and temperatures over 40°C will kill the organism. Infection is found in all age groups, but peaks in the pre-school and early school age groups.

Diagnosis

Patients with pulmonary symptoms and peripheral eosinophilia should be considered as potentially having ascaris infection. The adult female worm puts out a large number of eggs each day, so that stool examination is frequently sufficient to make the diagnosis. Serological tests are of little use.

Treatment

Either pyrantel pamoate (11 mg/kg orally, a single dose) or mebendazole (100 mg/dose given two times a day for 3 days) is effective. Mebendazole is not recommended for children less than 2 years of age. Piperazine citrate (75 mg/kg/day divided into four doses for 2 days) is an alternative which is very effective for intestinal obstruction. Stools should be re-examined about 3 to 4 weeks after treatment.

Sequelae and Complications

The incidence of intestinal obstruction is about 2 per 1000 cases. Most of these cases respond to medical management making surgical intervention only infrequently necessary. Less frequently, intestinal perforation or bile duct obstruction may occur. Worms have also been found escaping via aberrant sites such as umbilical fistules, hernial fistulas, the urinary bladder and the falopian tubes.

PLASMODIA

Clinical Manifestations

Periodic fever, chills, sweating, headaches and abdominal pain are characteristic of malaria. In between these paroxysms, the patient may be relatively symptom free. Paroxysms may last 3 to 6 hours, and often occur at regular intervals. *REMEMBER:* Malaria can mimic other diseases. For that reason, diagnosis should be made only if there is suspicion of the infection. Patients frequently will have hepatomegaly and splenomegaly. *REMEMBER:* Lymphadenopathy is not a finding in patients with malaria.

Less common clinical findings include a tender abdomen, jaundice, rash and scattered rales. High temperature and anemia may result in a flow murmur. Central nervous system symptoms may occur, especially in patients with *P. falciparum* cerebral malaria. Spinal fluid findings do not fit into any specific pattern.

Infants have less characteristic symptoms. Non-specific findings of irritability, anorexia, vomiting, diarrhea and restlessness may be the only clues to the diagnosis.

Etiology and Epidemiology

Plasmodia are obligate intracellular protozoa responsible for causing malaria. The life cycle includes a sexual reproductive phase in a mosquito and an asexual reproductive phase in man. The four species of plasmodia that most commonly infect man are: *P. vivax, P. falciparum, P. malariae* and *P. ovale.*

Sporozoites (the infective stage) are injected into the humans by a mosquito bite. They travel to the liver and invade hepatic cells. Replication in the liver produces exoerythrocytic schizonts. These schizonts rupture releasing merozoites which enter the circulatory system where they invade erythrocytes. After the parasites leave the liver they do not return; however, in *P. vivax* and *P. ovale* infections, not all the schizonts initially rupture so that there is an acute phase and a latent phase which may not rupture for months to years. Once the merozoite enters the erythrocyte it develops into a trophozoite, and once cell division occurs it forms schizonts. Once the schizont matures it ruptures releasing merozoites into the circulation which once again invade erythrocytes.

Malaria is acquired from an infected female Anopheles mosquito. Less frequently the infection occurs as a result of transfusion with contaminated blood or congenitally. The disease is predominantly found in tropical and subtropical areas. It is estimated that the prevalence of malaria worldwide is about 100 million cases. As many as 1 million victims in Africa die each year from malaria. In the U.S. and most of Europe, malaria is not endemic. Most cases in these regions are imported. *P. vivax* and *P. falciparum* are the most common causes of malaria.

Diagnosis

In areas of the world where malaria is endemic, suspicion of malaria is common. In the U.S., where malaria is seen infrequently, the diagnosis is frequently missed or delayed.

Patients with fever, chills, splenomegaly, or anemia and who have an appropriate geographic history should be evaluated for malaria. The diagnosis is made by examining both thick and thin blood smears for the parasites. Thick smears are used to find the parasites when few are present. Thin smears are helpful for determining which plasmodium is involved. Either Giemsa or Wright stain should be used for staining. In non-falciparum infections, only 2% or less of the erythrocytes are infected. In falciparum malaria the number of infected erythrocytes may exceed 60%. *REMEMBER:* Parasitemia is not a continuous process and several samples of blood taken at various intervals will increase chances of finding the parasite. Although usually not necessary, serologic tests are also available to detect malaria antibody.

In addition, routine CBC may help suggest the diagnosis. Normochromic normocytic hemolytic anemia, leukopenia and thrombocytopenia may be present. Eosinophilia does not occur.

Treatment

Treatment regimens are similar for all forms of plasmodia except for chloroquine-resistant *P. falciparum.* In uncomplicated cases, chloroquine phosphate is the treatment of choice. The recommended dose is 10 mg/kg of chloroquine base, as a first dose, followed by 5 mg/kg of base 6 hours, 24 hours and 48 hours later. Chloroquine is given orally.

In more severe attacks, quinine dihydrochloride can be given orally or by intravenous administration. If given I.V., pulse and blood pressure must be watched carefully. Arrhythmias and hypotension may occur.

If the infection is due to *P. vivax* or *P. ovale* there may be latent exoery-throcytic forms in the liver. Relapses will occur unless additional therapy is provided for these exoerythrocytic forms. The recommended "radical" cure is primaquine phosphate given 0.3 mg base per kg/day for 14 days, or 0.9 mg base/kg/week for 8 weeks. Glucose 6-phosphate dehydrogenase deficiency; seen most commonly in blacks, Orientals and people of Mediter-ranean origins; may result in a hemolytic anemia if affected patients receive primaquine. *REMEMBER:* Patients who become infected as a result of blood transfusions do not have an exoerythrocytic stage and, therefore, do not require "radical" cure.

If patients with *P. falciparum* infection do not show a good response to chloroquine therapy within 72 hours, chloroquine resistance should be suspected. Patients from areas where chloroquine resistance is known to exist and patients who do not get a good response to chloroquine should be treated with alternative therapy. In uncomplicated chloroquine-resistant malaria, quinine sulfate should be given orally 25 mg/kg/day divided into three doses per day and given for three days. In addition, pyrimethamine and sulfadiazine should also be given. Pyrimethamine is given 0.5 mg/kg twice a day for 3 days (maximum 25 mg/dose) and sulfadiazine is given as 100–200 mg/kg/day divided into 4 doses, for 5 days (maximum 2 gms/day). In patients with severe infection resistant to chloroquine, quinine dihydrochloride is given intravenously until the patient is able to tolerate oral therapy.

Travelers to areas where malaria is endemic are advised to take chemo-prophylaxis. In areas where chloroquine resistance is not a problem, chloro-quine phosphate, 5 mg base/kg is given once a week beginning 1 week before arriving in endemic areas and continuing weekly while in endemic areas and for 6 weeks after leaving endemic areas. If *P. ovale* or *P. vivax* are also endemic to the areas being visited, primaquine should be given 0.3 mg/kg/day for the last 2 weeks of chloroquine prophylaxis. Travelers to areas where chloroquine-resistant *P. falciparum* is present should receive pyrimethamine plus sulfadoxine (available as a fixed dose combination called Fansidar) once weekly for one week before arriving in the endemic area, until 6 weeks after exposure. Recommended doses are 1/8 tablet for infants less than 1 year; 1/4 tablet for children 1–3 years old; 1/2 tablet for children 4–8 years old; and 3/4 tablet for children 9–14 years old. *REMEM-BER:* Severe cutaneous reactions have been reported in individuals taking Fansidar. These include erythema multiforme, Stevens-Johnson syndrome and toxic epidermal necrolysis. Fatalities have been reported. Therefore, Fansidar should not be prescribed for individuals with a history of previous sulfanomide reaction and should be reserved for those travelers to rural areas where chloroquine-resistance occurs. Patients receiving Fansidar should also receive chloroquine to protect against other species of malaria. Fansidar resistance has also been reported in some areas.

Sequelae and Complications

Cerebral malaria occurs as a complication of *P. falciparum* infection. Nephrotic syndrome and acute tubular necrosis are also seen in severe cases of malaria. Abnormalities of liver function tests occur but usually a normal alkaline phosphatase is seen. Hypoglycemia has been reported, and falsely positive VDRL can be seen.

PNEUMOCYSTIS CARINII

Clinical Manifestations

In infants, onset is usually insidious. The infant is usually debilitated and between 2 and 6 months old. Prior to the development of respiratory symptoms, the infant may have diarrhea and weight loss. Respiratory symptoms include cough, tachypnea, dyspnea and cyanosis. Fever is usually absent or low-grade. Symptoms usually progress over 1 to 4 weeks. Untreated, the mortality is high.

In immunocompromised children, the onset is usually sudden. Initially, clinical manifestations include fever, cough, tachypnea and coryza. The cough is usually nonproductive and the fever, if present, is low-grade. Cyanosis usually occurs later in the course of the disease. Radiologic changes appear after clinical manifestations. Chest x-ray findings are variable. Most commonly bilateral diffuse parenchymal infiltrates are seen. As the disease progresses, the x-ray findings change from predominantly interstitial pattern to an aveolar pattern with air bronchograms. PaO_2 (arterial oxygen tension) is usually low in room air, and $PaCO_2$ is usually normal or low.

Etiology and Epidemiology

Pneumocystis carinii causes a pneumonitis predominantly in immunocompromised patients. *P. carinii* has a cystic and an extracystic form. Pleomorphic cells called sporozoites occupy the cyst. The extracystic form is referred to as a trophozoite. Pneumocystis is found worldwide and in a wide spectrum of animals. The major human victims are the immunocompromised host. Increasing incidence of disease due to *P. carinii* in children has paralleled advances in therapy for neoplastic disease and the longer survival of children with these underlying diseases.

In developing nations, *P. carinii* causes epidemic disease in malnourished children. In developed nations, *P. carinii* primarily affects children who are immunocompromised. Transmission is believed to be person-to-person. In addition, it is thought that disease in immunocompromised patients can occur as a result of reactivation of latent infections. Serologic studies indicate that about 2/3 of normal children ages 2–4 years have acquired antibody to *P. carinii.*

Diagnosis

Diagnosis depends on observing clinical manifestations consistant with *P. carinii* infection in a patient at risk. Effective diagnostic procedures include bronchoscopic brush biopsy, open lung biopsy and closed lung biopsy. Since pneumocystis infection is often present as a mixed infection, it is important to obtain an adequate specimen not only to establish the diagnosis of pneumocystis but to exclude additional pathogens. Specimens can be stained with methenamine silver stain or toluidine blue O stain to identify cysts. Trophozoites can be identified using Giemsa, Wright or polychrome methylene blue stains.

Serologic methods are available, but are frequently hard to interpret because of the immune incompetence of many of these patients and because *P. carinii* can exist in a latent state. Counterimmunoelectrophoresis can detect circulating *P. carinii* antigen in the majority, but not all patients.

Treatment

Untreated, the immune incompetent patient with *P. carinii* will almost always die. The infant with pneumocystis has at least a 50% chance of dying if untreated. Trimethoprim-sulfamethoxazole (TMS) is the treatment of choice. Pneumocystis resistant to trimethoprim-sulfamethoxazole occurs, especially in patients with the acquired immunodeficiency syndrome (AIDS). In these patients, pentamidine isethionate may be a suitable alternative. Patients with AIDS that are treated with TMS have a high incidence of rash, neutropenia, diarrhea and fever. Side effects associated with pentamidine include renal and liver dysfunction and hematological disorders.

Prophylaxis for *P. carinii* can be effectively done by giving TMS orally daily. This regimen has proved to be highly effective in high risk patients where the risk from pneumocystis exceeds the risk of side effects from TMS.

Sequelae and Complications

Untreated, the mortality rate approaches 100%. Some patients who recover have radiologic evidence of interstitial fibrosis. Less frequently, pneumothorax and pneumomediastinum have been reported.

TOXOPLASMA GONDII

Clinical Manifestations

There are two major categories of *T.* gondii infection: congenital and acquired. The congenital infection is discussed in the chapter dealing with perinatal infections. Acquired infection is usually asymptomatic. If symptoms occur in the immune competent patient, they are usually non-specific. Symptoms may include fever, malaise, myalgias, lymphadenopathy, sore throat, hepatosplenomegaly and rash. The disease may resemble infectious mononucleosis. The disease is usually benign and self-limited in the immune competent patient.

The immunocompromised patient may develop clinical disease with primary or reactivation infection. Frequently, the central nervous system is involved. Pneumonitis and myocarditis may also occur. CSF findings usually include mononuclear cell pleocytosis, increased protein and normal or slightly low glucose. Toxoplasma can also infect the eye and cause chorioretinitis. Most cases of *T. gondii* chorioretinitis are a result of congenital infection although symptoms may not present for two to three decades. Relapses of chorioretinitis are common.

Etiology and Epidemiology

Toxoplasma gondii is an intracellular parasite that infects humans as well as a wide variety of animals. *T. gondii* can take three forms: tachyzoite, tissue cyst and oocyst. Tachyzoites are capable of invading most mammalian cells except for non-nucleated erythrocytes. Once in the cell the tachyzoite multiples. The tissue cyst is the form that is usually responsible for spread of the infection to humans. Ingestion of uncooked or poorly cooked meat containing cysts is followed by enzymatic disruption of the cyst wall in the host's digestive tract. Viable organisms are released which invade and spread throughout the body. Oocysts reside only in members of the cat family and are responsible for maintaining *T. gondii's* life cycle.

Toxoplasmosis is found worldwide. The cat family is the definitive host. The incidence of seropositivity for *T. gondii* increases with age. In some nations, like France, over 90% of the population has *T. gondii* antibody by the fourth decade of life. In the U.S. the incidence rate among healthy adults ranges from 20–70%.

Ingestion of contaminated, incompletely cooked meats or contact with cat feces are the major modes of acquiring toxoplasmosis. Transmission via blood products and infected transplant organs have also been reported.

Diagnosis

Acute infection with *T. gondii* can be diagnosed by recovery of the organism from blood or other body fluids or by demonstrating the presence of tachyzoites in tissue sections. Prior infection can be demonstrated by lymphocyte transformation to toxoplasma antigens. Enzyme-linked immunosorbent assay (ELISA) has been used to identify toxoplasma antigen in serum in acute infection. Detection of IgM antibody or a fourfold rise in IgG antibody may also be useful in diagnosing infection.

Treatment

Patients who are immunologically competent acquire toxoplasmosis and have few other manifestations than lymphadenopathy need not be treated. A sparsity of good controlled treatment trials has resulted in uncertainty as to the efficacy, indications, and optimal regimen for therapy. Nevertheless, therapy is frequently considered for severe acute acquired infections as well as infections in immunodeficient patients. Therapy may be necessary for 2–6 months, and in immunocompromised patients longer therapy is often needed. Therapy is indicated for the treatment of ocular toxoplasmosis. One month of therapy results in a favorable response in the majority of these patients.

Pyrimethamine appears to act synergistically with sulfadiazine against toxoplasma. After a loading dose of 2 mg/kg/day of pyrimethamine for up to 3 days, pyrimethamine is then given 1 mg/kg/day divided into two doses (25 mg per day maximum). Sulfadiazine (or trisulfapyrimidine) is given 120–150 mg/kg/day divided into four doses. Hematologic toxicity can be prevented by daily administration of folinic acid.

An alternative regimen for ocular disease is the use of clindamycin plus sulfadiazine. In severe disease involving the macular or optic nerve, head steroids may be of value.

Sequelae and Complications

Toxoplasmosis in the immune competent patient is usually a self-limited benign disease. Chronic lymphadenopathy has been described in association with toxoplasmosis. Infrequently, dissemination can occur resulting in pneumonitis, encephalitis, or myocarditis. The immunodeficient patient may also develop central nervous system involvement. Fatalities do occur.

REFERENCES

1. AAP: Parasitic Diseases. Report of the Committee on Infectious Diseases, 1982; 19th edition: pp 149–193.
2. CDC: Prevention of Malaria in travelers. MMWR (suppl) 1982; 31:25–28S.
3. CDC: Cryptosporidiosis among children attending day-care centers - Georgia, Pennsylvania, Michigan, California, New Mexico. MMWR 1984; 33:599–601.
4. CDC: Update: Treatment of Cryptosporidiosis in patients with acquired immunodeficiency syndrome (AIDS). MMWR 1984; 33:117–119.
5. Dashefsky B, Teele DW: Infectious disease problems in Indochinese refugees. Pediatric Annuals, 1983; 12:232–244.
6. Hoang GN, Erickson RV: Guidelines for providing medical care to Southeast Asian Refugees. JAMA, 1982; 248:710–714.
7. Kovaleski T, Malangoni MA, Wheat LJ: Treatment of an amoebic liver abscess with intravenous metronidazole. Arch Intern Med, 1981; 141:132–133.
8. Krogstad DJ, Spencer HC, Healy GR: Current Concepts in Parasitology. N Engl J Med, 1978; 298:262–265.
9. Lerman SJ, Walker RA: Treatment of Giardiasis-Literature review and recommendations. Clinical Pediatrics, 1982; 21:409–414.
10. Marsden PD: Current Concepts in Parasitology-Leishmaniasis. N Engl J Med, 1979; 300:350–352.
11. Masur H, Michelis MA, Greene JB, et al: An outlook of community acquired *Pneumocystis carinii* pneumonia. N. Engl J Med, 1981; 305:1431–1438.
12. Medical Letter, Drugs for parasitic infections. The Medical Letter on Drugs and Therapeutics, 1984; 26:27–34.

13. Merritt RJ, Couglin E, Thomas DW, et al: Spectrum of amebiasis in children. Am J Dis Child, 1982; 136:785–789.

14. Meyer EA, Jarroll EL: Reviews and Commentary-Giardiasis. Amer J Epidemiol, 1980; 111:1–12.

15. Most HL: Treatment of parasitic infections of travelers and immigrants. N Engl J Med, 1984; 310: 298–304.

16. Most H: Trichinosis-Preventable yet still with us. N Engl J Med, 1978; 298:1178–1180.

17. Pearson RD, Sousa AQ: Leishmania Species (Kala-Azar, Cutaneous and mucocutaneous). In: *Principles and Practices of Infectious Diseases,* Mandell GL, Douglas RG, and Bennett JE (eds); Wiley Medical Publication, NY 1985; pp 1522–1530.

18. Shantz PM, Glickman LT: Toxocaral Visceral Lava Migrans. N Engl J Med, 1978; 298:436–440.

19. Warren KS: The Relevance of Schistosomiasis. N Engl J Med, 1980; 303:203–206.

20. Wyler DJ: Malaria: Host pathogen biology. Rev Infect Dis, 1982; 4:785–797.

21. Wyler DJ: Malaria-Resurgence, Resistance, Research. N Engl J Med, 1983; 308:875–878, 934–940.

Selected Parasitic Diseases

Organism	Epidemiology	Symptoms	Diagnosis	Treatment	Comments
Giardia lamblia	Person-to-Person	*Diarrhea, *Abdominal cramps, flatulence, distension, nausea, foul smelling stools, no blood/pus in stools, *weight loss	1. Stool - cysts 2. Duodenal aspirate, string test (Enterotest) - trophs	1. Quinacrine (Atabrine) 2. Metronidazole* (Flagyl) 3. Furazolidone (Furoxone)	1. Most patients asymptomatic 2. Can have chronic malabsorptive syndrome 3. Failure rate with any treatment about 10-20% 4. Investigate and treat household contacts
Entamoeba histolytica (Amebiasis)	Fecal - oral	1. Mild to severe diarrhea, may be bloody/painful 2. Invasive dis - dysentery d with (100%) pain with blood (95%) with mucous 3. Liver abscess, increased temperature, tender large liver 4. Can invade lung, heart, CNS	1. Stool - cysts trophs 2. Serology 3. Abscess drainage (Aspirate)	1. Diodohydroxyquin (diodoquin) 2. (Flagyl)- Metronidazole 3. Tetracycline 4. Surgical drainage	1. Can be asymptomatic 2. Liver abscess frequently present with no GI symptoms and no parasites in stool
Ascaris lumbracoides	Fecal - oral Killed by T 40 Survives cold Resistant to chemical disinfectants About 1 billion cases	1. Pneumonitis (if present usually lasts about 7 days) 2. Intestinal obstruction/ perforation 3. Bile duct obstruction 4. Most people asymptomatic	1. Peripheral eosinophils 2. Stool - eggs	1. Pyrantel Pamoate 2. Mebendazole 3. Piperazine citrate- (Intestinal obstruction)	1. In rural So. U.S.A. about 20-60% prevalence rate

*not FDA approved

Organism	Epidemiology	Symptoms	Diagnosis	Treatment	Comments
Plasmodium 1. faciparum 2. vivax 3. malariae 4. ovale (malaria)	1. Female anopheline mosquito 2. Blood transfusions 3. Transplacental spread	1. Paroxysms of chills and fever: q 48 hours -vivax, falciparum ovale: q 72 hours - malariae. 2. Tachycardia 3. Nausea/vomiting 4. Increased micturation 5. Headache 6. Anemia	Blood smears - thick and thin Serology	1. Chloroquine 2. Primaquine 3. Fansidar (pyrimethamine-sulfadoxine)	1. Isolation of patients not necessary except for blood precautions and exposure to mosquitos 2. Facliparum tends to have less typical presentation-cerebral malaria, blackwater fever 3. Relapses don't usually occur with falciparum 4. Congenital malaria-increased temp, jaundice, enlarged liver, enlarged spleen, hemolytic anemia 5. Primaquine used to treat exoerythrocytic phase
Shistosoma 1. mansoni 2. japonicum 3. haematobium	1. Affects 200 million people 2. Contaminated water - penetrates skin	1. Dermatitis 2. Katayama fever 3. Anorexia, diarrhea, abdominal discomfort 4. Hepatosplenic involvement (scarring) (enlarged liver and spleen) (varices) 5. Respiratory symptoms 6. Urinary symptoms 7. CNC symptoms	Viable eggs from stool, urine, Bx specimen	1. Praziquantel 40mg/kg x 1 for mansoni and haematobium, 20 mg/kg tid x 1 day for japonicum 2. Antiban (antimony sodium dimercapto-succinate) 3. Niridazole (Ambilhar)	1. Many patients are asymptomatic 2. Praziquantel - new single day treatment

Organism	Epidemiology	Symptoms	Diagnosis	Treatment	Comments
Leishmania donovani tropica infantum mexicana braziliensis	**Visceral** - India and Mediterranian region as well Latin America **Cutaneous** - India, many Asian nations, north Africa, Central Texas **Mucocutaneous** - South and Central America Transmitted by sandfly The organism is a protozoa	**Visceral (Kala-Azar)** 1. Insidious onset 2. Febrile 3. Sweats, no chills 4. Lymphadenopathy, splenomegaly 5. Darkened skin regions, erythema hypopigmentation **Cutaneous** (oriental sore) 1. Papules ulcers granulomas 2. Most commonly seen on anus and face **Mucocutaneous-** Cutaneous plus lesions in the nasopharyngeal mucosa which may lead to deformaties	1. Organism can be identified by biopsy of skin lesion, bone marrow or from aspirate of lesions and nodes 2. Serologic tests are also available	1. Stibogluconate sodium 10 mg/kg/day for 10 days parenterally 2. Alternate drug: pentamidine isethionate 3 mg/kg/day IM 3. Amphoteracin B has been used for non-viseral disease	1. Control measures include eliminating reservoirs (dogs, rodents) and reducing the sandfly population 2. Infected patients are potentially contagious if the insect vector is present
Enterobius vermicularis (pinworm)	1. Caused by a nematode 2. Worldwide distribution 3. Estimates of about 10% of U.S. population infected 4. Young children, their mothers, and the institutionalized have high prevalence rates	1. Anal pruritis 2. Vulva pruritis	1. Apply transparent tape to perianal skin. Examine tape (after placing on slide) for eggs under low microscopic power 2. Tape test best done upon arising in morning	1. Pyrantel pamoate 11 mg/kg x 1 po or 2. Mebendazole 100 mg po x 1 then repeat in 2 weeks	1. Examine household members for pinworms and treat

Organism	Epidemiology	Symptoms	Diagnosis	Treatment	Comments
Trypanosoma (Chagas' Disease) -Cruzi -Brucei	1. Transmitted by reduviid bugs 2. Primarily a zoonosis 3. Prevalence due to T. cruzi estimated to be 10-12 million 4. T. cruzi is primary etiology in the Americas	**Acute** 1. Mild, non-specific (sometimes) 2. Chagoma-indurated area of erythema and swelling with lymphadenopathy at the site where the parasite has penetrated the skin 3. Romama's sign - painless edema of the palpebra and periocular tissues-occurs when conjunctiva is portal of entry 4. Fever, anorexia, malaise and edema, lymphadenopathy, hepatosplenomegaly 5. Infrequently meningo-encephalitis occurs 6. Rarely myocarditis occurs **Chronic** 1. Years after initial infection 2. Primarily a cardiac disease arrhythimias congestive failure thromboembolisms	Examination of blood or buffy coat for parasite in acute infection 2. Culture techniques are avilable 3. Serology available and is useful for diagnosing chronic disease	1. Initial therapy nifurtimox (5 mg/kg/day po divided in 4 doses 2. Increase dose by 2 mg/kg/day q 2 weeks until maximum dose of 16 mg/kg/day is reached x 4 month	1. Homes of infected patients should be examined for the vector 2. Patients' family members should also be examined for infection

Organism	Epidemiology	Symptoms	Diagnosis	Treatment	Comments
Cryptosporidium species	1. Protozoan 2. Primarily an animal pathogen causing diarrhea 3. Causes diarrhea in children in day-care center environment, transient 4. In immunocompromised patients causes a severe diarrhea unresponsive to therapy	**Normal host** 1. Transient diarrhea 2. Watery stools 3. Abdominal cramps 4. Occasional fever and nausea 5. 1-10 day duration 6. Asymptomatic infection also occurs **Immunocompromised host** 1. Prolonged, often irreversible diarrhea 2. Malabsorption 3. Fluid and electrolyte abn. 4. Usually unresponsive to therapy	1. Identification of oocyst in stool 2. Small bowel biopsy 3. The parasite is iodine stain negative and acid fast stain positive	No effective therapy currently available	Major complications in patient with acquired immunodeficiency syndrome
Trichuris trichiura (whipworm)	1. Worldwide - ½ billion cases 2. 2 million cases in U.S. 3. Primarilily in poor rural communities and areas of poor hygiene 4. School age children have a high prevalence rate 5. Ingestion of embryonated ova leads to infection 6. Humans are major host	1. Usually asymptomatic 2. Mild anemia, bloody diarrhea, and rectal prolapse may occur 3. Malnutrition may develop	1. Examination of feces for ova will usually make diagnosis 2. The ova has been described as lemon shaped	Mebendazole (Vermox) po 100 mg bid x 3 days	Therapy is non-toxic and effective

Organism	Epidemiology	Symptoms	Diagnosis	Treatment	Comments
Trichinella spiralis (Trichinosis)	1. Nematode 2. Infection the result of eating insufficiently cooked meats containing the parasite - especially pork 3. Not transmitted human to human	1. Mild diarrhea 2. Fever 3. Myalgia 4. Periorbital edema 5. Urticarial rash 6. Hemorrhages (periorbital or subungual) 7. Myocardial failure and pneumonia may lead to death	1. Eosinophilia up to 70% 2. Serologic tests 3. Muscle biopsy	1. Steroids may decrease symptoms 2. Thiabendazole (25 mg/kg bid) for a week will kill adult worms but not encysted larvae	1. Adequate cooking of pork - i.e. no longer pink 2. 10 days of freezing pork will kill the larvae
Toxocara canis catis (visceral larva migraes)	1. Found in worms of dogs and cats 2. Most cases in North America and Great Britain 3. Contaminated soil or fomites can cause human infection 4. Usually occurs in children 1-4 years of age c a history of pica	1. Usually asymptomatic 2. Fever, hepatomegaly, malaise, cough 3. Leukocytosis, eosinophilia 4. Hypergamma-globulinemia 5. Ocular involvement can occur, retinal granulomas, endophthalmitis 6. Myocarditis	1. Hypergamma-globulimenia 2. Hypereosinophilia 3. Elevated iso-hemagglutinins 4. Serology 5. Liver biopsy may occasionally be useful	1. Steroids may help in severe cases 2. Thiabendazole (25 mg/kg bid x 1 week) or 3. Diethylcarbanazine	Effectiveness of therapy is controversial

KEY POINTS

1. *Entamoeba histolytica* is the protozoa responsible for amebiasis. Symptoms vary and asymptomatic cases occur, but serious manifestations like liver abscesses, cerebral abscesses, intestinal perforation and necrotizing colitis may be fatal.
2. *Giardia lamblia* is a fairly common intestinal parasite in the U.S. The infection can present as an acute gastroenteritis or as a chronic illness associated with malabsorption, diarrhea and weight loss.
3. As many as 1 billion cases of *Ascaris lumbracoides* may be present worldwide. Symptoms, when present, are primarily respiratory and gastrointestinal.
4. Prevention of malaria is accomplished by avoidance of mosquito bites, and the appropriate use of antimalarial agents (chloroquine, primaquine and pyrimethamine-sulfadoxine) before, during and after travel to endemic areas.
5. Untreated, *Pneumocystis carinii* can cause fatal pneumonitis in most patients.
6. The definitive host for *Toxoplasma gondii* is the cat. Pregnant women should avoid contact with cats to reduce the chances of acquiring the infection and passing it on to the fetus.

REVIEW QUESTIONS

Match the description in Column A with the appropriate disease in Column B (entries in Column B may be used more than once.)

A

1.) Extraintestinal disease may *not* be accompanied by gastrointestinal symptoms. Abscess fluid frequently described as "anchovy paste."

2.) Most commonly identified intestinal parasite in U.S.

3.) Approximately 1 billion cases worldwide. Therapy is pyrantel pamoate or mebendazole.

4.) Diagnosis is made by examination of stool for ova and parasites, by the "string test", by duodenal aspirate or duodenal biopsy.

5.) Transmitted by the female anopheles mosquito.

6.) Acquisition of the infection is usually related to ingestion of contaminated, incompletely cooked meats or contact with cat feces.

7. Treat with trimethoprim-sulfamethoxazole. Usually fatal in the immunocompromised patient if not treated. Symptoms are usually respiratory.

8.) Exoerythrocytic stage is treated with primaquine.

B

A. Malaria
B. Toxoplasmosis
C. Giardiasis
D. Amoebiasis
E. Pneumocystis
F. Ascaris

16

MISCELLANEOUS INFECTIONS I

This chapter deals with a variety of pediatric infections that used to be known as the common childhood infections. As a result of significant progress made in the past twenty to thirty years, many of the common pediatric infections have become distinctly uncommon. Measles, for example, has decreased from over half a million cases twenty-five to thirty years ago to 1 to 2 thousand cases per year. Congenital rubella has decreased from twenty to thirty thousand cases a year to less than 10 cases per year. Some of the infections that are discussed in this chapter will hopefully be of only historic interest because we will continue to maintain high levels of protection as a result of very successful immunization programs. Unfortunately, many of these diseases still have a significant mortality and morbidity in many other areas of the world.

MUMPS

Clinical Manifestations.

Mumps is frequently asymptomatic or subclinical and the patient may become infected and not have any obvious clinical manifestations. Nevertheless, a sizeable number of patients do have symptoms associated with mumps. In general, parotid swelling is the first sign of the illness. This may be unilateral or bilateral. In some cases, one side may swell up and then two to three days later the opposite side may become involved. Submandibular glands may also be involved. It is often accompanied by a moderate elevation in fever although usually not many other systemic symptoms are seen. The parotid swelling may produce a considerable amount of discomfort, especially if the child attempts to eat acidic type foods. Meningeal symptoms are not uncommon. Particularly in older children, complaints of headaches, photophobia and signs of meningeal irritation such as nuchal rigidity are not uncommon. Encephalitis, however, is not common. Meningoencephalitis due to mumps virus may occur without any evidence of parotid involvement. Pancreatic involvement occurs and may result in abdominal pain or anorexia and serum amylase levels may be elevated. Renal involvement may occur with mumps and may be manifested by hematuria and polyuria. The parotid swelling, if present, usually lasts 7 to 10 days. In most children the disease is self-limited and completely resolves within 10 to 14 days.

Etiology and Epidemilogy

Mumps is caused by a paramyxovirus which is an RNA virus. Mumps is primarily spread by the respiratory route and is fairly contagious. The introduction of the virus into a family setting frequently results in infection in all susceptible members of that family. The incubation period is about 16 to 18 days and the disease is probably communicable for up to three weeks. As many as 40% of the patients who are infected with the mumps virus may be asymptomatic. Mumps is primarily an illness of childhood and is most frequently seen in the winter and early spring months. It is estimated that as many as 95% of adults have had mumps and therefore are protected;

nevertheless, a much smaller percentage have a history compatible with mumps.

Diagnosis

In general the diagnosis of mumps is made on clinical grounds. It is important to remember that not all parotid swelling is due to mumps and that not all mumps has parotid swelling. Therefore, a certain percentage of false positive and false negative diagnoses will be made when based solely on clinical ground. If a definitive diagnosis is necessary, viral cultures may be obtained. The virus can be propagated in embryonated eggs and fibroblast tissue culture as well as other cultured cells. The virus is best cultured from throat swabs and can be found as early as two days before onset of parotid swelling and as late as 7 days after the onset of swelling. In addition, virus can also be isolated from spinal fluid and from urine. In routine cases, there is probably no indication for viral cultures provided that the clinical manifestations and clinical course are relatively routine.

Treatment

There is no antiviral therapy that is currently available for the treatment of mumps. It is generally an outpatient disease, not requiring hospitalization. Conservative management includes maintaining adequate hydration, analgesics for the discomfort associated with the parotid gland swelling and for any associated headache. Mumps is usually self-limited and almost invariably will respond to conservative therapy as just described. Mumps is preventible using the mumps vaccine. The vaccine is routinely given along with the measles and rubella vaccine at 15 months of age. It is highly effective and safe. With routine use of the vaccine, the incidence of mumps should continue to decrease resulting in fewer cases and a decreased morbidity and mortality.

Sequelae and Complications

Infrequently, mumps is a fatal illness. In past years approximately 40 cases have been fatal. Complications of mumps do occur. These include orchitis most frequently seen in post-pubertal males, but can be seen during the first few years of life. In teenagers and young adults the incidence of orchitis approaches 40% in those who develop mumps. Symptoms of orchitis include fever, severe pain, tenderness and swelling. Orchitis may be present without parotitis and in all cases of orchitis, mumps should be considered in the differential. Usually the involvement is unilateral. Atrophy of the testes may occur and sterility has resulted following cases of bilateral orchitis. Affected testes may be more likely to develop malignancy. Therapy is supportive with appropriate analgesics. Oophritis has also occasionally occurred in association with mumps. Mumps may also be involved in the development of thyroiditis. As previously mentioned, mumps meningoencephalitis does occur, although infrequently. It, in general, has a good prognosis. The spinal fluid from these patients usually has a pleocytosis, normal or slightly elevated protein, as well as a slightly decreased or normal glucose. The cells involved are usually lymphocytes and virus can usually be recovered from the spinal fluid if the tap is done early in the disease. Other complications include deafness, transverse myelitis and arthritis. The association between diabetes mellitus and mumps is not clear. Because of the higher incidence of complications from mumps in teenagers and adults, a strong emphasis should be placed on immunizing adolescents and adults who were not immunized as children and who did not have mumps during childhood.

MEASLES

Clinical Manifestations

The classic case of measles usually occurs after an incubation period of 10 days. The initial symptoms usually last about 3 days. The classic prodromal symptoms of cough, coryza, conjunctivitis, and koplik's spots in association with fever is strongly suggestive of measles as a diagnosis. Initially, respiratory symptoms are prominent. Symptoms usually increase in severity over the first 2 to 4 days of illness. Koplik's spots are pathognomonic for measles. These lesions are bluish white specks on the mucosal surface in the mouth. To some observers these lesions may just appear white. Classically the lesions are about 1 mm in size. Only a few may appear initially, but the numbers usually increase during the first day and may coalesce. The area surrounding the koplik's spots are red. Maculopapular lesions may also occur and these may occur on the palate during the prodromal period. In these patients the pharyngeal wall is often erythematous and injected and complaints of sore throat are common. The next stage of the illness is the exanthem period. The typical rash of measles usually appears around the fourteenth day after exposure. This is usually the peak period for respiratory symptoms, fever and koplik's spots and during the next three days, koplik's spots will frequently disappear. Typically the measles rash first appears behind the ears and on the forehead and then spread of the rash is centrifugal from the head to the feet. The rash is erythematous and maculopapular and over the first few days becomes confluent. The confluence is predominant on the face. After three or four days, the rash begins to fade and disappears in the same direction in which it came. As the rash fades, desquamation may occur and a brownish discoloration may be present. The rash usually lasts about a week. The fever usually persists two or three days beyond the appearance of the rash. Conjunctivitis and the nasal symptoms usually disappear about the same time. The cough also begins to fade, however, the cough may persist much longer than the other symptoms. Pharyngitis, lymphadenopathy, and splenomegaly are also occasionally seen. Younger children may have diarrhea, vomiting and signs of laryngitis and croup. Although not usually severe, abdominal pain is also reported.

Patients who are partially immune to measles may develop modified measles which is usually a mild illness that follows the normal sequence of events in regular measles, with a shorter duration of the prodromal period and koplik's spots may be few or missing. The rash is considerably more mild and there is no confluence. This form of the disease can be seen in infants usually during the first 6 to 9 months of age when they may still have maternal antibodies present, or in children who receive gamma globulin as a result of being exposed to susceptible children. The presence of antibodies in both those situations modifies the disease. In addition, it may occur in certain patients who do not have an optimal response to the live vaccine. Another form of measles is called atypical measles. This usually occurs in persons who received the inactivated measles virus vaccine. Those patients immunized against measles in the early to mid 1960's may have received the inactivated form of the vaccine and these patients were not adequately protected. The incubation period for atypical measles is about 7 to 14 days and there is a prodromal period in which the patient has fever and headache. In addition, abdominal pain is reported. Cough and vomiting have also been noted. Chest pain and weakness are frequently reported and koplik's spots are infrequently seen. The rash of atypical measles usually appears on the extremities first and progresses in a cephalad manner. The rash is usually erythematous and maculopapular and involves the palms and soles. The rash is particularly prominent on the ankles and wrists. The rash frequently also may have a component of petechiae. Other symptoms commonly found in regular measles such as conjunctivitis and coryza are infrequently seen in atypical measles. However, hilar adenopathy and pneumonia are common findings in this form of the disease. The illness may last up to 2 weeks in many patients. Serologic studies are useful in making the diagnosis of atypical measles. Initially low titers become very high during the first ten to 14 days of illness and frequently reach levels by day 10 considerably higher than those that are seen in regular measles.

Etiology and Epidemiology

The incidence of measles 25 to 30 years ago approached 1/2 million cases. In the past two to three years the incidence was approximately 2,000 cases per year and it is the goal in the United States to eliminate measles by 1990. This is possible with a conscientious use of measles vaccine and the rapid identification and isolation of the cases that occur. Most cases in the United States in recent years have either been imported or have been in teenagers or young adults who were not immunized during the initial immunization process when they were children. Measles virus is an RNA virus that closely resembles the virus that causes canine distemper. It is in the family of viruses known as paramyxoviruses. In this country, measles has predominantly been a disease of children. With the use of the measles vaccine, the age distribution of measles has increased so that the disease has become more common in the adolescent age group and considerably less frequent during the first few years of life. In developing countries, the majority of cases occur under two years of age. Measles is a winter and spring disease in the temperate climates, and can occur in epidemics. Although the incidence of disease is equal between males and females, it appears that complications may be more common in males. Death from measles does occur and seems to be related to age and nutritional state of the patient. Those young children under 2 years of age and adults with measles, are more likely to die from the disease than are patients in the intermediate age groups. Similarly, malnourished patients are more likely to die from measles than are well nourished children. The disease is spread by the respiratory route and is highly contagious. Measles has a variety of effects upon the immune system. Among them are defective neutrophil motility, leukopenia, thrombocytopenia, depressed cutaneous delayed hypersensitivity and reduction in certain components of the complement system.

Diagnosis

In patients who present with classic measles, koplik's spots, the typical prodromal symptoms, and classic measles rash, diagnosis of the disease is not difficult. Unfortunately, measles is not the only virus that causes exanthems in children. Other infections such as rubella, erythema infectiosum, roseola, infectious mononucleosis, mycoplasma and enteroviral infections may cause similar appearing rashes. There is greater difficulty in diagnosing atypical measles because it occurs infrequently and in various forms. A very accurate and detailed immunication history may provide significant clues to the diagnosis of atypical measles. This illness may appear very similar to Rocky Mountain Spotted Fever and meningiococcemia. Viral diagnosis of measles can be done in selected patients if felt to be necessary. The virus can be isolated in tissue culture, or measles antigen can be demonstrated by a variety of techniques. In addition, antibody to measles can be measured. In general, the simpliest way to make the diagnosis would be serial sera separated by a week, looking for a rise in titer to measles.

Treatment

There is not any specific treatment for measles. Treatment consists of support and appropriate uses of fluids. Antipyretic and antitussives will make the patient feel more comfortable. One must be cautious in returning too rapidly to normal activity as measles may damage ciliated epithelium and therefore render the host susceptible to secondary infection. No specific antiviral therapy is currently available.

Sequelae and Complications

Complications of measles include otitis media, pneumonia, larnygeal trachitis, appendicitis and encephalitis. The organism responsible for otitis media in patients with measles are the same as those in normal children and should be treated with appropriate antibiotics. Pneumonia may be either viral or may be a superimposed bacterial infection. It is usually appropriate to treat the pneumonia with antibiotics as pneumonia is the leading cause of death in patients with measles. Encephalitis infrequently occurs and may occur in association with seizures or prolonged states of coma. The clinical course is highly variable and close monitoring and intervention is frequently necessary. Although appendicitis does occur in patients with measles, acute abdominal pain may also be secondary to mesenteric adenitis due to the measles virus. When appendicitis occurs, it is the result of viral involvement in the appendix and the treatment is surgical. Infrequently, myocarditis and pericarditis have been associated with measles. Other infrequent complications are black measles which is characterized by confluent hemorrhagic skin eruptions in association with pneumonia, encephalitis, and disseminated intravascular coagulation. Thrombocytopenia has also been reported. A very rare complication of measles is subacute sclerosing panencephalitis (SSPE). This is a rare degenerative CNS disease, due to the persistence of measles virus in the patient. These patients have a high titer of measles virus antigens in the brain and may have high levels of measles antibody in sera and spinal fluid. Measles virus can be cultured from the brain in these patients. The apparent risk of developing SSPE in children who have had natural measles is about 1 per 100,000 infections. This risk is greater in children who are very young when they get their natural measles. This risk of SSPE in patients immunized against measles is about 1 per 1,000,000. The disease is insidious with progressive behavioral changes. Intellectual deterioration may be the initial symptom. In addition, patients may have psychological difficulties, motor incoordination, and seizures. Visual impairment and difficulties in speech have also been reported. As the disease progresses, the patient becomes stuperous. Dementia, mutism and central blindness are also found. Eventually the patient develops decorticate rigidity and ultimately dies. Progression of the disease may take 6 to 9 months or longer. In contrast to the relatively benign presentation of measles in the United States, the problem of measles in developing countries is significant, with mortality rates approaching 10% in some parts of Africa. These children may develop a fulminant, toxic illness without the classical localizing complications or symptoms that we are familiar with. Secondary infection and persistence of the measle virus infection are frequent. Immunocompromised hosts are another group of patients in which measles can be severe and fatal. These patients require aggressive supportive therapy.

It is a real possibility in the next decade for measles to be eliminated from the United States and be of only essentially historic interest. Nevertheless, because of the persistence of the virus throughout most of the rest of the world, elimination of the disease from the United States will only be accomplished and will only last with maximum immunization efforts. As the disease becomes less and less frequent in this country, missed diagnosis because of physicians' unfamiliarity with the clinical presentation could result in unwanted spread of the disease. It is therefore important that physicians become familiar with the presentation and symptoms so that should a case occur, the patient can be rapidly isolated to prevent its spread.

RUBELLA

Clinical Manifestations

Rubella presents two distinct clinical syndromes. The first is postnatal rubella which is usually a mild systemic illness. The patients classically have an erythematous maculopapular rash and lymphadenopathy. Posterior auricular nodes are commonly involved. Young children with postnatal infection usually present with rash. Older children, adolescents and adults may have a prodrome that includes eye pain, sore throat, headache and less frequently, swollen glands, fever and nausea. The prodrome may last one to five days and will be followed by the rash. The rash typically involves the entire body during the first day and begins to fade so that it is usually gone by the third day. Pruritis is seen more commonly in adults than in children. Infection without the rash occurs. Patients may be totally asymptomatic or may just have lymphadenopathy. As mentioned previously, posterior auricular nodes are primarily involved. Suboccipital nodes may also be involved. Large lymph nodes may be present for about a week. Fever is not a consistent finding in rubella. The duration of illness is variable but, in general, patients recover within three days of the onset of the rash.

The other clinical presentation for rubella is that of the congenital rubella syndrome. Clinical manifestations of this syndrome include low birthweight, cataracts, deafness, purpura, cardiac involvement, hepatosplenomegaly, jaundice, microcephaly, pneumonia and death. Most commonly these babies are small for dates. Despite being fullterm, up to 85% of them may have weights less than 2,500 grams. This growth retardation may continue after birth. Failure-to-thrive is not uncommon in congenital rubella babies. Death during the first year of life is often secondary to pneumonia, heart defects, hepatitis, thrombocytopenia, encephalitis or immune deficiency. *REMEMBER:* The most common cardiovascular abnormality in patients with congenital rubella syndrome is patent ductus arteriosus. Second in frequency are the pulmonary valvular abnormalities. It is also important to remember that some babies with congenital rubella syndrome may have immunological abnormalities resulting in a decreased ability to fight infection.

Etiology and Epidemilogy

Rubella virus is an RNA virus; a member of the togavirus family. Human beings appear to be the sole source of infection and transmission postnatally is primarily through direct and droplet contact from nasal pharmygeal secretions. The current rubella immunization program has been dramatically successful in reducing the incidence of congenital rubella in the United States from as much as 20,000 to 30,000 cases per year down to 3 or 4 cases per year, in the United States. The infection is communicable from a few days before to a few days after the appearance of the rash. The incubation period is 2 to 3 weeks. It is important to remember that infants with the congenital rubella syndrome may shed virus in nasopharyngeal secretions and in urine for many months to years after birth, and are therefore potential sources of infection to other children and pregnant women. Rubella is most frequently seen in the winter and spring and the disease appears to be present throughout the world.

The risk and extent of congenital rubella syndrome appears at least in part to be related to when during pregnancy maternal infection occurs. Infection during the first trimester usually results in a persistent rubella infection throughout the pregnancy with the resulting involvement of a variety of organs. Maternal infection during the second or third trimester may lead to fetal infection, but is usually not associated with significant abnormalities, although cultures from the baby at birth may be positive for rubella.

Diagnosis

It is frequently difficult, based on clinical grounds, to diagnose postnatally acquired rubella. There are no pathognomonic findings. Because rubella tends to be an epidemic disease, diagnosis can frequently be made based on a good history of contact and the appropriate season. Certain enteroviral exanthems may look very similar to rubella, however, in general enteroviral infections are a summer and fall disease whereas rubella tends to be winter and spring. *REMEMBER:* Since itching may be a major component of the clinical manifestations in adults, rubella may frequently be confused with an allergic reaction in adolescent and adult patients. In those adults or teenagers that also have fever, lymphadenopathy, headache or eye pain, the diagnosis of rubella becomes a little bit easier.

In those cases of congenital rubella where maternal infection during pregnancy is documented, the diagnosis of congenital rubella is relatively easy. Additionally, in those infants born with classical signs and symptoms of congenital rubella, the diagnosis can usually be made without much difficulty. Definitive diagnosis in these babies can be made by viral isolation. Specimens for culture can be obtained from urine, nose, throat, bluffy coat of blood and cerebral spinal fluid. If rubella I_gM antibody titers are available at your medical center, then that may also assist in making the diagnosis. In postnatally acquired rubella it is usually not necessary to make a definitive diagnosis. The exception to this is in the pregnant female in which case the virologic studies as well as serologic studies should be done to make the diagnosis. Fourfold elevations in antibody titer to rubella, evidence of rubella specific I_gM antibody, or positive viral cultures are all diagnostic of rubella in these women.

Treatment

There is no specific therapy for rubella. In most postnatally acquired disease no intervention is necessary. In rare cases of serious rubella such as encephalitis, appropriate supportive measures should be instituted. Children with congenital rubella syndrome present a different problem. Because of the variety of organ systems involved, these patients often require close follow-up and occasional intervention by appropriate subspecialists. These children should be thoroughly evaluated to identify all malformations and abnormalities that are present.

The goal of eliminating congenital rubella from the United States is achievable if the high rate of compliance with the immunization program continues. High priority needs to be given to those women in child bearing years who do not have antibody to rubella. These women should be immunized if not pregnant. Inadvertent administration of rubella vaccine during pregnancy does not appear to create a significant risk to the fetus. Nevertheless it should not be done intentionally.

Sequelae and Complications

Joint involvement is a common complication of rubella. It appears to be more common in adolescents and adults than in children and more common in women than in men. Either arthritis or arthralgia may be present. Fingers, knee and wrist are most commonly involved. The arthritis may last up to four weeks after onset. The joint symptoms usually begin shortly after the appearance of the rash. Most neurologic manifestations are uncommon.

Encephalitis is a rare complication of rubella. It is similar to, but less severe than, the encephalitis associated with measles and usually occurs shortly after the appearance of the rash. Thrombocytopenia has been reported in association with rubella. This complication is more common in children than in adults and in girls more so than boys. About four days after the appearance of the rash, thrombocytopenia may occur. This is usually a self limited complication. Infrequently myocarditis and pericarditis have been reported and some patients have reported testicular pain. In children with a normal immune system, postnatal rubella is very infrequently fatal.

CHICKENPOX (VARICELLA)

Clinical Manifestations

In normal healthy children varicella is an illness that is normally characterized by a generalized vesicular eruption and mild systemic manifestations. The rash is usually pruritic and is frequently accompanied by mild to moderate fever. Classically the rash starts on the scalp or trunk. These lesions are superficial and may appear in different stages of evolution in various parts of the body. Lesions may also appear on the mucous membranes of the mouth and conjunctiva. The rash spreads from the head and trunk out to the extremities. Eventually the vesicles crust over. In immune compromised patients, varicella can be severe and life threatening. Lesions in patients who are immune compromised may be umbilicated and often appear to be deeper than the classic superficial lesions found in varicella in healthy children. Visceral involvement is also more common in children who are immune compromised, and in leukemic patients the mortality from chickenpox approaches 7%. The illness is usually more severe in adults than in children. Varicella may also present as a congenital infection. In the classic congenital varicella syndrome, limb atrophy and scaring of the skin on the extremities is seen. The central nervous system and the eyes may also become involved.

Etiology and Epidemiology

Varicella zoster virus is a member of the herpes group of viruses. Varicella is typically a disease of the late winter and early spring. The disease is highly contagious and spreads rapidly within households. Well over 90% of exposed susceptible patients will develop the disease. The incubation period appears to be about 12 to 14 days. The virus may produce a latent infection and will remain in the body in this latent form without producing any clinical symptoms. Reactivation of the virus produces zoster; also known as shingles. It appears that the virus is dormant in the dorsal root ganglia since zoster usually occurs in the distribution of sensory nerve roots. The disease is transmitted person-to-person and because the virus is very labile it is unlikely to be transmitted by fomites. Patients are probably infectious for at least 24 hours prior to the occurrence of the rash and probably remain infectious until all lesions have crusted over.

Diagnosis

In patients who present with a known exposure and the classic rash, diagnosis of varicella is usually straight forward. In immune compromised patients, one needs a high index of suspicion for the disease and although the disease may often be strongly suggestive by the clinical manifestations, confirmation using virologic studies may sometimes be necessary in these patients. A sample of vesicular fluid is adequate for viral culture. The yield is usually greatest if the vesicular fluid is obtained during the first three days following the onset of disease. Acute and convalescent sera may also be obtained to look for an antibody rise as another way of making the diagnosis.

Treatment

In healthy immunocompetent patients, treatment of varicella infection is rarely indicated. In these patients the disease is almost uniformly self-limited and only supportive care is necessary. However, in the immune compromised patient, this disease may be life threatening. In immune compromised patients with known exposure, the disease may be prevented or aborted using zoster immune globulin. In general, zoster immune globulin is most effective if it is given to the patient within 72 hours of exposure to the disease. Zoster immune globulin should be given to newborn infants whose mother had the first signs of varicella less than 5 days before delivery or within 48 hours after delivery; as in this age group, varicella can be potentially life threatening. In immune compromised patients who present with clinical symptoms, the use of acyclovir or Ara-A may be effective in preventing the dissemination of the disease and in reducing the duration of time of infection. Varicella vaccine has been proven effective in leukemic children in preventing infection. The vaccine is not yet licensed although it is expected to be so in the near future and appears to be safe and effective. The incidence of zoster following varicella vaccine appears to be approximately the same as after natural infection. It is the initial primary infection, the varicella disease, that is potentially life threatening to immune compromised patients and not the recurrence of infection, the zoster infection. The vaccine, therefore, serves a useful purpose.

Sequelae and Complications

In the normal healthy patient, complications from varicella are infrequent. Superinfection of the skin lesions may occur especially in patients who scratch their lesions. Central nervous system manifestations of varicella can occur. These can include aseptic meningitis and fulminating encephalitis. More common than either of those two manifestations is cerebellitis which occurs toward the end of the first week of illness. These patients are usually ataxic. The prognosis is usually good. Less frequently, transverse myelitis, Guillain-Barre syndrome and myositis have been reported. Bleeding may occur with varicella, and idiopathic thrombocytopenia purpura has been reported. Other infrequent manifestations include nephritis, myocarditis and arthritis. There appears to be a strong association between varicella infection and the development of Reyes syndrome in children. Varicella gangrenosa, purpura fulminans, varicella pneumonia and hepatitis may occur. The key to preventing complications in immune compromised children appears to be either administration of zoster immune globulin after exposure or the early institution of appropriate antiviral therapy.

ROSEOLA INFANTUM (EXANTHEM SUBITUM)

Clinical Manifestations

Roseola is a febrile illness in children which is associated with a transient rash and convulsions. Infrequently, encephalitis may occur. Classically the illness begins with three to five days of high fevers. The patient defervesces and then the rash appears which usually lasts a day or two. During the period of high fever, convulsions may occur. Although the patient is febrile, the patient looks toxic infrequently and usually is quite active and alert. Associated symptoms are usually quite mild and may include some respiratory symptoms as well as some gastrointestinal symptoms. Prior to the appearance of the rash, palpebral edema may be present and may be a good diagnostic clue to roseola prior to the appearance of the rash. The rash is an erythematous one and is usually macular or maculopapular. The lesions are usually discrete and blanch with pressure. Sometimes the lesions are surrounded by whitish rings and the rash is usually most prominent over the neck and trunks. The white blood cell count may be useful in suggesting the diagnosis as it is usually low with as few as three thousand cells per cubic millimeter and as many as 90% lymphocytes. This is certainly not pathognomonic but is suggestive of the disease in an otherwise healthy child with a high fever.

Etiology and Epidemiology

Roseola is believed to be of viral origin. In general, roseola is an illness of children between the ages of 3 months and 4 years, with the majority of cases occurring during the first two years of life. The illness appears to occur year round and occurs equally amongst boys and girls. Much remains to be learned about the epidemiology of roseola. The period of communicability, the duration of incubation and the mode of spread have not been well worked out. The incubation period appears to be somewhere between 5 and 15 days however.

Diagnosis

The diagnosis is a clinical one and is usually not too difficult to make in those patients who have the classical clinical course of high fevers, followed by defervescence and the appearance of the rash. No doubt, many cases are missed that do not fit into this classic pattern. There are however no tests available at this time to make a definitive diagnosis.

Treatment

There is no specific treatment for roseola. In those patients who develop complications such as febrile seizures or encephalitis appropriate measures should be taken to support them.

Sequelae and Complications

The most common complication of roseola is convulsions. Abnormalities of the cerebral spinal fluid have also been reported, although infrequently. In most of the cerebral spinal fluids examined, findings have been essentially within normal limits. Encephalitis can occur secondary to roseola and while most patients recover, sequelae have been reported including hemiplegia, paresis and mental retardation. Infrequently, thrombocytopenia purpura has been reported.

ERYTHEMA INFECTIOSUM (FIFTH DISEASE)

Clinical Manifestations

Erythema infectiosum classically presents as a rash on the face. There are very few systemic symptoms or prodromal symptoms prior to the appearance of the rash. Occasionally fever, headache and malaise may be present shortly before the appearance of the exanthem. Initially the rash appears on the face and the appearance is frequently described as the "slapped face" appearance. The cheeks are fiery red. There is circumoral pallor. The rash then progresses to involve the proximal extremities and has the appearance of being erythematous and maculopapular. It then spreads to the trunk and the buttocks and becomes confluent with a lace-like appearance. The intensity of the rash may vary over the next several days to weeks and may completely disappear and then re-appear in relatively short periods of time. Certain factors such as temperature and exposure to sunlight may affect the frequency of recurrences. Adults with this disease frequently complain of significant pruritus.

Etiology and Epidemiology

Erythema infectiosum occurs throughout the world although it appears to be most common in those areas that are not tropical. It usually occurs in epidemics and appears to be most frequent in the winter and spring months. The incubation period is between 4 and 14 days. It is believed that the mode of spread is as a droplet respiratory infection. The disease is most common in school age children and there does not seem to be a preference for one sex. The etiologic agent of erythema infectiosum is thought to be parvovirus.

Diagnosis

Patients presenting with the classical rash are usually not difficult to diagnose and during epidemics one usually has a high index of suspicion. The differential diagnosis should include rubella and scarlet fever. Scarlet fever can usually be ruled out by the lack of pharyngitis or the lack of a positive throat culture for streptococcus.

Treatment

There is no specific treatment for erythema infectiosum and because it is, in general, a mild disease, symptomatic therapy is usually not indicated. No vaccine is currently available to prevent the infection.

Sequelae and Complications

The most common complication is arthritis which is much more common in adults than children and may occur in as many as 50% of the adult cases. Infrequently encephalitis has been reported in association with this infection.

KEY POINTS

1. The common finding in patients with mumps, parotid swelling, need not always be present. Involvement of the central nervous system is not uncommon and may occur in the absence of parotid swelling. Orchitis may occur in association with mumps, most commonly in postpubertal males.

2. The classic prodromal symptoms of measles are cough, coryza, conjunctivitis and koplik's spots. The decreasing frequency of measles in this country makes the likelihood of missing a case of measles and failure to rapidly isolate the patient a potentially serious problem.

3. Symptoms of rubella, if present, include an erythematous maculopapular rash and lymphadenopathy, often posterior auricular nodes. Adults and older children may have eye pain, a sore throat and headache. Congenital rubella has multiple abnormalities associated with it and can result in death in infancy.

4. Varicella is a potentially fatal disease to immunocompromised patients, such as those with leukemia. Aggressive, appropriate use of zoster immune globulin and acyclovir has helped decrease the mortality in these high-risk patients. The varicella vaccine should further reduce the risk.

5. Roseola typically presents as high fever (sometimes associated with convulsions) followed by defervescence and a rash.

6. Fifth's Disease is also known as slapped face syndrome because of the red maculopapular appearance on the face.

REFERENCES

1. ACIP: Report of the Committee on Infectious Diseases, AAP, 1982, pp 76, 133–139, 142–145, 227–228, 229–235.
2. ACIP: Rubella prevention. MMWR 1984; 33:301–310, 315–318.
3. Brunell PA: Mumps. In Feigin RD, Cherry JD(eds): Textbook of Pediatric Infectious Disease. Philadelphia, WB Saunders, 1981, pp. 1231–1235.
4. CDC: Elimination of rubella and congenital rubella syndrome-United States. MMWR 1985; 34:65–66.
5. CDC: Multiple Measles outbreaks on college campuses - Ohio, Massachusetts, Illinois. MMWR 1985; 34:129–130.
6. CDC: Mumps-United States, 1983–1984. MMWR 1984; 33:533–535.
7. CDC: Rubella vaccination during pregnancy. MMWR 1984; 33:365–372.
8. Cherry JD: Roseola Infantum. In Feigin RD, Cherry JD(eds): *Textbook of Pediatric Infectious Disease.* Philadelphia, WB Saunders, 1981, pp 1404–1408.
9. Hilleman MR, Buynak EB, Weibel RE, et al: Live, attenuated mumps virus vaccine. N. Engl J. Med 1968; 278:227–232.
10. Lerman SJ, Gold E: Measles in children previously vaccinated against measles. JAMA 1971; 216:1311–4.
11. Mortimer PP: Fifth Disease and parvovirus. Brit Med J 1984; 289:338–339.
12. Preblud SR, Steler HC, Frank JA, et al: Fetal risk associated with rubella vaccine. JAMA 1981; 246: 1413–1417.

REVIEW QUESTIONS

Match items in Column A with choices in Column B. (Choices in Column B may be used more than once.)

A	B
1.) Slapped face	A. Measles
2.) Fever, seizure, rash	B. Mumps
3.) Orchitis	C. Varicella
4.) May respond to acyclovir	D. Shingles
5.) Posterior auricular nodes	E. Rubella
6.) Reactivation of latent herpes virus infection	F. Roseola
	G. Fifth's Disease
7.) Degenerative CNS disease related to the persistance of measles virus in the patient	H. Subacute sclerosing panencephalitis
8.) Use of inactivated vaccine does not protect but does result in atypical presentation of the illness	
9.) Joint involvement is a common complication, especially in female teenagers and adults	
10.) Vesicular lesions usually starting on the head and trunk; the lesions typically itch; the lesions eventually crust over	

17

MISCELLANEOUS INFECTIONS II

ACQUIRED IMMUNE DEFICIENCY SYNDROME

Clinical Manifestations

In the pediatric patient, acquired immune deficiency syndrome (AIDS) is defined as a patient with evidence of a cellular immune deficiency in whom no specific cause of the decreased cellular immune function is known. Certain diseases known to occur in infants without AIDS are excluded as being adequate evidence for impaired cellular immune function. These include the congenital infections like toxoplasmosis and Herpes simplex infection during the first month of life, and cytomegalovirus during the first six months of life. In order to make the diagnosis of AIDS, primary immune deficiencies such as severe combined immunodeficiency, DiGeorge syndrome, Wiscott-Aldrich, graft versus host reactions, hypogammaglobulinemia, agammaglobulinemia and neutrophil abnormalities must be ruled out. Secondary immune deficiency as a result of suppressive drugs, malignancy or starvation need also to be ruled out.

Major manifestations include interstitial pneumonia, oral thrush, bacterial sepsis or meningitis, and salivary gland enlargement. The presence of AIDS or AIDS related virus in the mother is also a major criteria. Minor manifestations include hepatosplenomegaly, failure-to-thrive, diarrhea, lymphadenopathy and recurrent bacterial infections.

Etiology and Epidemiology

By the end of 1986 there were about 28,000 cases of AIDS reported to the CDC. It is expected that this number will double in the next year unless means of prevention are found. Of these 28,000 cases, half of the adults have died, and about two thirds of the children have died. Of those patients diagnosed before 1983, three-fourths are dead. Slightly more than 1% of all AIDS patients are less than 13 years old. Most pediatric cases are in patients less than 1 year old at diagnosis. The incubation period is 1 month to 5 or more years.

In adult patients *Pneumocystis carinii* and Kaposi's sarcoma are the major manifestations of AIDS. In pediatric patients, Kaposi's sarcoma is an infrequent finding.

Most children with AIDS come from families where one or both parents are at increased risk for AIDS or actually have AIDS. Other risk factors include blood transfusions and hemophilia. In adults, primary risk groups include homosexual or bisexual males, intravenous drug abusers, blood product recipients and other miscellaneous groups.

The etiologic agent for AIDS appears to be a retrovirus. The virus has been designated as lymphadenopathy virus (LAV), human T-cell leukemia virus (HTLV III) and AIDS associated virus (AAV). Infection with this virus results in decreased numbers of helper T-cells and a decreased helper/suppressor T-cell ratio. Other effects of the infection include altered *in vitro* T-cell function, polyclonal B-cell activation with increased levels of total serum immunoglobulin but decreased ability to mount *de novo* antibody responses to specific antigen, and increased alpha-interferon.

Diagnosis

The diagnosis of AIDS depends primarily on the appropriate evidence of immune deficiency in a patient without another explanation for cellular immune dysfunction. In addition, demonstrating evidence of AIDS associated virus infection helps substantiate the diagnosis. Many laboratories are now able to test for the presence of antibody to AAV. It is not yet clear what significance the presence of antibody has in an otherwise asymptomatic host.

Treatment

At this time there is no proven therapy against the virus that causes AIDS. Ribavirin, among other antivirals, are currently being evaluated. The use of interferon as well as intravenous gammaglobulin are also being evaluated.

Current therapy is directed at the opportunistic infections AIDS patients get. Prophylactic use of trimethoprim-sulfamethoxazole may help decrease the incidence of *Pneumocystis carinii* infections in AIDS patients. Efforts are currently underway to develop a vaccine against the virus causing AIDS.

Sequelae and Complications

Cryptosporidium infection may lead to a protracted debilitating diarrhea which, in AIDS patients, may be fatal. A wide variety of infections including *P. carinii* and other parasites, CMV, Herpes, fungi and bacteria have been reported in these patients. Close surveillance and early intervention are essential to keep these patients alive.

BRUCELLOSIS

Clinical Manifestations

Brucellosis can present as an insidious disease with nonspecific symptoms, or as an acute infection with the sudden onset of signs and symptoms of the disease. Symptoms include fever, chills, sweats, weakness, arthralgias, headaches and backaches. Lymphadenopathy and hepatosplenomegaly are often present. Other findings include anorexia, testicular pain, dysuria, hematuria, eye pain and dizziness.

Etiology and Epidemiology

Brucellosis is caused by a small gram-negative rod that is non-motile and non-spore forming. Several organisms in the genus Brucella are responsible for this disease. These include *B. suis, B. abortus,* and *B. melitensis.*

Brucella primarily infects animals. The organism is fairly hardy and can survive in water for four to five weeks, in damp soil for up to 10 weeks, and may survive on fomites for 3 or 4 days. It has been found in sterile milk and its survival time is prolonged when refrigerated. In milk it concentrates in the cream fraction, and has been found in ice cream. Goat's cheese can also contain Brucella.

Transmission to humans may occur by direct animal contact (most common way in the United States), respiratory spread and via blood transfusions from infected donors. People dealing with livestock or meat processing are at highest risk. The incubation period is 1 to 3 weeks. Eradication programs have been successful in cows in the United States. Swine remain a major source of infection in the United States.

Diagnosis

Suspicion of a possible case of Brucellosis can result from appropriate symptoms and a suggestive history. A history of animal contacts or fresh goat's cheese ingestion helps make the diagnosis.

Laboratory diagnosis can be made by culture. The organism can live inside leukocytes so blood cultures and bone marrow cultures may be valuable. In addition, cultures may be obtained from lymph nodes, cerebrospinal fluid and other sites containing granulomatous lesions. The organisms may be in low quantity in the blood so large samples are desirable.

When culture is not available or not successful, serologic techniques are valuable. The brucella agglutination test will detect the disease as early as the first week of illness. There is cross-reactivity in the test with *F. tularensis* and *Vibrio cholerae*. While the agglutination test may remain positive for months to years, other tests are available to determine the acuteness of the infection.

Treatment

Three weeks of tetracycline therapy is curative in most cases. Streptomycin is added in seriously ill children. Trimethoprim-sulfamethoxazole may be substituted for tetracycline. Herxheimer reactions have been reported in severe cases. This reaction can be avoided if oral steroids are administered.

Sequelae and Complications

Complications may occur in about 10% of infected patients. The list of complications include: meningoencephalitis, ruptured mycotic aneurysm, endocarditis, osteomyelitis, arthritis, pneumonitis, renal abscess and nephritis. Most fatalities are associated with endocarditis.

EPSTEIN-BARR VIRUS INFECTION

Clinical Manifestations

Epstein-Barr Virus (EBV) infection is most frequently diagnosed as the mononucleosis syndrome (mono). Mono is usually a self-limited illness. It is typically characterized by fever, adenopathy, tonsillitis and malaise. Splenomegaly is common. In a small number of patients the clinical course becomes chronic or recurrent. EBV can also cause asymptomatic infection or non-specific symptoms in infants and children. In those patients who do have clinical disease, symptoms may be very different from the typical mono syndrome.

EBV primarily infects the B-lymphocyte and can, therefore, set up infection in a variety of sites to which the B-lymphocyte travels. A variety of illnesses have been associated with EBV infection, primarily based on serologic evidence. These include pneumonia, lymphoma, Reye's syndrome, Kawasaki disease, AIDS, Guillain-Barre syndrome and Gianotti-Crosti syndrome, among others. How real some of these associations are is still not clear.

Etiology and Epidemiology

EBV virus is a member of the Herpes virus group. In children, primary infection is usually asymptomatic. In adolescents and young adults, primary infection usually presents as the "mono" syndrome. The virus remains latent in the B-lymphocyte and oropharyngeal tissue and may recur as a recurrent EBV infection, or may cause Burkitt's lymphoma or nasopharyngeal carcinoma. The virus, which may survive in the oropharynx for 18 months after clinical infection, is transmitted by saliva. Close contact is usually required and spread through casual contact is not frequent. Antibodies are more rapidly acquired in tropical areas than in industrialized countries. In the U.S., about 50% of all children seronconvert by age 5 years.

Diagnosis

Laboratory indications of EBV infection include a lymphocytosis with about 30% of the white blood cells being atypical lymphocytes at the peak of the illness. Atypical lymphocytes are not unique to EBV infection however. Thrombocytopenia may also occur.

Agglutinating antibodies (heterophile antibodies) are present in about 90% of older children and adults with EBV infection. Monospot tests are a reliable quick method of demonstrating the presence of heterophile antibodies. In younger children, heterophile antibody detection is not a reliable way to diagnose EBV infections as many false negative tests occur.

The detection of EBV specific antibodies is a more reliable diagnostic method in the younger patient. Antibodies to viral capsid antigen (VCA) are usually detected at the beginning of the clinical course of the infection. IgM antibodies persist for 4 to 8 weeks, IgG antibodies are lifelong. Serum antibodies to early antigen (EA) are of two types. Anti-D EA peaks at 3 to 4 weeks after onset and lasts up to 6 months. Anti-R EA is rarely seen in mono, except in severe illness. It is associated more with African Burkitt's lymphoma. Anti-D EA is present in about 70% of cases. The presence of EA and VCA-IgG suggests recent infection. The presence of VCA-IgM also suggests recent infection. Epstein-Barr nuclear antibody (EBNA) occurs later in the disease, usually a month or more after onset. This antibody persists for life and its appearance suggests the convalescent stage of the illness or past infections.

The virus may also be cultured, however, this is not routinely available in most laboratories.

Treatment

Treatment is supportive. The use of steroids remains controversial. Their use, in general, is limited to those patients with potentially obstructed airways, those with significant thrombocytopenia or hemolytic anemia, and perhaps those with cardiac or CNS involvement. There is currently no available antiviral therapy for EBV infection.

Sequelae and Complications

Many complications of EBV infection have been reported. These include hepatitis, carditis, pneumonitis, laryngeal obstruction, ruptured spleen, and transverse myelitis, among others. Complications are not frequent.

INFANT BOTULISM

Clinical Manifestations

The classic presentation is of a previously well infant who becomes constipated. This is followed by symmetric weakness which descends. Facial weakness, decreased suck or a weak cry may be the initial clues. Progression may be rapid and involvement of cranial nerves is often followed by involvement of the rest of the body. Examinations usually reveal an infant who has a weak cry and little spontaneous movement but who does not otherwise appear acutely ill. The child is usually alert, with good perfusion and is afebrile. Motor responses are poor or absent. There is abnormalities of sensation in some infants. Autonomic dysfunction is frequently manifested as bladder and abdominal distension and decreased salivation. The average duration of hospitalization for these infants is about one month.

Etiology and Epidemiology

Botulism is caused by toxin producing *Clostridium botulinum.* Group 1 C. botulinum are proteolytic strains that produce toxins that are responsible for virtually all infantile botulism. The toxins produced are extremely neurotoxic and primarily affect transmission at all peripheral cholinergic junctions by preventing the normal release of acetylcholine after depolarization at neural terminals. The toxin is bound irreversibly but recovery is possible by the formation of new motor end plates.

Initial reports of infantile botulism were associated with spore ingestion from honey. The majority of cases, however, are probably related to spores found in the environment. In general, those areas of the United States with the highest spore counts in the soil have a correspondingly high incidence of infantile botulism.

Ingestion of spores in adults does not lead to botulism. In infants the intestine is not resistant to the spores, and they survive. *REMEMBER:* Breastfeeding is strongly associated with the development of botulism. The intestine of breast fed infants differs from that of bottle fed (formula-fed) infants in several respects including that their intestinal flora is different.

The differences in microbial flora may account for the ability of *C. botulinum* to grow in the breast fed infant's intestine.

Epidemiologic markers for infants at risk for botulism includes being full-term, white, previously healthy and, as previously stated, purely or predominantly breast-fed. Other common characteristics are that these babies' immunizations are up to date, they have two parent families and that mom is a homemaker.

Diagnosis

The diagnosis can strongly be suspected based on clinical presentation and appropriate historical data. Certain tests may assist in diagnosis. Electromyography demonstrates motor unit action potentials that are short and of small amplitude and excessive for the amount of power exerted (BSAP pattern). Rapid repetitive nerve stimulation will result in enhancement of compound action potential. Nerve condition is at normal speed. Edrophonium chloride or neostigmine injection does not result in a significant clinical response. *C. botulinum* toxin in the stool or isolation of *C. botulinum* confirms the diagnosis.

Treatment

The essence of treatment is supportive care. As deterioration frequently continues over the first week, hospitalization is essential. Respiratory support including use of respirators is frequently required. The syndrome of inappropriate antidiuretic hormone (SIADH) secretion occurs, most often in infants on the respirator.

The role of antibiotics and antitoxin is not clear. Recovery usually occurs without specific therapy and despite the persistence of the toxin and organism in stool for weeks to months. Penicillin does not appear to effect the course nor does use of antitoxin. *REMEMBER:* Use of aminoglycosides in suspected cases of botulism is contraindicated because these antibiotics contribute to neuromuscular blockade and may result in respiratory failure.

Sequelae and Complications

Infant botulism is rarely fatal. Complications include respiratory failures, otitis media, SIADH, and pneumonia. Less frequently, autonomic instability, the adult respiratory distress syndrome, and convulsions occur.

KAWASAKI SYNDROME (KS)

Clinical Manifestations

Symptoms of KS include: fever, conjunctival injection; mucous membrane changes including dry, cracked lips, "strawberry" tongue, and injected pharynx; abnormalities of the peripheral extremities including edema of the hands and feet, erythema of palms and soles, and desquamation; lymphadenopathy and rash. Associated findings include sterile pyuria, arthralgias, arthritis, liver function abnormalities, gallbladder distension and cardiac disease.

Classically the illness occurs in three phases. The first phase usually lasts 8–12 days. The child usually has fever unresponsive to antibiotics. Shortly after the onset of fever, conjunctival injection is found along with dry, cracking lips. Pharyngeal injection and a "strawberry" tongue (protuberance of the tongue papillae) often are seen and occur shortly after the onset of fever. This phase of the illness is often also characterized by lymphadenopathy (cervical) and rash. Typically the rash is morbilliform, scarlatiniform, or erythema multiforme-like.

The second phase of the illness is the subacute phase. During this phase, the patient usually defervesces. Desquamation of fingers and toes usually occurs and in some patients arthralgias or arthritis may occur. Usually the larger joints are involved. Thrombocytosis is also seen. It is during this stage that carditis occurs. This is the most significant finding in KS. It is carditis that is responsible for the 2% mortality rate in this illness. Aneurysm, sudden death, myocarditis, myocardial infarction, arrhythmias and mitral insuffiency may occur. Clinically apparent cardiac involvement is present in about 20% of KS patients.

The final phase of illness is the convalescent phase and is characterized by the disappearance of symptoms and a fall in the erythrocyte sedimentation rate. Cardiac involvement may not become apparent until late in the illness.

Less frequent clinical findings include diarrhea, abdominal pain, abdominal organ necrosis, urethritis, meatal stenosis, testicular necrosis, otitis, uveitis, myositis and hypertension.

Etiology and Epidemiology

KS was first described in 1967 by the Japanese. Since 1971, the disease has been recognized in the United States. Cases have been reported from many countries worldwide. The disease was originally called mucocutaneous lymph node syndrome. Over 900 cases had been reported to the CDC by 1983. There is a slight male predominance and the disease usually occurs under 8 years of age. Most patients are 3 years old or less. Both sporadic cases and epidemics have been reported. No etiology has been found although many infectious and non-infectious etiologies have been proposed. The illness may appear all year round, but, in the United States, most cases occur in winter or spring.

Diagnosis

The diagnosis of KS is made on clinical grounds. Criteria have been established by the CDC. The diagnosis can be made in patients with fever for five or more days that does not respond to antibiotics, and in whom other likely causes have been ruled out if 4 or 5 criteria are present: 1) Bilateral conjunctival injection, 2) Mucous membrane changes, 3) Extremity changes, 4) Rash, 5) Cervical lymphadenopathy (greater than 1.5 cm).

Treatment

Because the specific etiology has not been identified, definitive therapy can not be recommended at this time. Most authorities recommend aspirin therapy. Steroids are not recommended and may be associated with an increased risk of aneurysm formation. Some preliminary data suggest that high dose intravenous gammaglobulin may reduce the risk of coronary artery formation.

Sequelae and Complications

The major complications are the cardiac ones. Close follow-up of KS patients is necessary for months to years following the acute illness. The cardiac complications may not appear during the acute illness.

LEPTOSPIROSIS

Clinical Manifestations

Leptospirosis is a biphasic illness. The first stage (septicemic) usually lasts a week or less and is characterized by fever, conjunctival injection, myalgias, abdominal pain, vomiting and headache. In mild cases, after the patient becomes afebrile no additional symptoms may occur. In others, after a few days without fever the patient develops meningitis symptoms, uveitis, rash and again develops fever (immune stage). Symptoms usually last a week or less, but in rare cases a more chronic meningitis may occur. Not all patients develop all symptoms or have the second stage of the illness.

A much less frequent form of the disease is icteric leptospirosis (Weil's syndrome). Jaundice, hemorrhage, myocarditis and renal failure may occur. Most fatalities associated with leptospirosis occur in patients with Weil's syndrome.

Etiology and Epidemiology

Leptospirosis is caused by infection with leptospiras which are spirochetes similar to treponema. Contact with infected animals results in human infection. Rats and other rodents served as important hosts for human infection in the past. More recently in the U.S., dogs have become a major source of infection. Occupational exposure to infected livestock is another source of human infection.

The disease is found worldwide but is most common in moist, semitropical and tropical regions. Only about 100 cases per year are reported in the U.S. Asymptomatic cases also occur.

Diagnosis

During the first phase of the illness, leptospira are recoverable from blood and CSF. During the second stage, the organisms are primarily found in urine.

Agglutination tests will become positive by the sixth to twelfth day of illness. Serial samples demonstrating a rising titer helps substantiate the diagnosis, especially where culture is not available.

Treatment

Leptospirosis is usually a self-limited disease. Early institution of penicillin or tetracycline therapy may help shorten the course.

Sequelae and Complications

In children, acalculous cholecystitis has been reported. Iridocyclitis, pneumonia, encephalitis and adult respiratory distress syndrome have also been reported. Renal failure occurs, and in patients with the icteric form of the disease, may lead to death.

LYME DISEASE

Clinical Manifestations

Lyme Disease (LD) is characterized by a distinctive rash. Initially a red macule or papule form. The lesion grows and expands to become annular. The lesion, known as erythema chronicum migrans, may eventually reach up to 70 cm in diameter and have central clearing. Although usually a single lesion is present, multiple lesions can be seen. Associated findings sometimes seen include fever, headache, neck stiffness, myalgias, malaise, fatigue, arthralgias, and lymphadenopathy. Cardiac, neurologic, and arthritic complications may not develop for weeks to months after the appearance of the initial skin lesion. Cardiac complications include myocarditis and conduction defects. Neurologic complications include meningoencephalitis, peripheral neuritis, and Bell's palsy. Arthritis may develop even later than the cardiac and neurologic complications, and may recur over several years. Erosion of bone and cartilage may occur. The arthritis is usually monoarticular or oligoarticular and usually involves large joints.

Etiology and Epidemiology

LD is a tick-borne illness. It usually occurs in the summer months. The organism is transmitted by Ixodes ticks. Both *I. pacificus* and *I. dammini* ticks are vectors. *I. dammini* is primarily seen in the northeast and midwest parts of the U.S. and *I. pacificus* is found in the western U.S. The infecting organism appears to be a spirochete. Spirochetes have been isolated from Ixodes ticks, and from the skin lesions, blood and CSF of infected patients. The spirochete has been classified as a Borrelia. The illness has been reported in both adults and children. Most cases have been reported from the coastal Northeast, the Midwest, and the West. Isolated cases have been reported in the South and Southeast.

Diagnosis

The diagnosis can often be made on clinical grounds. This is especially true in patients with the classic erythema chronicum migrans rash. Diagnosis may be more difficult in patients who present with the later manifestations. Serologic diagnostic tests are available and appear to be more reliable in late disease than when only the rash is present. *REMEMBER:* Antibodies for LD cross-react with some of the other spirochetal diseases, especially treponemal infections, but patients with LD will have a negative VDRL. Rheumatoid factor is usually negative. Joint fluid has an average white cell count of 25,000 but there is a wide range. Most of these cells are polymorphonuclear cells. Protein is frequently around 5 g/dl. Glucose is usually over 2/3 of serum glucose. In general, the reaction within the affected joint is similar to that seen in rheumatoid arthritis.

Treatment

Early treatment with penicillin, tetracycline or erythromycin is relatively effective. Tetracycline and penicillin appear to be more effective in preventing late major complications. In children, 10–20 days of therapy with penicillin is effective in treating symptoms and usually in preventing most major complications if therapy is started early. Most patients with arthritis will respond to high dose penicillin therapy.

Sequelae and Complications

Recurrent arthritis, recurrent cardiac involvement, and prolonged neurologic abnormalities have been reported. Recurrent joint involvement can lead to chronic changes in bone and cartilage. Cardiac involvement may last days to months. Neurologic complications may run a prolonged course but usually resolve.

PLAGUE

Clinical Manifestations

Plague usually presents as a sudden onset of fever, chills and malaise. Tender adenopathy, usually in the groin, results in the formation of bubo. An inoculation site near the bubo may be seen but its not always evident. Lymph node suppration is common. CNS manifestations are believed to be the result of toxin. Memory loss, vertigo, speech disorders, altered state of consciousness, and abnormal gait have all been reported. Meningitis has infrequently been reported. Pneumonic plague has similar symptoms but is rapidly progressive and frequently fatal.

Etiology and Epidemiology

Plague is caused by *Yersinia pestis,* a gram-negative bipolar staining rod (using carbolfuchsin - methylene blue stain). The bite of an infected flea is the most common way for humans to acquire the infection. Droplet inhalation from patients with pneumonic plague may also lead to disease. The organism can survive in the soil and this may serve as another source of infection. Plague outbreaks have occurred worldwide. In the United States, the endemic areas are in the western half of the country.

Diagnosis

History of a bite or physical evidence of a bite associated with localized adenopathy (bubo) accompanied by fever, malaise and sometimes chills should suggest the diagnosis. In addition, a history of living in or visiting an endemic area supports the diagnosis. Laboratory confirmation is achieved by culture of blood and aspirate of infected lymph nodes. In patients with pulmonic involvement, sputum samples may be helpful. Culturing of *Y. pestis* carries a risk of spread to laboratory personnel. Demonstrating the presence of antibody to *Y. pestis* by passive agglutination with sensitized sheep red blood cells is an alternative method of confirming your clinical diagnosis.

Treatment

Antibiotic therapy should begin promptly. Streptomycin is the drug of choice. Because of the possibility of resistant organisms, chloramphenicol or tetracycline should also be used. Plague meningitis is rare but when it occurs, chloramphenicol should be used in the treatment. Contacts of patients with plague should receive either tetracycline or sulfadiazine for 1 week.

Sequelae and Complications

With prompt therapy about 95% of patients survive. Untreated plague pneumonia is almost always fatal; and bubonic plague carries a mortality of around 50%. Superinfection of infected nodes may occur. Both *Staphylococcus aureus* and pseudomonas species can cause superinfection. Arthritis and liver abscesses have been reported.

ROCKY MOUNTAIN SPOTTED FEVER

Clinical Manifestations

The major findings in Rocky Mountain Spotted Fever (RMSF) are rash and fever. The patient frequently complains of headache and may be confused. Myalgias and edema often occur, and the patient may appear toxic. *REMEMBER:* RMSF without the rash can also occur although it is less common than RMSF with the rash.

The typical rash of RMSF initially is a macular rash that blanches with pressure. These lesions usually evolve into maculopapules or petechiae. The rash may eventually become hemorrhagic. Typically the rash appears on day two or three of illness, and spreads from the pheriphery toward the trunk. It frequently is found on the palms and soles.

A variety of central nervous system manifestations may occur. These include confusion, headache, meningismus, coma, seizures, ataxia and spastic paralysis.

Gastrointestinal symptoms often appear early in the disease. Gastrointestinal involvement is most commonly manifested as abdominal pain and vomiting. In some patients the abdominal pain has been reported to resemble appendicitis.

Etiology and Epidemiology

RMSF is caused by Rickettsia rickettsii. It is primarily an infection that occurs in the western hemisphere and is transmitted by the bite of a tick. The dog, wood and Lone Star ticks are common vectors. Most cases occur from April to September. In the U.S., most cases occur in children less than 15 years of age. The incidence of RMSF in the eastern U.S. is much bigger than the number of cases found in the West.

Diagnosis

Diagnosis of RMSF is primarily based on the clinical manifestations. Associated findings include a leukopenia during the first few days of illness and thrombocytopenia.

The confirmation of the diagnosis can be made by immunofluorescent technique of a skin biopsy obtained early in the disease. Weil-Felix serologic testing may be positive during the second week of illness in the untreated patient. A single high titer or serial rising titers will further support the diagnosis. Specific RMSF serologic tests are available with varying degrees of sensitivity. Positive tests, in general, are quite specific.

Treatment

RMSF can be treated with chloramphenicol or tetracycline. Therapy should begin as soon as possible. Treatment should continue for at least two or three days beyond when the temperature returns to and stays normal. If treatment is provided early in the course of the illness and if appropriate supportive care is provided, the patient usually recovers. Death is usually the result of delayed diagnosis and treatment.

Sequelae and Complications

Complications are not frequent. Superinfection occasionally occurs. Bronchopneumonia is infrequently seen.

TULAREMIA

Clinical Manifestations

Tularemia usually presents as one of six different forms: ulceroglandular, oropharyngeal, typhoidal, glandular, oculoglandular and pneumonic. Ulceroglandular is the type most frequently seen. The first clinical manifestation is usually tender swollen lymph nodes. At the site where the bacteria penetrates the skin, a papule often appears. The papule may rupture, resulting in the formation of an ulcer. Glandular tularemia does not have an obvious entry site lesion but is otherwise similar to the ulceroglandular form. Inguinal node involvement is most commonly seen. In oculoglandular disease, the conjunctival space is believed to be the portal of entry. There is eye pain and inflammation and edema of the involved eye. Small yellow nodules may form on the sclerae and palpebral conjunctiva. Ulcerations may also be present. Typhoidal tularemia presents as sepsis. High fevers, headaches, chills, aching and vomiting are frequently present. Symptoms usually begin abruptly. Non-specific skin rashes and diarrhea may also be seen. Hepatosplenomegaly is seen. This form of the disease can be seen after ingesting contaminated food. Oropharyngeal tularemia is also a result of eating contaminated food. Pseudomembranes may form over the tonsils. The cervical nodes often are involved. Pneumonic tularemia is infrequently seen in children. It is seen in infected laboratory personnel and can be lethal. Secondary pneumonias can be seen as a result of hematogenous spread in patients with one of the other forms of tularemia. *REMEMBER:* Suppurative nodes are potentially infectious and if a drainage procedure is done, appropriate precautions including wearing a mask should be taken.

Etiology and Epidemiology

Tularemia is caused by a small gram-negative pleomorphic coccobacillus called *Francisella tularensis.* The organism is an intracellular pathogen. The organism can survive freezing for up to three weeks. Thorough cooking of infected meat will make the meat safe for consumption. Incubation varies from 3 to 21 days.

Infection may be contracted through ticks, fleas, mites, or infected animal bites. Rabbits are a major reservoir of infection. In the U.S., ticks play a major role in the spread of tularemia. Spring and summer are peak seasons for tularemia.

Diagnosis

Patients presenting with clinical manifestations compatible with any of the types of tularemia should be evaluated for the infection. History of a tick bite or contact with a potentially infected animal is also a valuable clue. Laboratory confirmation is usually accomplished by serologic test. Agglutination tests are commonly done. Antibodies can be detected by week two of the illness. Demonstrating a four-fold rise in titer of serial specimens (acute and convalescent) makes the diagnosis. *REMEMBER:* Cross-reactivity may occur with Brucella and in patients in whom Brucella is in the differential, additional serologic testing may be needed. Because the organism may infect laboratory personnel if it is aerosolized resulting in a potentially lethal pneumonia, many laboratories will not attempt to isolate *F. tularensis* in culture.

Treatment

The drug of choice is streptomycin. Therapy is usually given for seven days, but is extended based on clinical considerations. Gentamicin also appears to be effective therapy. Less effective are chloramphenicol and tetracycline. Both result in prompt clinical improvement, but because they are bacteriostatic, relapses can occur. Streptomycin resistant *F. tularensis* exist but are rare. With appropriate therapy response is clinically apparent within a few days.

Sequelae and Complications

In appropriately diagnosed and treated cases, complications are infrequent. Relapses occur, especially in patients treated with bacteriostatic antibiotics. Mortality is low and is primarily associated with the pneumonic and typhoidal forms of tularemia.

KEY POINTS

1. Kawasaki syndrome is diagnosed by the presence of fever, mucous membrane changes, abnormalities of the extremities, lymphadenopathy and rash.

2. Cardiac involvement is responsible for the mortality associated with KS.

3. The typical lesion of Lyme Disease is erythema chronicum migrans which starts as a macule or papule and expands forming an annular lesion with central clearing.

4. Streptomycin is the drug of choice for the treatment of tularemia. Less effective are chloramphenicol and tetracycline; both of which produce clinical improvement but frequently relapses occur.

5. Constipation and weakness in an alert, afebrile child should suggest the possibility of infant botulism.

6. Plague is endemic in areas of the western U.S. Treatment with streptomycin (either with or without chloramphenicol or tetracycline) is effective in eliminating the infection.

7. Symptoms of brucellosis are non-specific. A detailed history is therefore important to determine if animal contacts, or relevant ingestions occurred.

8. Early institution of therapy is important. The patient must be closely monitored for complications. Therapy should be continued for 3 weeks.

9. HTLV-III, a retrovirus appears to be responsible for AIDS. Infection causes a derangement of the cellular immune system in some patients resulting in increased susceptibility to opportunistic infections.

10. RMSF may occur with or without a rash. The rash, when present, begins on the extremities and moves centrally. The palms and soles are often involved.

11. EBV infection commonly results in the infectious mononucleosis syndrome. However, there are many atypical presentations of EBV infection, especially in infants and young children.

12. Leptospirosis is typically a biphasic illness which is usually self-limited.

REFERENCES

Andiman WA: Epstein-Barr virus-associated syndromes: A critical reexamination. Pediatr Infect Dis 1984; 3: 198–203.

Arnon SS, Damus K, Thompson B, et al: Protective role of human milk against sudden death from infant botulism. J Pediatr 1982; 100: 568–573.

Bell, DM, Brink EW, Nitzkin JL, et al: Kawasaki Syndrome: Description of two outbreaks in the United States. N. Engl J. Med. 1981; 304:-1568–1575.

Bells DM, Moren DM, Holam RC, et al: Kawaski Syndrome in the United States 1976 to 1980. Am J Dis Child 1983; 137: 211–214.

Bernard KW, Helmick CG, Kaplan JE, et al: Surveillance of Rocky Mountain Spotted Fever in the U.S. 1978–1980. J Infect Dis 1982; 146:297–299.

Boyce, JM: Francisella tularensis (tularemia). In: Mondell GL, Douglas RG, Bennett JE (eds). *Principles and Practice of Infectious Diseases* (2nd edition). New York: John Wiley and Sons, 1985; 1290–1294.

CDC: Kawasaki Syndrome - United States. MMWR 1983; 32:98–100.

CDC: Rocky Mountain Spotted Fever - United States 1980. MMWR 1981; 30:318–320.

CDC: Update: Acquired Immunodeficiency Syndrome - United States. MMWR 1985; 34:245–248.

CDC: Update: Lyme Disease - United States. MMWR 1984; 33:268-270.

Davis, AE, Bradford WD: Abdominal pain resembling acute appendicitis in Rocky Mountain Spotted Fever. JAMA 1982; 247:2811–2812.

Evans AS, Niederman JC, McCollum RW: Seroepidemiological studies of infectious mononucleosis with EBV virus. N Engl J Med 1968; 279:1121–1127.

Fleischer G, Henle W, Henle G, et al: Primary infection with Epstein-Barr virus in infants in the United States: Clinical and serologic observations. J Infect Dis 1979; 139:553–558.

Furusho K, Sato K, Soeda T, et al: High-dose Intravenous gammaglobulin for Kawasaki Disease. Lancet 1983; 111:1359.

Giunchi G, deRosa R, Fabiani R: Trimethoprim-sulfamethoxazole combination in the treatment of acute human brucellosis. Chemotherapy 1971; 16:332–335.

Haynes, RE, Sanders DY, and Cramblatt HG: Rocky Mountain Spotted Fever in Children. J. Pediatr 1970; 76:685–693.

Henle W, Henle G, Niederman JC, et al: Antibodies to early antigens induced by Epstein-Barr virus in infectious mononucleosis. J Infect Dis 1971; 124:58–63.

Jacobs, RF. Tularemia. In: Nelson JD, McCracken GH (eds.) *Clinical Reviews in Pediatric Infections.* Philadelphia: BC Decker Inc, 1985; 165–170.

Long SS: Botulism in infancy. In Nelson JD, McCracken GH (eds.): *Clinical Reviews in Pediatric Infectious Disease.* Philadelphia: CV Mosby Co, 1985; 181–186.

Long SS: Epidemiologic Study of infant botulism in Pennsylvania: Report of the infant botulism study group. Pediatric, 1985; 75:928–934.

Long SS: Gajewski JL, Brown LW, et al: Clinical laboratory and environmental features of botulism in southeastern Pennsylvania. Pediatrics, 1985; 75:935–941.

Martone WJ, Kaufman AF: Leptospirosis in humans in the U.S. 1974 to 1978. J Infect Dis 1979; 140:1020–1022.

Mason WL, Eigelsbach HT, Little SF, et al: Treatment of tularemia, including pulmonary tularemia, with gentamicin. Am Rev Resp Dis 1980; 121:39–45.

McClain JBL, Ballou WR, Harrison SM, et al: Doxycycline therapy for leptospirosis Ann Intern Med 1984; 100:696–698.

Meissner HC, Gellis SE, Milliken JF: Lyme disease first observed to be aseptic meningitis. Am J Dis Child 1982; 136:465–467.

Peters G. Leptospirosis: A zoonosis of protein manifestations. Ped Infect Dis 1981; 1:282–288.

Pickett J, Berg B, Chaplin E, et al: Syndrome of botulism in infancy. Clinical and electrophysiologic study. N Engl J Med 1976; 295:770–772.

Polin RA, Brown LW: Infant Botulism. Pediatr Clin North Am 1979; 26:345–354.

Radford DJ, Sondheimer HM, Williams CJ et al: Mucocutaneous lymphnode syndrome with coronary artery aneurysms. Am J Dis Child 1976; 130:596–598.

Rogers MF: AIDS in children: A review of the clinical epidemiological and public health aspects. Ped. Infectious Dis 1985; 4:230–236.

Russell H, Sampson JS, Schmid GP, et al: Enzyme-linked immunosorbent assay and indirect immunofluorescence assay for Lyme disease. J Infect Dis 1984; 149:465–470.

Selikoff IJ, Teirstein, AS, Hirschman SZ (eds): Acquired Immune Deficiency Syndrome. New York: The New York Academy of Sciences, 1984.

Steere AC, Bartenhagen NH, Craft JE, et al: The early clinical manifestations of Lyme disease. Ann Intern Med 1983; 99:76–82.

Steere AC, Gibofsky A, Pattarroyo ME, et al: Chronic Lyme arthritis: Clinical and immunogenetic differentiation from rheumatoid arthritis. Ann Intern Med 1979; 90:896–901.

Steere AC, Grodzicki RL, Kornblatt AN, et al: The spirochetal etiology of Lyme Disease. N Engl J Med 1983; 308:733–740.

Street L, Granth WW, Alva JD: Brucellosis in childhood. Pediatrics 1975; 55:416–421.

Tarplay M: Tularemic pharyngitis. Pediatr Infect Dis 1983; 2:266.

Westerman EL: Rocky Mountain Spotless Fever - a dilemma for the clinican. Arch Intern Med 1982; 142:1106–1107.

Young EJ: Human Brucellosis. Rev. Infect Dis 1983; 5:821–842.

Yow MD: Brucellosis. In Feigin RD and Cherry JD (eds) *Textbook of Pediatric Infectious Diseases,* Philadelphia, WB Saunders Co, 1981, pp828–833.

Yow MD: Tularemia. In: Feigin RD, Cherry JD (eds). *Textbook of Pediatric Infectious Diseases.* Philadelphia. WB Sauncers Co. 1981; 1005-1011.

REVIEW QUESTIONS

Match the description from Column A with the appropriate choice in Column B

A

1.) Maculopapular, petechial rash spreading from periphery centrally; lesions found on hands and soles; leukopenia and thrombocytopenia

2.) Constipation, decreasing symmetric weakness, weak cry, little spontaneous movement

3.) Erythema chronicum migram, arthritis, carditis, tick borne illness

4.) Most common in children less than 3 years of age, fever unresponsive to antibiotics, conjunctival injection, mucous membrane changes, extremity changes, rash, cervical adenopathy

5.) Serologically cross-reacts with Brucella, responds to streptomycin therapy, organism is a small gram-negative coccobacillus

6.) Frequently presents as tender groin adenopathy associated with fever, organism is a Gram negative bipolar staining rod

7.) Fresh goat cheese injection, small Gram-negative rod, eradication programs in cows have been successful in controlling the spread of infection in the U.S.

8.) Caused by a member of the Herpes virus family, this infection has a variety of clinical presentations; older children and adults will usually have heterophile antibodies

9.) Spirochete infection, often biphasic, dogs are a reservoir for infection

10.) Retrovirus infection associated with multiple immunologic abnormalities including decreased numbers of helper T cells, altered *in vitro* T cell function, and polyclonal B cell activation

B

A. Kawasaki Syndrome
B. Lyme Disease
C. Tularemia
D. Infant Botulism
E. Plague
F. Brucellosis
G. AIDS
H. Rocky Mountain Spotted Fever
I. Epstein-Barr Virus Infection
J. Leptospirosis

18

PREVENTION OF INFECTION

The discipline of infectious diseases deals with three major areas: the diagnosis of infection, the treatment of infection, and the prevention of infection. This chapter deals with the third of these areas, infection prevention. The four broad categories into which we can divide prevention are: immunizations, passive antibodies, sterile techniques and isolation, and antibiotics. Each play very important roles in reducing the incidence of infection and controlling the spread of infection.

Immunizations

The charts on the following pages contain information on standard immunizations routinely given to children as well as information about immunizations which are given for specific indications; and information on some newer and experimental vaccines. Less frequently used vaccines are not included. *REMEMBER:* Be extremely cautious in administering active immunization to immunocompromised patients. (See chart at the end of chapter.)

Passive Antibody

Immunity is to a large extent a result of the presence of specific antibody. Specific antibody combines with the specific antigen resulting in either modification or elimination of the effect of that antigen. Factors involved in determining the success of antibody administration include: administration of adequate amount of antibody to neutralize the antigen, administration of antibody soon enough to be effective, and that the antigen is able to be neutralized by the specific antibody. Effective passive immunization requires that the side effects from antibody administration not be worse than the effects of the disease being prevented.

Immune globulin (IG) is also known as gamma globulin, immune serum globulin or normal serum immune globulin. It is prepared from pooled human plasma, and is approximately 95% IgG. The half-life is three to four weeks, and effective serum levels are maintained for 2–3 months. This pooled IG contains antibody reflective of the infectious disease history of the donors and therefore should provide some protection against a variety of infections. *REMEMBER:* IG is hepatitis B free and, therefore, should not place recipients at risk of acquiring hepatitis B. IG is available as an intramuscular or intravenous preparation.

IG has been used in many circumstances. It has been used in antibody deficiency (congenital or acquired), prophylaxis against measles, hepatitis (A or B) and varicella. Other indications are more controversial. There is no evidence that IG is beneficial in infants who are malnourished or failures to thrive, infants with frequent infections, infants with allergic disorders, or in premature newborns, unless there is evidence for a defect in IgG production.

In addition to IG, specific immunoglobulins are available. Useful specific IGs include hepatitis B, varicella-zoster, tetanus and rabies. These preparations contain high-titer antibody against the specific pathogen and, when available, are preferred to normal IG for known exposures to the above diseases.

Passive antibody protection does not depend on the patient having an intact immune system. Their use is therefore particularly important in the immunocompromised patient. Passive antibody protection lasts only 2–3 months. Repeat infections are therefore possible. (See chart at the end of chapter.)

Sterile Techniques and Isolation Procedures

The use of sterile techniques and the implementation of appropriate isolation procedures play a major role in controlling infections in hospitals. Direct and indirect contact is a major route for the spread of infections, and the single most important intervention in preventing spread is handwashing. Spread of infections within nurseries, intensive care units, and to immunocompromised patients is often the result of poor or non-existent handwashing practices. The additional use of gowns, masks and gloves may assist in interrupting the spread of infections.

Isolation procedures are valuable in preventing the spread of infection when the appropriate form of isolation is used. The chart summaries the different types of isolation and when each is appropriately used. There is little evidence that standard reverse isolation practices are of any value and have, in general, been abandoned. (See chart at the end of chapter.)

Antibiotics

Antibiotics play an important role in preventing infection. The prophylactic uses of antibiotics include:
1) exposures to patients with *Neisseria meningitidis* infection - rifampin, sulfonamides.
2) families with children under 4 years of age, exposed to household contacts with serious *Haemophilus influenzae* infection - rifampin.
3) exposures to patients with pertussis-erythromycin.
4) immunocompromised patients at risk for pneumocystis disease-trimethoprim-sulfamethoxazole.
5) rheumatic fever - penicillin, erythromycin.
6) endocarditis - penicillin; erythromycin, vancomycin.
7) tuberculosis - isoniazid.
8) a variety of abdominal surgical procedures - many choices.
9) recurrent otitis - trimethoprim - sulfamethoxazole and others.
10) recurrent urinary tract infections - many choices.
11) traveler's diarrhea - (in adults) - doxycycline.

*It is important to use antibiotics judiciously. Misuse of antibiotics can lead to infection with more virulent organisms, the development of resistant organisms, and undesirable toxicities from the antibiotic used.

KEY POINTS

1. Infections are prevented by the appropriate use of vaccines, antibiotics, isolation technique and sterile technique.
2. Passive antibody administration provides temporary protection against an infection.
3. Active antibody production usually results from natural infection as well as from immunization. Protection usually is of long duration.
4. In specific circumstances, the appropriate use of antibiotics can prevent disease. Misuse may result in the emergence of resistant strains and more serious pathogens.
5. The single most important intervention in preventing the spread of infection within institutions, day care centers and hospitals is good handwashing.

REFERENCES

Benenson AS: *Control of Communicable Disease in Man* (12 edition). The American Public Health Association. Washington, DC 1981.

CDC: Recommendations for protection against viral hepatitis. MMWR 1985; 34:313–335.

Fulginiti, VA: *Immunization in Clinical Practice.* J.B. Lippincott Company. Philadelphia, 1982.

Harris AA, Levin S, Trenhomer GM: Selected Aspects of Nosocomial Infections in the 1980s. The American Journal of Medicine 77(1B): 3–10, 1984.

Hirschmann JV: Rational Antibiotic Prophylaxis. Hospital Practice 1980; 105–123,

Moffet HL: Pediatric Nosocomial Infections in the Community Hospital. Pediatric Infectious Disease 1982 1:430–442,

Pizzo PA: Isolation Techniques in the Hospital. Pediatric Infectious Diseases 1983; 2:94–98,

Report of the Committee on Infectious Diseases (19th edition). American Academy of Pediatrics, Evanston, Illinois, 1982.

ROUTINE IMMUNIZATIONS

Disease	Reason For Vaccine	Type Of Vaccine	Immunization Schedule	Route	Side Effects	Comments	Rx
Diphtheria	Mortality 10% despite antibiotics & supportive care - about 50 cases/year in the U.S.A.	Inactivated toxin (toxoid)	2, 4, 6, 18 mos. preschool every 10 years	IM	Increase with age usually attributed to other components of DPT- usually mild. Acute hemolytic anemia - RARE.	2 levels of potency. D-child. <7 y/o d- >7 y/o d contains – ¼ dose of D.	Infected pt-PCN & anti-toxin if not immunized. Close contact - PCN/erythro x 7 days c̄ F/up cults. Td & toxin if close F/up not possible & patient unimmunized.
Tetanus	50% of cases occur c̄ minor wound - no medical care was sought - about 100 cases/year in the U.S.A.	Toxoid (tetanospasmin)	2, 4, 6, 18 mos. Preschool every 10 yrs.	IM	Increase with age correlates c̄ level of circulating anti-toxin -Usually mild local reaction -Anaphylaxis- very rare.	1st dose produces little or no antibody. Vaccine can be given with TIG	-TIG should be given in all tetanus-prone injuries. -Booster given

Disease	Reason For Vaccine	Type Of Vaccine	Immunization Schedule	Route	Side Effects	Other	Rx
Pertussis	-10% of cases occur in 1st yr. of life. -¾ of deaths during 1st year.	Inactivated whole bacterial suspension. (formalin/phenol) killed	2, 4, 6, 18 mos. Preschool	IM	↑T (–50%) -Sore nodule (–50%) -Seizures (gen'lized) -"Screaming episodes" (–6%) -Encepalopathy 24-28 hrs. post immunization) Adverse reactions increase $\bar{c}$ age Don't use in > 7 y/o, pt., $\bar{c}$ hx of bad reaction pt $\bar{c}$ evolving CNS disease.	Immunity post disease good-immunity post immunization-short lived. Contraindications: previous convulsion, screaming episodes, collapse, anaphylaxis thrombocytopenia, T > 105° or "hard" CNS Sx's	-Supportive -Erythromycin therapy decreases infectivity -Close contacts erythromycin
Measles	-U.S. goal to eliminate disease by 1990 -1960 - ½ million cases/year -1980- 15,000 cases/year	live (LMV) (attenuated)	15 months old. If given prior to 12 mos. old, should be repeated.	SQ	↑T, rash-15% Depressed cell mediated immunity Seizures usually associated with ↑T and usually benign	-LMV may give false negative PPD -Egg allergy not contrain-dication -Can give to TB pt. on anti-TB treatment. -Do not give to 1. un-Rx'd TB 2. High T 3. Immunodef (decreased CMI) 4. 2-3 mos.	-LMV given c in 48 hrs. of ex-posure may modify/abort disease -IG will abort/ modify dis. if given c /in 6 da. of exposure

Disease	Reason For Vaccine	Type Of Vaccine	Immunization Schedule	Route	Side Effects	Other	Rx
Mumps	-Highly contagious -Aseptic meningitis Orchitis 15% Oophoritis	Live attenuated	15 mos.	SQ	↑T Rash Parotitis-CNS rare	-Not recommended in preg. -Can have meningitis w/o parotitis -Should immunize all w/o hx of mumps	Ig if pregnant or immuno-compromised.
Rubella	Congenital rubella	Live-attenuated	15 mos.	SQ	-Rash 10% -Lymphadenopathy 20% -↑T 4% -Joint pain (most common in adults) -Peripheral neuropathy-rare	-Contraindications 1. Pregnancy 2. Altered immunity -May be given to: 1. children of preg. women 2. nursing mothers -Ig can be used in immunocompromised host & pregnancy -Reinfection after disease/immun. occurs but does not cause viremia & not detrimental to fetus.	Ig if pregnant or immuno-compromised.

Disease	Reason For Vaccine	Type Of Vaccine	Immunization Schedule	Route	Side Effects	Other	Rx
Polio	-Paralytic polio develops in 1-2% of pt's infected	Salk-killed IPV	2, 4, 6, 18 mos. & Preschool	SQ	-None	-IPV preferred for adults -Premies get OPV @ 2 mos. post birth (if still in hosp. give on discharge) -IPV prevents dis. not infection or intestinal carriage -OPV shed in GI tract resulting in possible 2° immunization of non-immune contacts -OPV shed in oro-pharynx 1-3 weeks -OPV contraindicated in immuno-suppressed and their household contacts-give *them* IPV -avoid in preg. if possible adults get salk vaccine	
		Sabin-live attenuated (OPV)	2, 4 18 mos. Preschool	Oral	-Vaccine associated Paralytic disease -Transient suppressor of TB sensitivity		
Haemophilus H. influenzae type B	Important cause of meningitis, epiglottitis, arthritis, pneumonia and cellulitis in young children	Polysaccharide	24 mos. of age	IM	Local reactions: fever anaphylactoid reaction-rare	-Vaccine not protec-tive under 18 months of age -Protection best if vaccinated at or after 24 months of age	

SPECIFICALLY INDICATED IMMUNIZATIONS

Disease	Reason For Vaccine	Type Of Vaccine	Immunization Schedule	Route	Side Effects	Other	Rx
Pneumococcal Infection	-Asplenia -Splenic Dysf. -Chronic Dis. predisposing to pneumo. inf. -Institutionalization	Polyvalent Polysaccharide	1 dose (in adults) > 2 yr. old	SQ/IM	Erythema - 50% Mild pain - 50% Anaphylaxis $5/16^6$ 2nd dose causes reactions in adults	Contains 23 types responsible for 90% of pn. dis. in U.S. -Respond to vaccine in 2-3 weeks -Booster **not** recommended -Safety in pregnancy not known -Avoid in 1st trimester -Recommended for CHD chronic lung dis. chronic renal dis. Diabetes Mellitus chronic severe anemia compromised immune system	PCN

Disease	Reason For Vaccine	Type Of Vaccine	Immunization Schedule	Route	Side Effects	Other	Rx
Meningococcal Dis	-Not routinely used in U.S.	Polysaccharide	single dose	SQ	- ↑ T - rarely	-Vac. against A & C -C Dis. most common in infants but C vac. not effective B causes most dis. but no vaccine against B	PCN
Hepatitis B	High risk groups 1. Homosexuals 2. Dialysis pts/ workers 3. Medical personnel	Inactivated HB_sAg	3 doses	IM	Local Rx "Flu-like" symptoms	Not assoc. with AIDS No effect on Hb_sAg pts. or pts. with antibody to HB_sAg May abort/modify illness if given post-exposure Can be given with Hepatitis B immune globulin	
Yellow Fever	Endemic in much of Africa, Central and S. America Mortality 5-40%	Live-attenuated 1. 17 D vaccine 2. Dakar vaccine (not used in U.S.)	1 dose	SQ	17 D 1. Headache 5-10% 2. Myalgia 5-10% 3. Slight T 5-10% 4. Encephalitis-rare Dakar 1-5 % develop encephalitis	Should not be administered to children < 6 mos. old Appears to be effective for at least 15 years Should not be given to egg-sensitive individuals	

Disease	Reason For Vaccine	Type Of Vaccine	Immunization Schedule	Route	Side Effects	Other	Rx
Influenza	-High infectivity -High mortality	Killed	Adults - 1 dose whole virus vaccine 12 yr. - 1 dose split if previous vaccinated -Rec. changes ea. year 6 mos.-3 yrs.- ½ dose split		↑T Allergic Rx-rare Guillaine-Barre Risk increases with age		Prophylaxis Amantadine HC1 70% effective against Inf A taken daily for duration of epidemic or 10-14 days after immunization
Rabies	-Fatal -No effective Rx	Killed	HDCV - days 0, 3, 7, 14, 28 If had pre-exposure immunization then give 2 doses, 3 days apart	IM	-Local reaction 44% -Mild systemic 20%	-Can be given during pregnancy -HRIG given c̄ 1st shot -Duck embryo vac. alternative SQ 21 doses high rate of side effects	None successful
BCG	-Not routinely used in U.S.	Live Attenuated	< 1 mo. ½ dose > 1 yr. 1 dose	Intra-dermal	-Most common in infants -Ulcers -Lymphadenopathy	-BCG - results in loss of skin test -Don't give to immunocom-promised -Avoid in pregnancy -Recent study suggests not as effective as originally thought	INH Rifampin PAS Ethambutol etc.

NEW AND EXPERIMENTAL VACCINES

Diseases	Reason For Vaccine	Type Of Vaccine	Comments	Treatment
Varicella	Can be life-threatening in immuno-compromised patients (e.g. A.L.L.)	Live Attenuated	Effective in preventing or modifying disease in children with leukemia who are in remission Does not appear to result in increased incidence of zoster	ARA-A Acyclovir
Rotavirus	Major source of morbidity/ mortality in infants in third world nations	Oral	Initial trials suggest it is effective in reducing infection rate and incidence of clinically significant diarrhea.	Supportive

IMMUNE GLOBULINS

<table>
<tr><th>Specific IG</th><th>Dose</th></tr>
<tr><td>Hepatitis B Immune Globulin</td><td>Neonate with HBsAg positive mother-0.5 ml as soon after the birth as possible, then begin hepatitis B vaccine regimen

Other individuals exposed to Hepatitis B 0.06 ml/kg as soon as possible after exposure</td></tr>
<tr><td>Varicella-Zoster Immune Globulin
Used in patients with leukemia, lymphoma, immunosuppressive therapy (> 2 mg/Kg/day prednisone or equivalent), immune deficient states, and infants born to mothers whose first clinical sign of varicella occured 5 days or less before delivery or 48 hours or less after delivery.</td><td>125 units/10Kg weight
(minimum dose 125 units)
(maximum dose 625 units)</td></tr>
<tr><td>Tetanus Immune Globulin</td><td>250-500 IU for all significant wounds in patients who have received 2 or fewer doses of vaccine (infiltrate part of dose around wound)

3,000 IU for clinical tetanus</td></tr>
<tr><td>Rabies Immune Globulin</td><td>20 IU/Kg

give 1st does of vaccine at same time part of dose of immune globulin should be infiltrated around bite site</td></tr>
</table>

ISOLATION PROCEDURES

Type of Isolation	Examples of Applicable Diseases	Procedure
Strict	Rubella (congenital) Varicella	Private room Gowns and masks Good hand washing Gloves desirable (If parents are not susceptible consideration can be given to allowing them to visit without precautions as long as they do not come into contact with other patients)
Contact	Herpes simplex Scalded Skin syndrome	Private room Gowns, mask, gloves for those coming into contact with patient Good hand washing
Respiratory	Pertussis Measles Mumps	Private room Mask - if person is susceptible to the illness Good hand washing
Drainage and Secretion	draining wounds conjunctivitis zoster	Private room Gowns and gloves for direct patient contact Good hand washing
Enteric	Salmonella Shigella Cholera Hepatitis Viral Meningitis AIDS	Private room not necessary (can put hepatitis patient in private room) Good hand washing
Blood	Malaria AIDS Hepatitis B, non A-non B	Label blood "isolation" Clean blood spills promptly Handle needles, syringes and blood stained items with special care Good hand washing Gloves

REVIEW QUESTIONS

1.) Match Column A with answers in Column B. (Each answer can be used more than once.)

A
1. DPT vaccine
2. OPV vaccine
3. MMR vaccine
4. H. influenzae vaccine
5. Pneumococcal vaccine
6. Hepatitis vaccine
7. Varicella vaccine

B
A. 3 shot regimen should begin soon after birth if mother is a carrier
B. Most side effects attributable to one component of this combined vaccine
C. Live attenuated, given around 15 months of age
D. Valuable in children with leukemia, this vaccine is live attenuated
E. Not very effective during first 2 years of life
F. Live attenuated vaccine which is associated rarely with paralysis and death

2.) High titer antibody is available against _________, _________, _________, and _________.

3.) Rifampin appears to be reasonably effective prophylaxis for household contacts of patients with _________ and _________ infections.

4.) Match Column A with Column B

A
A. Contact isolation
B. Secretion and drainage isolation
C. Strict isolation
D. Respiratory isolation
E. Blood precautions
F. Enteric isolation

B
1. Herpes simplex
2. Varicella
3. Pertusis
4. Zoster
5. Malaria
6. Viral meningitis

ABBREVIATIONS

OPV	oral polio vaccine
IPV	inactivated polio vaccine
preg	pregnancy
c̄	with
w/o	without
mo	months
—	negative
+	positive
↑ T	fever
hx	history
Ig	immune globulin
PCN	penicillin
erythro	erythromycin
⋈	anti
Tig	tetanus immune globulin
IM	intramuscularly
Sq	subcutaneously
pn	pneumococcal
Inf	influenzae
HDCV	human diploid cell vaccine
HRIG	human rabies immune globulin

LABORATORY DIAGNOSIS OF INFECTION

Medicine has become increasingly dependent on the laboratory for assistance in making diagnoses. The identification of infectious disease etiologies depends on efficient, reliable, and experienced microbiological, viral and serological laboratories.

This chapter will cover some of the essentials of laboratory diagnosis. It is not designed to make the reader competent at performing all of these methods. Rather this chapter is intended to provide a basic understanding of the tests to order as a clinician, of the limitations of various tests and of their appropriateness in a given clinical situation.

ROUTINE LABORATORY DIAGNOSTIC TOOLS

Bacterial Cultures

The gold standard of laboratory diagnosis of infection is the culture. In experienced hands cultures are reliable, reproducible and consistent.

In the microbiology laboratory three different types of media are used to culture bacteria. Enrichment media allow the growth of fastidious organisms. They contain growth factors which are needed by certain bacteria. Thus, blood agar is used to grow streptococci and certain anaerobes; and heated blood agar (chocolate) is used for Neisseria and Haemophilus. Selective media contain inhibitors of bacterial growth. Inhibitors used include salts, antibiotics and dyes. Examples of selective media include Thayer-Martin agar which allows the growth of *Neisseria gonorrhea* but inhibits the growth of most other bacteria of the genitourinary tract and yeast, selenite which allows the growth of Salmonellae species but not most other bacteria; and phenylethyl alcohol which allows the growth of Gram positive but not Gram negative bacteria. The third type of medium is differential media. This allows a degree of differentiation between various bacteria growing on the same plate. MacConkey agar is a differential medium that uses lactose fermentation to distinguish between bacteria. Lactose fermenters (like *E. coli*) turn pink while non-fermenters like staphylococcus are colorless. Certain bacteria do not grow well or at all on the routine type media discussed so far. These require highly specialized media. Examples are Bordet-Gengou agar for *Bordetella pertussis,* Fletcher's medium for Leptospira, Lowenstein-Jensen for *Mycobacterium tuberculosis* and Loeffler's medium for *Corynebacterium diphtheriae.*

Chlamydia can be difficult to grow. It has intracellular growth requirements and therefore, cannot be cultured on routine culture media. In the past, the most common method of diagnosing chlamydia was by inoculation of chick embryo yolk sacs. This procedure was tedious, and subject to contamination. Recently, cell culture lines have been identified that can support the growth of chlamydia. Hela cells and McCoy cells are now used and are more sensitive than the yolk sac cultures. After incubation, the cells are then stained with iodine or fluorescent conjugate to identify the chlamydial inclusions.

Viral Cultures

Viruses are, in general, cultured in cell cultures. Diagnosis can usually be made based on the cell lines in which the virus grows and the type of cytopathic effect (CPE) the virus has. CMV, for example, may take up to four weeks to grow. Infected cells will appear rounded and refractile and can be seen to grow in plaques on top of the cell sheet. Lysis does not occur. In contrast, varicella zoster virus will frequently grow in 4-21 days and cause plaque areas of large granular cells with lysis in the center of the plaque. *Herpes simplex* is a rapidly growing virus and cytopathology can often be seen in 24 hours. Characteristically, there is ballooning of infected cells. Plaque formation is followed by lysis of the cells. Rubella virus does not cause any cytopathic effect in the cell cultures that are routinely used. Identification of rubella is therefore made by challenging with echo 11 virus the cells infected with what is suspected to be rubella. If CPE occurs (rounded refractible cells 1–4 days after echo challenge) the culture is negative for rubella.

Not all hospitals have viral culture capabilities. Where available, the information obtained can be very useful. When used in combination with some of the rapid diagnostic techniques available, viral diagnoses can frequently be made within 48–72 hours. As more anti-viral agents become available, the importance of an accurate viral diagnosis will increase.

Fungal Culture

The diagnosis of fungal infections can be critical, especially to immunocompromised patients. Some fungi will stain Gram positive with Gram stain, but can be distinguished based on their larger size. India ink, potassium hydroxide and antigen detection methods can also be useful. Confirmation of suspected diagnoses is best done with fungal cultures. Culture media used include Sabouraud's dextrose agar, inhibitory mold agar that contains chloramphenicol to surpress bacteria, brain heart infusion agar with chloramphenicol and cyclohexamide (prevents growth of contaminating fungi and cryptococci) and biphasic blood culture medium (for filamentous fungi, like aspergilla). Some fungi are slow growers and may take two or more weeks to grow.

Stool Examination for Ova and Parasites

Stool for parasites should be examined as freshly as possible. Stool should be examined unstained in a saline preparation, and stained with various iodine solutions. If the parasite is not successfully visualized, various concentration methods are available to increase the yield. Both the zinc sulfate method and the formol-ether method can be used to concentrate the specimen. Iron hematoxylin or trichrome stain can be used to increase the amount of detail one can see and also will make the preparation permanent. Identification is made by recognition of characteristic ova, cysts or worms in feces.

NON-SPECIFIC TESTS FOR INFECTION

Many tests are available which can assist in deciding whether or not we are dealing with an infection in a given patient. Other tests may help us decide whether or not we are dealing with a bacterial etiology. None of these non-specific tests for infection are foolproof and therefore the results obtained from them must be used in conjunction with other laboratory tests, clinical assessment and history.

Nitro Blue Tetrazolium Dye Test (NBT)

This is a test of neutrophil function and activity. NBT dye is yellow, and when phagocytized *in vitro* by neutrophils, is reduced to a blue-black deposit. In the unstimulated NBT test, there will be an increased number of neutrophils that reduce NBT when infection is present. The test is more frequently used to look for neutrophil dysfunction such as is seen in chronic granulomatous disease (CGD). When CGD is suspected, a stimulated NBT test is done. Decreased numbers of neutrophils that reduce NBT are seen.

In evaluating patients for infection with the NBT test, false positives can occur in patients with acute myocardial infarction, inflammatory bowel disease, and neoplasms. False negatives can be seen in bacterial arthritis, meningitis, sickle-cell anemia patients, patients with lupus erythematosus as well as patients taking salicylates or corticosteroids.

Limulus Lysate Assay (LLA)

In vitro, endotoxin causes gelling of lysates of amebocytes from limulus polyphemus (horseshoe crab). The detection of endotoxin could screen for Gram negative infection. While the test is not reliable when using sera, it appears to provide a reasonably reliable indication of the presence of endotoxin in the cerebrospinal fluid. The test is reasonably fast, practical and easy to do. From Gram negative meningitis, it appears to be as reliable as the Gram stain.

Erythrocyte Sedimentation Rate (ESR)

ESR is a non-specific measure of active disease. In general, it is of more value in following the response to therapy or progress of the disease than in making specific diagnoses.

Erythrocytes will normally sediment in plasma because of their density. Red cell aggregates will increase the rate of sedimentation. The ESR is the distance that the red cells fall per unit of time, usually millimeters/hours. Red cells usually do not aggregate because they repel one another due to their negative charge. However, in the presence of certain plasma proteins, the change is decreased and aggregation occurs. The presence of fibrinogen, alpha globulins or gamma globulins will result in red cell aggregation and an increased ESR. Abnormally shaped red cells will not effectively aggregate; thus the ESR may not increase if sickle cells, anisocytosis, spherocytosis or acanthocytosis is present. *REMEMBER:* Anemia often results in an elevated ESR and polycytemia may falsely lower the ESR. Blood sugar, calcium or phosphorous does not affect the ESR. Bile salts and an increased blood urea nitrogen decrease the ESR and cholesterol increases the ESR. Anti-inflammatory drugs can decrease the ESR. An elevated ESR can be seen in a wide variety of diseases, infectious and non-infectious. In general, the ESR is elevated during the acute or active phases of disease, then tapers off toward normal during therapy or during remissions. Non-infectious diseases associated with elevated ESR include anemias, neoplasms, inflammatory bowel disease, collagen vascular diseases, glomerulonephritis, nephrosis, hemolyticuremic syndrome, thyroid disease, burns and surgery.

Many clinicians use ESR less frequently for making diagnoses than for following the diseases. For example, patients with acute osteomyelitis or endocarditis will frequently show a decreased ESR if given effective treatment. A modification of the ESR called the zeta sedimentation rate requires less blood and is more rapid. It correlates well with the ESR.

C-reactive Protein (CRP)

C-reactive protein is an abnormal alpha globulin found in patients with infections, as well as in patients with non-infectious inflammatory diseases. This protein disappears when the infection or inflammatory process has subsided. There appears to be increasing evidence for its usefulness in certain situations to distinguish bacterial from viral infection. CRP rises rapidly with the onset of neonatal bacterial sepsis and meningitis and parallels the course of the disease. It has been suggested that a return of the CRP occurs in treatment failures and relapses. CRP is rapid and relatively inexpensive. CRP should not be used as the sole criteria for diagnosis of bacterial disease, nor is it wise to base duration of therapy solely on this one test. Nevertheless, in conjunction with other clinical and laboratory data, CRP may be useful, especially in the neonate.

Orosomucoid (O) and Prealbumin (PreA)

Both orosomucoid and prealbumin are acute phase reactants; that is, like CRP they are proteins that respond to inflammation. Measurement of O and PreA may be useful in evaluations of neonates for sepsis. PreA is actually a "negative acute phase reactant" because in the septic neonate, the levels of PreA fall. PreA is also a reflection of nutritional status. O increases in the presence of inflammation. Available data suggests that CRP is a more rapid acute phase reactant than either O or PreA. These proteins may be useful in following the course of the disease and the response to therapy.

White Blood Cell Count (WBC), Hemolysis, Thrombocytopenia

There are many causes of hemolysis. Infected patients may show evidence of hemolysis. This is especially true of patients with mycoplasma or *Haemophilus influenzae* infections. The WBC count has been used extensively to assist in the diagnosis of infection. Total white cell count, ratios of bands to total neutrophils, and neutrophil counts have all been used to assess for infection. While a rise in total WBC and an increase in the percentage of bands frequently suggest bacterial infection, it is important to remember that low-total white cell counts can also occur, especially in the presence of overwhelming or serious infection. In contrast, viral infections frequently cause a modest WBC depression or are found in normal numbers. The distinction is not cut and dry. Occasionally viral infections may have an elevated WBC, especially early in their course. White cell morphology may also be helpful, especially in neonates. Vacuolization and toxic granulations can be seen in the blood from neonates with bacterial infection. Thrombocytopenia is also seen in infected infants and children. It is most strongly associated with septicemia. None of these blood determinants make the diagnosis of infection. They must be used in conjunction with other laboratory studies and with clinical data in deciding the likelihood that a patient is infected.

Gram Stain

The Gram stain is an easy rapid method of determining the presence of bacteria in body fluids. It can also be useful to determine the type of bacteria when the staining technique is done properly.

The first step is to make a thin smear of the material to be examined onto a slide. It is then air dried and heat fixed. The slide is then covered with crystal violet for at least 10 seconds. This dye will stain all bacteria and yeast. Rinse the slide with tap water and then flood the slide with Gram's iodine and allow to stand for at least 10 seconds. The iodine will make the crystal violet permanent on the Gram positive bacteria. After rinsing the slide again, decolorize with 95% ethanol until the ethanol is colorless. Rinse again and cover the slide for 10 seconds with safranin which stains all bacteria and yeast. Rinse, blot dry and examine on a microscope. Those bacteria that are Gram positive will appear purple. Those that are Gram negative will appear red. In experienced hands the test is rapid and reliable. *REMEMBER:* Negative Gram stains do not rule out bacterial infection.

Acridine Orange Stain

Acridine orange is a fluorochrome. It stains nucleic acids of somatic cells, bacteria and other microorganisms. At the proper pH, bacteria will stain orange. The stain has also been used to identify *Trichimonas vaginalis* and malarial parasites. The prepared stain is flooded over an air dried heat fixed slide and allowed to sit for 2 minutes. It is then rinsed, dried and examined under a microscope. This technique provides less information than the Gram stain, but at least in some hands is significantly more sensitive for the detection of the presence of bacteria in a specimen.

RAPID METHODS OF DIAGNOSING INFECTION

The gold standard for laboratory diagnosis of infections in most situations are the culture techniques. In most situations, traditional culture techniques require at least 24 hours before a reliable identification of the organism can be made. As clinicians, we seek faster yet reliable ways of making the diagnosis. The result has been the emergence of many rapid laboratory tests that are designed to provide valuable information sooner than can be provided by routine cultures. This section will deal with some of the more practical and available methods.

Counterimmunoelectrophoresis (CIE)

CIE is one of the most widely used forms of rapid diagnosis. The test is used to identify antigen in body fluids. Its primary clinical use has been to identify bacterial antigen in cerebrospinal fluid, urine and blood using commercially available antisera. The basic principle of CIE is migration of antigen (negatively changed) and antibody to opposite poles in an electric field on a buffered semisolid gel. Where they meet, a precipitin band will form if the antibody is specific for the antigen being tested. Unfortunately, false negatives result from insufficient antigen concentration, insufficient negative charge on the antigen, or high molecular weight. False positives may result from epitopes (similar antibody-combining sites) among different bacteria. CIE is most frequently used to identify *Haemophilus influenzae, Streptococcus pneumoniae, Neisseria meningitidis* and Group B streptococcus. Osmotically concentrated urine appears to give the best yield. Blood, CSF, and other body fluids may also be used.

Latex Agglutination (LA) and Coagglutination (CA)

Both LA and bacterial CA are antigen detecting techniques. LA is done by using antibody coated latex particles. In the presence of specific antigen, the latex particles will agglutinate upon incubation. LA may be more sensitive than CIE. False positives related to the presence of rheumatoid factor have been reported. Common uses include the identification of *H. influenzae, Strep. pneumoniae, N. meningitides,* Group B streptococcus, *Cryptococcus neoformans* and Group A streptococcus. Recently T.B. meningitis has been successfully diagnosed using LA.

Bacterial coagglutination makes use of Protein A, a protein found in the cell wall of *staphylococcus aureus.* This protein binds the Fc fragment of many IgG immunoglobulins. Thus, heat-inactivated *S. aureus* that is coated with antibody will bind antigen to the Fab sites resulting in the agglutination of the staphylococci. The sensitivity of this test appears to be similar to that of LA.

Immunofluorescent Assays (IFA)

IFA is a sensitive test used primarily for viral detection, identification of Rocky Mountain Spotted Fever and pertussis. The test uses antibody conjugated to a fluorescent dye like fluorescein or rhodamine. The conjugated antibody is allowed to react with the specimen being tested. After free conjugated antibody is washed away, the presence of specific fluorescence indicates the presence of the antigen. This test has been particularly useful in diagnosing diseases caused by the herpes group of viruses, respiratory viruses and *B. pertussis* among others. The test, when done by well trained personnel, is very sensitive. False results are not uncommon with inexperienced personnel. In addition, the test requires some expensive equipment which will further limit its availability. Fluorescent methods can be used to detect antibody as well as antigen, and is therefore useful in quantitative antibody determinations.

Radioimmunassay (RIA) and Enzyme-Linked Immunosorbent Assay (ELISA)

RIA and ELISA are both very sensitive methods to identify small quantities of antigen and to measure antibody titers. Antigen is detected by RIA by tagging antibody with a radioisotope and then allowing it to react with the specimen suspected of containing the antigen being sought. ELISA is an antibody-enzyme system. If the antigen being sought is present, an antigen-antibody-enzyme complex will form. When substrate is added, it will react with the enzyme producing a color change which indicates the presence of the antigen. ELISA appears to be as sensitive as RIA and has gradually replaced RIA in many instances. ELISA is commonly used for the diagnosis of *Herpes simplex,* hepatitis A and B, respiratory syncytical virus, Epstein-Barr virus, varicella-zoster, candida, and *H. influenzae.*

Acid-Fast Staining (AFS)

Acid-fast staining is done to identify mycobacteria. More than one method exists to do AFS. Basically, the slide with the smear is stained with carbolfuchsin solution for 30 minutes and then drained and decolorized with 1% acid alcohol for an additional 30 minutes. The slide is rinsed and then counterstained with methylene blue. Acid-fast organisms stain red. Another standard method (Ziehl-Neelson) requires heating of the slide. The results are the same.

Mycobacterial cultures may need to be incubated for weeks before they become positive thus making AFS important in making a presumptive diagnosis. Sputums and gastric aspirates are the most common sources of specimens for suspected pulmonary tuberculosis.

India Ink

Sediment from centrifuged CSF can be stained with India Ink to make a presumptive diagnosis of cryptococcal meningitis. CSF fluid sediment is mixed with an equal volume of India Ink on a slide. By this technique, about 50% of patients with cryptococcal meningitis will demonstrate the presence of cryptococcus. The organism appears to have a doubly refractile cell wall, well outlined capsule, and refractile cytoplasmic inclusions. Latex agglutination methods are available for diagnosing cryptococcal meningitis and are more sensitive than India Ink.

REFERENCES

Bennish M, Beem MO, Ormiste V: C-reactive protein and zeta sedimentation ratio as indicators of bacteremia in pediatric patients. J Pediatr 1984; 104:729–732.

Bennish M, Vardiman J, Beem M: The zeta sedimentation ratio in children. J Pediatr 1984; 104:249–251.

Chmel H: Rapid methods for the diagnosis of infectious diseases: An overview. Clinical Microbiology, 1981; 3:138–140.

Cornall CJ, Pepple JM, Moxon ER, et al: C-reactive protein in spinal fluid of children with meningitis. J Pediatr 1981; 99:365–369.

Friedman AD, Ray CG: Rapid laboratory diagnosis of infection. Pediatric Infectious Disease, 1982; 1:366–373.

Hanson LA, Jodal U, Sabel KG, et al: The diagnostic value of C-reative protein. Pediatric Infectious Diseases, 1983; 2:87–90.

Kleiman MB, Reynolds JK, Watts NH, et al: Superiority of acridine orange stain versus Gram stain in partially treated bacterial meningitis. J Pediatr 1984; 104:401–404.

Lascari AD: The erythrocyte sedimentation rate. Pediatric Clinics of North America, 1972; 19(4):1113–1120.

Minnich L, Ray CG: Comparison of direct immunofluorescent staining of clinical specimens for respiratory virus antigens with conventional isolation techniques. Journal of Clinical Microbiology, 1980; 12:391–394.

Naiman HC, Albritton WL: Counterimmunoelectrophoresis in the diagnosis of acute infection. Journal of Infectious Diseases, 1980; 142:524–531.

Philip A: Acute-phase proteins in neonatal infection. J Pediatr 1984; 105:-940–942.

Richman D, Schmidt N, Plotkin S, et al: Summary of a workshop on new and useful methods in rapid viral diagnosis. Journal of Infectious Diseases, 1984; 150:941–951.

Sann L, Bienvenu F, Bienvenu J, et al: Evolution of serum prealbumin, C-reative protein, and orosomucoid in neonates with bacterial infection. J Pediatr 1984; 105:977-981.

Whittle HC, Tugwell P, Egler LJ, et al: Rapid bacteriological diagnosis of pyogenic meningitis by latex agglutination. Lancet 1974; 1:619–621.

Yolken R: Enzyme-linked immunosorbent assay (ELISA): A practical tool for rapid diagnosis of viruses and other infectious agents. Yale Journal of Biol. Med., 1980; 53:85–92.

KEY POINTS

1. The gold standard for laboratory identification of the etiology of infection is the culture.
2. Antigen detection techniques offer the advantages of being rapid and of being able to determine etiology in patients already on antimicrobial therapy, but false positive and false negative results occur.
3. The identification of viral etiologies can be done reliably and quickly with the combined use of viral cultures and antigen detection methods. As more viral infections become treatable, this ability for rapid, reliable viral detection will increase in importance.
4. The primary use for the nitrobluetetrazolium dye test is in demonstrating neutrophil dysfunction as is seen in chronic granulomatous disease.
5. The erythrocyte sedimentation rate is, in general, more valuable when used to follow the course of a disease or the response to therapy than it is in the diagnosis of disease.

6. In skilled hands, the Gram stain is a rapid method that provides information as to whether bacteria are present; whether they are Gram positive or negative; and based on morphology a preliminary identification of what organism is involved. In unskilled hands, much misinformation may result. Whenever possible, Gram stain results should be confirmed by culture or other methods.

REVIEW QUESTIONS

1.) Most rapid diagnostic techniques used to identify pathogens are designed to detect ______________.

2.) The three major classifications of bacterial media are ______________, ______________, ______________ .

3.) The presence of virus in cell cultures (tissue cultures) is usually detected by the presence of ______________.

4.) A stimulated nitro blue tetrazolium test is useful to detect ______________.

5.) ______________ detects the presence of endotoxin.

6.) For each of the conditions listed below, identify whether the affect would be to increase or decrease the sedimentation rate:
A) Anemias ______________
B) Burns ______________
C) Bile salts ______________
D) Cholesterol ______________
E) Collagen vascular disease ______________
F) Polycythemia ______________

7.) Match the test from column A with the appropriate description in column B

A	B
A. Counterimmunoelectrophoresis	1. Gram positive and negative bacteria appear the same color
B. Gram stain	2. *E. coli* appears red
C. Limulus Lysate	3. Migration of antibody and antigen through an electric field
D. Acidine Orange	4. Stains for cryptococcus
E. Latex Agglutination	5. Detects endotoxin
F. Potassium hydroxide	6. Useful in detection of yeast and fungi
G. India ink	7. Rapid sensitive method of antigen detection using antibody coated particles

20

ANTIMICROBIAL AGENTS

ANTIBIOTICS

This chapter is intended to give the reader a basic understanding of some of the commonly used antibiotics, as well as some of the newer antibiotics. Indications for use, potential indications for use, precautions and toxicities will be discussed.

CHLORAMPHENICOL

Indications

Choramphenicol is a broad-spectrum antibiotic that has played a major role in the treatment of pediatric patients with serious infections. Several broad generalizations can be made regarding the spectrum of coverage of chloramphenicol. With the exception of *Pseudomonas,* most aerobic bacteria are sensitive to chloramphenicol; although within each species of bacteria there is wide variability. In addition, over 90% of anaerobes are sensitive. Chloramphenicol has also been demonstrated to be effective against some mycoplasma, chlamydia, rickettsia and schistosomes. It has little or no activity against fungi, mycobacteria, viruses and protozoa. In general, the drug is bacteriostatic although it appears to be bacteriocidal against *Haemophilus influenzae, Streptococcous pneumoniae* and *Neisseria meningitidis* in the appropriate dose.

There are oral and parental forms of chloramphenicol. The oral form is absorbed very well resulting in serum levels equal to or greater than that achieved parenterally. The drug is metabolized in the liver and excreted primarily by the kidneys. The metabolism of the drug varies greatly from individual to individual. The half-life has been reported to vary from two hours to twelve hours. Desirable peak serum levels are 10 to 25 ug/ml. This is usually achieved with doses of 75 mg/kg/day divided into four doses, except in the neonate where smaller doses are usually given. After an intravenous dose of chloramphencol, peak serum levels are seen within 1 to 2 hours of the dose; after oral therapy the peak is usually reached in 2 to 3 hours. *REMEMBER:* Because of the individual variation in chloramphenicol metabolism, especially in neonates and infants, it is important to monitor chloramphenicol serum levels. Chloramphenicol distributes to virtually all body tissues. It crosses the placenta and can also be found in breast milk. The drug crosses into the cerebrospinal fluid and can achieve levels of 35% to 65% of serum levels, regardless of the degree of meningeal inflammation. It also enters the white blood cell and is active intracellularly.

In pediatrics, the primary use for chloramphenicol is in meningitis patients beyond the neonatal period. The most common organisms encountered in bacterial meningitis in children are *H. influenzae, N. meningiditis* and *S. pneumoniae;* all of which are sensitive to chloramphenicol. Chloramphenicol is usually used in combination with penicillin or ampicillin pending culture and sensitivity results. Recently, several new cephalosporins have been approved which may serve as alternatives to this standard antibiotic combination. Ampicillin resistant *H. influenzae* is not uncommon, and there have been infrequent reports of chloramphenicol resistant *H. influenzae.* Thus the combination of ampicillin and chloramphenicol is desirable initial therapy until sensitivities are known.

Other uses of chloramphenicol include serious *H. influenzae, S. pneumoniae* or *N. meningiditis* infection in penicillin allergic patients; brain abscesses; anaerobic infections and intraocular infections. Chloramphenicol is lipid soluble and therefore penetrates into aqueous and vitreous humors. This can occur even after topical application. Its penetration intraocularly is superior to penicillin, cephalosporins and aminoglycosides.

Adverse Reactions

Chloramphenicol interacts with other drugs that are also liver metabolized. Examples include phenobarbitol which will stimulate liver microsomal enzyme activity and decrease the chloramphenicol serum level; and acetominophen which will increase the half-life of chloramphenicol. Patients on dilantin who receive chloramphenicol may demonstrate increased dilantin levels.

Chloramphenicol may also have hematologic effects. Aplastic anemia is often fatal and is not dose related. It often does not occur immediately and can occur after therapy has been discontinued. The actual incidence is controversial but may be about 1 per 25,000 patients receiving the drug. While this complication has occurred in identical twins, it is not yet clear whether there is a genetic predisposition. *REMEMBER:* Aplastic anemia has been reported with topical ocular application of chloramphenicol, therefore it should be reserved for therapy of intraocular infections and not used for bacterial conjunctivitis when other suitable antibiotics are available. The second type of hematologic side effect is inhibition of mitochondrial protein synthesis in the bone marrow cells. First this leads to a depression of erythropoesis and then a decrease in the myeloid cells. Rarely does this reaction lead to aplastic anemia. Usually it is reversible. Finally, in patients with G-6-PD deficiency, acute hemolytic anemia has been reported after administration of chloramphenicol.

The gray baby syndrome is seen infrequently now because we are able to monitor serum levels of chloramphenicol in neonates. The syndrome consists of vasomotor collapse, abdominal distension, a fall in blood pressure, and gray skin. The syndrome can be seen with chloramphenicol concentration of over 70 ug/ml. Exchange transfusion and charcoal column hemoperfusion have been tried to treat the syndrome; the results have been mixed.

Chloramphenicol may also cause neurologic side effects. Delirium, nightmares, encephalopathy, optic neuritis, peripheral neuropathy and asterixis have all been reported. Most of these side effects disappear with discontinuation of therapy.

Nausea, vomiting and diarrhea occur, primarily with oral therapy. Vomiting can be reduced by giving the medicine on an empty stomach. Other gastrointestinal symptoms include glossitis, mucosal candida, and very rarely, hepatitis.

In vitro chloramphenicol decreases lymphocyte tranformation and *in vivo* antibody synthesis is decreased. It is not clear if these immunologic changes are of clinical significance. Other side effects include allergic skin rashes, anaphylaxis, delayed wound healing, growth arrest and alopecia.

Chloramphenicol can be a life-saving drug when used in treatment of serious infections caused by susceptible organisms. The side effects of therapy are potentially severe; therefore, chloramphenicol should be reserved for serious infections where the risk of treatment failure outweighs the risk of toxicity.

RIFAMPIN

Indications

Rifampin was originally isolated from a mold *Streptomyces mediteranei;* found in the soil of a french pine forest. It has a wide spectrum of activity. Rifampin is considered to be one of the most active antibiotics available for the treatment of coagulase positive and negative staphylococci. Against most other Gram positive cocci it is less active than penicillin. It has antimicrobial activity against *N. meningiditis, N. gonorrhea* and *H. influenzae.* It is very active against *Legionella pneumophilia,* and has good activity against *Clostridia difficile.* Rifampin also has very good antimycobacterial activity.

Rifampin is used for the prophylaxis against *N. meningiditis* infection and it is currently recommended for prophylaxis against *H. influenzae.* Rifampin has become a first line drug as part of combination therapy against mycobacterial infection. It has been used as part of the treatment regimen for ventricular shunt infections due to coagulase negative staphylococci and for staphylococcal endocarditis. Although rifampin has no antifungal activity alone, it enhances the activity of amphoteracin B and miconazole against candida. In the treatment of leprosy, rifampin is used in combination with Dapsone.

The drug works by inhibiting the synthesis of RNA. RNA polymerases of mammalian cells are relatively resistant to rifampin. Rifampin is relatively well absorbed after an oral dose except immediately after a meal. Blood levels tend to be somewhat lower in children than adults. The major limitation of the drug is the rapid emergence of resistance. It is because of this problem of resistance that rifampin is usually used in combination with another antibiotic in all but the shortest treatment courses.

Excretion of rifampin is about two thirds bile and one third into urine. Hepatic disease prolongs the half-life of rifampin. It is 55% protein bound. Peak levels usually occur 2 to 4 hours after the dose and blood levels are detectable even after 24 hours. The drug gets into the cerebrospinal fluid and is found in breast milk.

Adverse Reactions

Rifampin is a strong inducer of microsomal enzymes in the liver decreasing the half-life of certain drugs. Rifampin interacts with oral contraceptives increasing the risk of pregnancy while on therapy. Menstrual irregularities and amenorrhea are also seen. Rifampin also increases the rate of degradation of warfarin and other oral anticoagulants. It decreases the biological activity of glucocorticoids and can ameliorate the symptoms of Cushing's Syndrome by inducing hepatic cortisol-6-hydroxylase. Rifampin may cause symptoms of narcotic withdrawal in patients on methadone. It decreases the half-life of digitoxin. *REMEMBER:* Rifampin is excreted in urine and turns urine red. This is not an indication to stop therapy. In addition, rifampin is secreted in tears and will stain soft contact lenses.

Other side effects include mild rashes, gastrointestinal complaints including cramping, transient elevation of liver function tests, light chain proteinuria and, rarely, purpura or hepatitis.

Rifampin is immunosuppressive. Both cell-mediated immunity and antibody responses are decreased but this does not seem to be clinically significant.

High doses and intermittant doses appear to be associated with increased side effects and a flu-like illness. Patients who have tried to commit suicide by taking doses as high as 12 grams survive but their skin turns lobster-red for a few days. The dose of rifampin is 10–20 mg/kg/day divided into 1 or 2 doses per day orally.

VANCOMYCIN

Indications

Vancomycin was introduced in the 1950's as an effective anti-staphylococcal antibiotic. The drug is derived from *Streptomyces orientales.* It inhibits biosynthesis of cell wall phopholipids and peptidoglycan polymers. It also inhibits RNA synthesis. The drug is bacteriocidal in multiplying organisms.

Vancomycin is effective therapy for *Staphylococcus aureus* and *S. epidermidis* Those organisms deficient in autolysis may be relatively tolerant to the bacteriocidal action of vancomycin. In patients with tolerant organisms, the addition of other antibiotics such as rifampin may be necessary.

Other organisms sensitive to vancomycin include *Streptococcus pyogenes, Str. pneumoniae,* and microaerophilic streptococci. In addition, *Clostridia, Neisseria gonorrhoeae* and *Corynebacterium diphtheriae* are also usually susceptible at clinically obtainable concentrations. Mycobacteria, Gram negative organisms and fungi are not susceptible.

In pediatrics, the most common indications for the use of vancomycin include infections due to strains resistant to beta-lactamase-resistant penicillins and cephalosporins; patients with penicillin or cephalosporin allergy; patients who do not adequately respond to other treatment regimens when the organism is vancomycin sensitive; and certain special situations such as shunt infections or antibiotic associated pseudomembranous colitis.

Vancomycin is given intravenously. There is not a satisfactory intramuscular preparation available. Vancomycin is absorbed poorly from the gastrointestinal tract but is given orally for antibiotic associated *Clostridia difficile* pseudomembranous colitis. The parenteral drug is eliminated from the body by glomerular filtration. It is over 80% eliminated within 24 hours of dose administration. The elimination half-life varies from 2 to 10 hours with longer half-lives associated with neonates and infants.

In newborns, the recommended dose is 30 mg/kg/day divided into 2 doses during the first week of life. After that, the dose can be increased to 45 mg/kg/day divided into three doses. After the first month of life, 40 to 60 mg/kg/day of vancomycin is given. The dose is divided into 4 doses/day. Orally, vancomycin is given as 10 to 50 mg/kg/day divided into four doses.

Vancomycin perfuses poorly across uninfected meninges. Vancomycin can be given in small doses intrathecally in patients with meningitis if there is not a good response to intravenous therapy.

Adverse Reactions

Side effects include phlebitis at the site of infusion, fever, chills, rashes, leukopenia, eosinophilia and rarely, shock. Neurotoxicity occurs and is manifested by auditory nerve damage and hearing loss. If serum levels are kept below 30 ug/ml neurotoxicity is rarely seen. Dosing in infants and neonates may be particularly difficult without the assistance of pharmokinetic studies. Nephrotoxicity occurs infrequently.

CLINDAMYCIN

Indications

Clindamycin inhibits bacterial protein synthesis. It is usually bacteriostatic. The drug is effective against a broad spectrum of Gram positive organisms excluding enterococcous and Nocardia. Most but not all *Staphylococcus auerus* are sensitive to clindamycin in clinically achievable serum concentration. At achievable serum concentrations essentially all Gram negative organisms are resistant. It inhibits strain of *Toxoplasma gondii* and has been reported to be effective as part of the treatment regimen for ocular toxoplasmosis. Most clinically significant anaerobes are sensitive to clindamycin. Infrequently strains of *Bacteroides fragilis* have been resistant.

Clindamycin is indicated for the therapy of many anaerobic infections. It is effective in treating aspiration pneumonias and lung abscesses. In combination with gentamicin it is effective against a wide spectrum of mixed flora infections. It is an effective antistaphylococcal drug and has been used effectively in osteomyelitis.

Clindamycin is rapidly absorbed after oral administration and does not seem to be significantly affected by the presence of food in the stomach.

It is metabolized mainly by the liver and primarily excreted in urine and in bile. It penetrates well into most body sites although data is lacking as to achievable concentrations in the human central nervous system. The drug readily crosses the placenta and significant levels of the antibiotic are found in the fetus. The half-life of clindamycin in adults is about three hours and is not significantly affected by decreased renal function. Patients who are functionally anephric, however, should have their clindamycin dose decreased by about fifty percent. Hepatic dysfunction prolongs the half-life of clindamycin and, when possible, drug levels should be monitored in patients with liver disease.

Adverse Reactions

Pseudomembranous colitis is the best known adverse reaction of clindamycin administration, although in pediatric patients it is an infrequent finding. Pseudomembranous colitis is characterized by diarrhea, abdominal pain, fever and mucous and blood in the stools. It is believed that the overgrowth of clindamycin-resistant *Clostridrium difficile* in the gastrointestinal tract is responsible for pseudomembranous colitis. The clostridial exotoxin elaborated apparently is directly responsible for the symptoms. This complication, although rare in pediatrics, can be fatal. Oral vancomycin is used to treat the condition. Metronidazole has also been used successfully. Diarrhea without other signs of pseudomembranous colitis is seen more frequently, yet in pediatrics is still a relatively infrequent side effect.

Ampicillin-like skin rashes can be seen in patients receiving clindamycin. Other reactions that have been reported include Stevens-Johnson syndrome (erythema multiforme major), itching, drug fever, pruritis, urticaria and hematologic abnormalities including thrombocytopenia and granulocytopenia. Anaphylaxis has also been reported. There have been occasional reports of elevation of serum liver enzymes in patients receiving clindamycin.

THE PENICILLINS

General Principles

Pencillins are, in general, active against bacteria that contains peptidoglycan in their cell wall that is accessible to the antibiotic. The penicillins interfere with the biosynthesis of cross-linkages between peptide chains in actively growing cells resulting in lysis of the cell. The penicillins (and cephalosporins) bind to protein beneath the cell wall and inhibit cell wall production.

Because many penicillins are inactivated or destroyed in the stomach, they are not suitable oral agents. Those penicillins that are resistant to gastric acid pass through the stomach and are absorbed in the duodenum. Peak serum levels after oral administration usually occur within an hour of administering the dose.

Most penicillins are excreted in an active form in the urine. Some are also excreted, in part, in the bile. In general, the half-life of the penicillins is short. Most of them are widely distributed throughout the body, including to variable extents, to the cerebrospinal fluid.

Naturally Occuring Penicillins

Aqueous Crystalline Penicillin G (ACPG)

ACPG comes as either a sodium or potassium preparation. It rapidly produces a high serum peak. Because of some degradation in the stomach it is not ideal as an oral preparation (phenoxymethyl penicillin is preferred for oral administration). Nevertheless, it is an effective parenteral drug. The half-life is approximately 30 minutes but increases with decreasing renal function. ACPG is about 50% bound to plasma proteins. Potassium ACPG contains 1.7 meq of potassium per million units ACPG and sodium ACPG contains 2.3 meq of sodium per million units. Patients with renal impairment should not receive the potassium preparation. *REMEMBER:* Too rapid infusion of potassium penicillin G intravenously may result in hyperkalemia and arrhythmias.

The addition of procaine to penicillin G results in a long-acting preparation. The peak serum concentration is not as high as ACPG without the procaine. Peak concentrations after an intramuscular injection of procaine penicillin G occur after one to two hours and detectable concentrations may persist in the blood for up to 24 hours (about four times that of ACPG alone). Procaine penicillin tends to produce side effects to a greater extent than does penicillin without the procaine. Hoigné Syndrome seen immediately after the intramuscular injection of procaine penicillin G is characterized by bizarre behavior and neurologic reactions which subside spontaneously and usually rapidly (within ten minutes) after the administration of the procaine penicillin.

Benzathine penicillin G has low peak serum values but may persist in the blood for as long as four weeks. While procaine penicillin is useful for the treatment of gonorrhea and pneumococcal pneumonia, benzathine penicillin G is more appropriate for syphilis and streptococcal pharyngitis.

Phenoxymethyl Penicillin (Penicillin V)

Penicillin V (Pen V) is relatively resistant to gastric acid and is, therefore, a suitable oral agent. Higher blood levels are achieved with Pen V than with ACPG. Pen V administration usually results in peak serum levels within 30 minutes. The drug is detectable in blood up to four hours later.

Semisynthetic Penicillins

Semisynthetic penicillins are penicillinase-resistant and include methicillin, oxacillin, Nafillin, cloxacillin and dicloxacillin. Cloxacillin and dicloxacillin are oral preparations. These penicillins are penicillinase-resistant probably secondary to an effect of their acyl side chain which prevents opening of the beta-lactam ring. These drugs are synergistic with the aminoglycosides against *S. aureus*.

Methicillin

Methicillin is the least protein bound in the group of antibiotics. It is inactivated by gastric acids and therefore is not an appropriate oral agent. After parenteral administration, maximum serum levels are achieved in about 30 minutes and about half the dose is excreted unchanged by the kidneys during the first 6 hours. The drug distributes to many body sites, but does not penetrate normal meninges, and penetrates inflamed meninges unpredictably. Methicillin is less effective than penicillin G for streptococcal infections, and most enterococci are methicillin resistant. Adverse reactions associated with methicillin use include interstitial nephritis, anemia, neutropenia and granulocytopenia.

Nafcillin

Nafcillin is about 70% protein bound. Unlike methicillin, nafcillin is primarily inactivated in the liver and about 10% of it is excreted in the bile. Although all semisynthetic penicillins cross the blood-brain barrier poorly and erratically, nafcillin appears to achieve greater CSF levels than the others, in general. Nafcillin does not accumulate in anuric patients and therefore, no alteration in drug dose is required in patients with renal impairment. Adverse reactions associated with nafcillin include thrombophlebitis and elevated serum glutamic oxalecetic transaminase (SGOT).

Oxacillin

Oxacillin is about 80% protein bound. When given orally only 30% is absorbed making it less well absorbed than cloxacillin or dicloxacillin.

It is metabolized by the liver to a greater extent than methicillin but not as much as nafcillin. As a result, patients with liver impairment will need to have their dose adjusted for either nafcillin or oxacillin. Oxacillin has been associated with elevated SGOT and with granulocytopenia.

Cloxacillin and Dicloxacillin

Approximately 50% of the orally administered dose is absorbed from the gastrointestinal tract. They are about 95% protein bound. Both are effected by the presence of food in the stomach to a lesser extent than is oxacillin and are metabolized to only a small extent.

Expanded Spectrum Penicillins

Ampicillin

Ampicillin is available as an oral or a parenteral preparation. It is active against some Gram negative bacteria in addition to many Gram positive organisms. It is effective against many strains of *Hemophilus influenzae* (most beta-lactamase negative strains), *Escherichia coli, Proteus mirabilis,* shigella and salmonella. It is effective, although in general somewhat less effective *in vitro* than penicillin G, against most streptococci (including pneumonococci), Neisseria, and clostridia although these differences are usually not clinically apparent. It is often more effective against enterococci. Ampicillin is often synergistic with aminoglycosides against enterococci.

Oral administration results in peak serum concentrations in two hours, and intramuscular injection will result in peak levels being reached in about one hour. Intravenous administration provides the highest serum concentrations, and oral administration provides the lowest; usually the peak after oral administration does not exceed 3 ug/ml. Renal dysfunction will prolong the half-life. Only 10% of ampicillin is protein bound. The antibiotic concentrates in bile and in urine. Taking oral ampicillin with food does not significantly decrease serum concentrations. Ampicillin crosses uninflamed meninges poorly but crosses inflamed meninges adequately enough to treat meningitis when the drug is given in high doses. Adverse reactions associated with ampicillin include diarrhea, skin rashes and pseudomembranous colitis.

Amoxicillin

In both spectrum of coverage and chemical structure, amoxicillin is very similar to ampicillin. It is an oral preparation in the U.S. Amoxicillin is better absorbed and, given the same dose, blood levels are approximately twice those achieved by ampicillin. The incidence of diarrhea, a common side effect of ampicillin, is less frequent with amoxicillin. Except for the treatment of shigella infection, amoxicillin may be substituted for oral ampicillin in essentially all other infections. Side effects from amoxicillin are essentially the same as from ampicillin except for less frequent diarrhea with amoxicillin. Amoxicillin is also available in combination with clavulonic acid, a beta-lactamase inhibitor. Sold under the name Augmentin, the drug broadens the spectrum of amoxicillin to include many beta-lactamase producing organisms.

Carbenicillin and Ticarcillin

These antibiotics have a similar spectrum of coverage as ampicillin. In addition, they are usually effective against indole-positive *Proteus,* Enterobacter, *Morganella* and many strains of *Pseudomonas aeruginosa.* Klebsiella and most Serratia are resistant. These drugs are not as active as either penicillin G or ampicillin against most Gram positive organisms. Ampicillin is at least twice as effective against *H. influenzae* than are either carbenicillin or ticarcillin. Beta-lactamase producing organisms are relatively resistant. In general, ticarcillin is more active against *P. aeruginosa* than is carbenicillin. These drugs are bacteriocidal and about 50–60% protein bound. They are not well absorbed orally and should, therefore, be given parenterally for systemic infections. The half-life of carbenicillin is about 1 hour, and that of ticarcillin about 20% longer. Renal failure will prolong the half-lives, and if both liver and renal failure are present, the half-lives are further prolonged.

The major value of these drugs is in fighting *P. aeruginosa* infections although they may also play a role in the treatment of indole-positive *Proteus* and *Morganella.* These agents work synergistically with the aminoglycosides, especially against *Pseudomonas.* They cross the meninges in patients with meningitis and have successfully treated Pseudomonas meningitis and abscesses when the minimal inhibitory concentration (MIC) is sufficiently low. The cerebrospinal fluid concentration of these drugs must be 32 times the MIC to achieve killing. In general, breast milk concentration of these drugs is low. In the absence of biliary obstruction, the concentration of carbenicillin and ticarcillin in the bile is several times the serum concentration.Clinical situations in which these agents are used include cystic fibrosis, osteomyelitis, urinary tract infections, infected burns or decubitis ulcers, and in the neutropenic patient. The combination of these drugs with an aminoglycoside or cephalosporin has proven to be effective empiric therapy in the febrile neutropenic patient.

Hypersensitivity reactions to these antibiotics are relatively uncommon. Rashes occur. Pseudomembranous colitis occurs less frequently than with ampicillin. Abnormal platelet aggregation occurs with high concentrations of either ticarcillin or carbenicillin. Interstitial nephritis occurs with carbenicillin but less frequently than with methicillin. Carbenicillin (more commonly than ticarcillin) may produce sodium overload and hypokalemia. Transient abnormality in liver function is seen more frequently with carbenicillin than with ticarcillin. Seizures, although rare, may occur with high doses, especially in the presence of renal function. Phlebitis at the site of infusion occurs with either antibiotic.

Mezlocillin, Azlocillin and Piperacillin

These semisynthetic pencillins are derived from ampicillin. They are monosodium salts (carbenicillin and ticarcillin are disodium salts) and have relatively low sodium content. Their structure enables enhanced penetration of the bacterial cell wall, resulting in enhanced inhibition of cell-wall synthesis of dividing bacteria, but also in increased susceptibility to beta-lactamase degradation. These antibiotics are given parenterally. Less protein binding, and a shorter half-life than carbenicillin or ticarcillin characterize these three antibiotics. About 10% of these drugs are metabolized and they are primarily excreted unchanged in the urine. Their concentration in bile exceeds that of carbenicillin or ticarcillin. Mezlocillin (MEZ), azlocillin (AZ) and piperacillin (PIP) are more active against most Gram positive organisms than either ticarcillin or carbenicillin. AZ is at least eight times more effective against *P. aeruginosa* than carbencillin. It is beta-lactamase sensitive and is thus inactivated by beta-lactamase producing organisms. MEZ inhibits about 75 percent of *Klebsiella* compared with 5 percent inhibition by carbenicillin. It also has superior *H. influenzae* and *B. fragilis* activity as compared to carbenicillin. It has good enterococcal coverage. PIP has very good coverage against *Hemophilus,* many *Enterobacteriaceae,* and many anaerobes. It also has very good *Pseudomonas* coverage. AZ has less chance of causing bleeding or platelet aggregation problems. Mezlocillin can precipitate hypokalemia. Neutropenia has been reported when piperacillin is administered for long periods of time. Many of the other side effects common to the other penicillins have been reported with AZ, MEZ and PIP.

Adverse Reactions to Penicillins

There are several reactions common to all or most penicillins. These include skin rashes; diarrhea; neurologic abnormalities including seizures; hematologic abnormalities including neutrophenia; allergic reactions including anaphylaxis; drug-induced fever; and serum-sickness type reactions.

REMEMBER: Certain reactions are associated particularly with specific penicillins. Potassium penicillin G is associated with hyperkalemia and arrhythmias. Procaine penicillin is associated with Hoigné Syndrome. Skin rash, diarrhea, and pseudomembranous colitis are seen with ampicillin. Interstitial nephritis and hematologic abnormalities are associated with methicillin. Oxacillin may cause granulocytopenia and nafcillin may cause thrombophlebitis. Carbenicillin has caused sodium overload and hypokalemia as well as platelet dysfunction; and piperacillin may cause neutropenia. It is important to keep these adverse reactions in mind and monitor for them appropriately.

The Problem of Penicillin Allergy

It is estimated that at least 5 percent of patients may be skin test positive (allergic) to the penicillins. Up to 20% of patients will give a positive history of penicillin allergy. In penicillin allergic patients life-threatening complications can occur in 2 to 3 percent of acute reactions. These life-threatening reactions include hypotension, laryngeal edema, bronchospasm and cardiac dysfunction. It is estimated that anaphylactic reactions are fatal in 3 to 9 percent of cases.

Several epidemologic generalizations can be made regarding penicillin allergy. Oral administration is safer than parenteral administration. Cross-reactions among the beta-lactam antibiotics occur. Most allergic reactions occur in patients with beta-lactam antibiotics but who had no reaction to that prior exposure. Although most anaphylactic reactions occur within 30 minutes of receiving the first dose, some cases of anaphylaxis have not occured for over one hour after the dose. Very young and very old patients have less of a chance of having fatal anaphylaxis than do other patients. Gender is not a risk factor. Most fatal anaphylactic reactions occured in patients who had had no previous adverse reactions to penicillin.

Sensitization by penicillins involves several factors. Antibodies form in response to antibiotic-protein couples formed as a result of the beta-lactam rings tendency to covalently couple to proteins. The result is that virtually all patients treated with penicillins have an immunologic response. IgM and IgG responses are detectable in at least 90 percent of treated patients. IgE antibody is less frequently detectable (2 to 5 percent). Those patients who do not actively suppress their IgE response become the "penicillin allergic" patients.

Skin testing appears to be an effective way to identify patients at risk for an allergic reaction. Systemic reactions to skin testing occur but they are usually mild and infrequent. The test is reliable in patients over 12 months of age. Data is not available on infants, but since IgE induced release of mediators from mast cells can occur at birth, it is possible that the test may be reliable even in infants. Two-thirds of patients with a positive skin test will have an acute reaction when penicillin is administered. False negatives are rare. (The test will identify at least 90% of allergic patients.) Three-fourths of patients who had an allergic reaction to penicillin still have a positive skin test one year later. Only 20 percent have a positive test ten years later. Patients who no longer express IgE antibodies to penicillin can be treated with beta-lactam antibiotics. *REMEMBER:* Although macular rashes commonly seen with antibiotics like ampicillin are usually nonallergic, pruritic macular rashes may indicate drug allergy. In one study, 45 percent of patients with pruritic macular rashes were skin test positive. It is also important to remember that serum sickness, although not IgE mediated, nevertheless seems to be a marker for patients who are at risk for an allergic reaction to administration of penicillin in the future. Cross-reactions between penicillin and other penicillins and cephalosporins are a major problem, however, the frequency and degree of cross-reaction is not certain in pediatric patients.

In patients who are skin test positive for penicillins, the first consideration should be given to using non-beta-lactam antibiotics whenever possible. When life-threatening infection exists to which the penicillins are clearly the best chance for survival, patients should be desensitized prior to the administration of therapeutic doses. Desensitization can be done orally or parenterally. Oral desensitization is felt to carry less risk for severe allergic reaction. Throughout the desensitization process, intravenous access must be maintained to provide emergency therapy should a serious reaction occur. The antibiotic is administered every fifteen minutes during the desensitization process. Cutaneous reactions are common and can be treated with antihistamines. Each oral dose is double the previous dose beginning with 100 units of penicillin (or its equivalent - the oral form of the specific penicillin to be used in therapy should be used for desenitization, if available). The thirteenth dose will be approximately 400,000 units of penicillin orally. The next dose is 200,000 units subcutaneously, then 400,000 units, then 800,000 units. The seventeenth dose is 1,000,000 units I.M. A similar regimen can be used for parenteral desensitization. *REMEMBER:* During desensitization the patient must be continuously monitored and the physician must be prepared to immediately intervene to control serious reactions. Once the penicillin therapy is instituted, it is important to avoid lapses in therapy that might enable anaphylactic sensitivity to reappear.

ERYTHROMYCIN

Indications

Erythromycin is a broad spectrum macrolide antibiotic. It is produced by *Streptomyces erythraeus.* It is available as oral and parenteral preparations. Its activity is less in acidic than in alkaline environments. Protein binding of erythromycin is greater than 40%. It binds ribosomes of susceptible organisms resulting in the inhibition of protein synthesis.

The oral preparation comes as erythromycin base, sterate, estolate and ethylsuccinate, and the intravenous preparations are gluceptate and lactobionate. Intramuscular administration of erythromycin is not recommended.

Erythromycin's spectrum of activity include many Gram positive organisms, including staphylococci; *Mycoplasma; Bordetella pertussis; Corynebacterium diphtheriae, Listeria; Chlamydia; Hemophilus; Neisseria;* many anaerobes; and some enterococci. It is also clinically useful against *Treponema pallidum,* many rickettsiae and some non-tuberculous mycobacteria (eg. kansasii and scrofulaceum).

This antibiotic is only moderately potent. It should not be used for serious or life-threatening infections. In general, its usefulness is in those patients with infections suitably treated as outpatients.

Erythromycin base and sterate are administered as enteric coated tablets so that they are not inactivated by the low gastric pH. They are absorbed in the upper small bowel. They should be administered on an empty stomach and peak values in serum are achieved about four hours after ingestion. The estolate is not affected by gastric acidity or food in the stomach. Peak concentrations occur about two hours after ingestion. The ethylsuccinate is adequately absorbed but is best given on an empty stomach. The intravenous preparations achieve peak serum levels about one hour after administration.

Erythromycin distributes to most body tissues except from the central nervous system. At best, four doses of erythromycin are needed to achieve levels in middle ear effusions of about 1 ug/ml. This level is insufficient to adequately treat many *H. influenzae* infections. Patients receiving erythromycin may not show a clinical response for at least 24 hours after initiating therapy. The same lag can be encountered in treating sinus infections.

The drug is concentrated in the liver and excreted in active form in the bile. Some demethylation occurs in the liver resulting in partial deactivation of the erythromycin. Erythromycin crosses the placenta. High concentrations are found in breast milk. Only a small amount of erythromycin is found in urine. In general, dose changes are not necessary in renal failure. The estolate is better absorbed, more effective, and better tolerated than the ethylsuccinate.

Adverse Reactions

Erythromycin is one of the safest antibiotics available. Gastrointestinal upset is one of the most common side effects. Symptoms include nausea, vomiting, diarrhea and epigastric distresses. Intravenous administration may cause thrombophlebitis. Infrequently hypersensitivity reactions occur. These include skin rash, fever and eosinophilia. Erythromycin estolate has been associated with cholestatic hepatitis. This toxicity is rare in children. The vast majority of patients with this complication have been at least 12 years old. Less frequently this complication is seen with ethylsuccinate. Sensorineural hearing loss occurs infrequently and is associated with high doses of erythromycin. It is reversible. Hypertrophic pyloric stenosis has been infrequently reported in infants receiving the estolate. Pseudomembranous colitis has rarely been reported. *REMEMBER:* Concomittant administration of erythromycin and theophylline may lead to theophylline toxicity. In addition, erythromycin may lower the maintenance dose of glucocorticoids needed by asthmatic patients.

Erythromycin may falsely elevate results for tests that assay for catecholamines and 17-hydroxycorticosteroids in the urine and for colorimetric measurement of SGOT. Serum folate and urinary estriols may be falsely decreased.

CEPHALOSPORINS

The term cephalosporin is used in the broad sense to include true cephalosporins as well as cephamycins and oxa-beta-lactams. They are semisynthetic derivatives of cephalosporin C, a compound elaborated by *Cephalosporium acremonium*. Cephalosporin are usually divided into three categories: first, second and third generation. In general, the first generation cephalosporin provides good Gram-positive coverage including staphylococci. They are usually not effective for enterococci. The second generation of cephalosporin are fairly beta-lactamase stable and are effective against many organisms including many strains of *Haemophilus influenzae, Neisseria gonorrhea* and *Bacteroides fragilis.* The third generation cephalosporins provide significantly improved Gram negative coverage, with varying degrees of Gram positive coverage.

First Generation Cephalosporins

Cephalosporins are closely related to the penicillins. They inhibit bacterial cell wall synthesis in a similar manner to the penicillins. The mechanism is to inhibit cross-linking of the linear peptidoglycan strands. These antibiotics, like the penicillins, have a beta-lactam ring. Alteration in side chains in the second and third generation cephalosporins protect the beta-lactam ring to a greater extent than in the first generation drugs resulting in a broader spectrum of coverage. Oral and parenteral preparations are available.

The first generation cephalosporins are active against most Gram positive aerobes and most anaerobes except *B. fragilis* and some Gram negative organisms. The two major Gram positive exceptions are the enterococcus and most methicillin resistant staphylococci. *REMEMBER:* Although methicillin resistant staphylococci may appear sensitive to the cephalosporins by disk susceptibility methods, the minimal inhibiting concentration as determined by tube dilution is sufficiently high as to usually make these antibiotics not very useful clinically against methicillin resistant staphylococci.

First generation cephalosporins penetrate poorly into the cerebrospinal fluid. They also usually do not achieve clinically useful levels in vitreous humor, aqueous humor and prostatic tissue. These antibiotics do cross the placenta and enter the fetal circulation. In addition, they are excreted in low concentrations in breast milk.

These antibiotics are extensively used, especially in general practice. Considering their wide use, it is impressive that serious side effects have been reported so rarely. Most of the reported adverse reactions are relatively mild. The common ones include rash, drug fever, transient elevations in liver function tests and positive Coombs tests (direct and indirect). Renal toxicity is rare and has primarily been associated with cephaloridine. There has been an occasional case of interstitial nephritis in patients treated with cephalothin. Treatment of patients with cephalosporin plus aminoglycoside may increase the risk of nephrotoxicity.

Cross-reactive antibodies for the penicillin and cephalosporins are not infrequently seen. Nevertheless, clinical allergic reactions happen infrequently. Patients with a history of an immediate type reaction to the penicillin should avoid cephalosporin therapy if possible.

Second Generation Cephalosporins

Second generation cephalosporins have somewhat less Gram positive activity as compared to first generation cephalosporins. However, they have expanded Gram negative coverage. This expanded Gram negative coverage includes greater resistance to beta-lactamases. Better coverage is provided against *H. influenzae, N. gonorrheae, B. fragilis* and other Gram negative organisms. In general, these antibiotics are not appropriate for the therapy of meningitis. Oral and parenteral preparations are available.

The side effects of the second generation cephalosporins are essentially the same as the first generation cephalosporins. Serious side effects are rare. Rash, drug fever and transient elevation of liver function tests are the most commonly recognized reactions.

Third Generation Cephalosporins

These antibiotics, as a group, have decreased activity against Gram positive organisms. Their Gram negative coverage is significantly enhanced over the first two generations of cephalosporins. Those organisms that are susceptible to these third generation cephalosporins, in general, have very low minimal inhibitory concentrations. Many of the third generation cephalosporins have better central nervous system penetration and because of the relatively low MIC's for many organisms, these drugs can be appropriate for the treatment of meningitis in certain situations. So far, third generation cephalosporins are available for parenteral use only.

The list of adverse reactions from third generation cephalosporins tends to be somewhat greater than with the previous generations of antibiotics. Local inflamation at the site of infection occurs. Hypersensitivity reactions have been reported. Gastrointestinal distress has been reported. Eosinophilia, a positive Coombs test, leukopenia, granulocytopenia and thrombocytopenia have all been reported. Transient elevations in liver function tests infrequently occur. Some of these antibiotics produce a disulfiram-like reaction and patients should therefore avoid alcohol. Some also cause disturbances in vitamin K-dependent clotting functions. Another potentially serious problem is superinfection with enterococci which has been seen in patients on third generation (and to a lesser extent second generation) cephalosporins. Antibiotic associated pseudomembranous colitis has been reported.

SELECTED CEPHALOSPORINS

Cephalothin

Cephalothin is one of the original first generation cephalosporins. It is a parenteral antibiotic and provides good coverage against Gram positive organisms as described previously in the chapter. It is given every four to six hours and the recommended dose in pediatrics is 75 to 125 mg/kg/day. It is known by the trade name of Keflin. The side effects are those described previously and in addition there have been a few cases of renal toxicity associated with its use.

Cefazolin

Cefazolin is another first generation cephalosporin that to a large extent has replaced cephalothin for parenteral administration. The drug is given every 8 hours in a dose of 50 to 100 mg/kg/day and this is an advantage over the more frequent dosing of cephalothin. Cefazolin is sold under the brand names of Ancef and Kefzol.

Cephalexin

Cephalexin is an oral first generation cephalosporin. It is given every 6 hours in a dose of 25 to 50 mg/kg/day. Its spectrum of coverage and toxicities are the same as the other first generation cephalosporins.

Cefadroxil

Cefadroxil is a first generation cephalosporin that is given orally every 12 hours. The dosage is 30 mg/kg/day. Its advantage over cephalexin is that it can be given less frequently and still achieve adequate levels in the blood. It is sold under the brand names of Duricef and Ultracef.

Cefamandole

Cefamandole is a parenteral second generation cephalosporin. It is effective against many ampicillin resistant strains of *Hemophilus influenzae* and has a much broader spectrum of Gram negative coverage than does the first generation cephalosporin. It does not get into the spinal fluid in adequate concentrations to treat meningitis. At least one study has demonstrated that infants on cefamandole who have a superficial *Hemophilus influenzae* infection (ie. pneumonias, skin infections, cellulitis) may develop meningitis while on therapy. Therefore, if cefamandole is to be used in children under 1 year of age, it must be used with extreme caution and the child must be monitored closely. Cefamandole is usually given parenterally every 4 to 6 hours. The dose is 100 to 150 mg/kg/day, and it is sold under the trade name of Mandole.

Cefoxitin

Cefoxitin is another second generation parenteral antibiotic. It is effective against a wide variety of Gram negative organisms including penicillin resistant *Neisseria gonorrhae* and many of the *Bacteroides fragilis* group. It is not appropriate therapy for meningitis and therefore must be used with caution in very small infants. Because of its good Gram negative coverage and its anaerobic coverage, the drug has been used frequently for intra-abdominal infection and post-surgical abdominal infection. Cefoxitin is given every 4 to 6 hours in a dose of 80 to 160 mg/kg/day. It is sold under the brand name of Mefoxin.

Cefaclor

Cefaclor is an oral second generation cephalosporin that is primarily used for the treatment of suspected ambulatory-type pediatric infections suspected to be due to *Hemophilus influenzae*. Not all *H. influenzae* are sensitive to cefaclor and, especially in the case of otitis which is one of the more common uses in pediatrics treatment, failures and relapses do occur on cefaclor. Cefaclor is given every 8 hours in a dose of 40 mg/kg/day. It is sold under the brand name of Ceclor.

Cefuroxime

Cefuroxime is a second generation cephalosporin that is given parenterally. It has both good Gram negative and Gram positive coverage and is effective against *H. influenzae. H. influenzae* resistance to cefuroxime is extremely rare. In contrast to the other second generation cephalosporins, cefuroxime is appropriate therapy for meningitis and has been approved for that purpose. In most situations, it would probably not be considered a first line drug of choice, but offers the advantage, at least theoretically, over the other second generation cephalosporins that are given parenterally, that it at least protects the meninges in infants who are being treated for non-meningeal *H. influenzae* infection. The drug is normally given every 8 hours except in the case of meningitis when it can be given every 6 hours. The dose in non-meningitis patients is 75 to 150 mg/kg/day and in meningitis the recommended dose is between 200 and 250 mg/kg/day. Cefuroxime is sold under the trade name of Zinacef.

Moxalactam

Moxalactam is a parenteral third generation cephalosporin. It achieves clinically useful levels in the cerebrospinal fluid and it is effective against a wide spectrum of *Hemophilus influenzae* and *Neisseria gonorrhea* as well as many other Gram negative organisms. It is useful against many Enterobacter. In general, moxalactam offers relatively poor coverage for the Gram positive organisms. In particular it is not good coverage for Group B streptococcus, *Streptococcus pneumoniae,* enterococcus, *Bacteroides fragilis, Clostridia, Staphylococcus* or *Pseudomonas.* In addition to the side effects associated with the other third generation cephalosporins, moxalactam also can cause a vitamin K dependent clotting abnormality which is reversible with the administration of vitamin K. In pediatrics, moxalactam's major use appears to be in neonatal meningitis. Moxalactam is effective therapy for *E. coli* meningitis in the newborn and, especially in ampicillin resistant *E. coli* meningitis, may be the drug of choice. The main disadvantage of moxalactam appears to be its inactivity against enterococcus and some of the anaerobic organisms. The result is that superinfection with enterococcus is not uncommon in patients being treated with moxalactam. The kidneys appear to be the major route of excretion of moxalactam although some of it is also excreted in the feces. Renal dysfunction therefore may require alteration in the dose of moxalactam. The half-life is somewhat prolonged in patients with hepatic dysfunction but not significantly so. Moxalactam is dosed every 6 to 8 hours and the dose is 150 to 200 mg/kg/day. The drug is sold under the brand name of Moxam.

Cefotaxime

Cefotaxime is active against most Gram negatives including *Neisseria gonorrhea* and *Hemophilus influenzae.* Cefotaxime offers better coverage of Gram positive organisms than moxalactam does. The drug penetrates into bile, bronchial secretions, lung tissue, cerebrospinal fluid, aciditic fluid and middle ear fluid. It is liver metabolized and therefore is less sensitive to renal dysfunction than is moxalactam. Vitamin K dependent clotting abnormalities seen with moxalactam has not been reported with cefotaxime. Because adequate concentrations of cefotaxime will get into the cerebrospinal fluid, this drug, like moxalactam, is appropriate therapy for meningitis. In pediatrics, its primary use is in the neonate with *E. coli* meningitis. Cefotaxime is not appropriate therapy for *Pseudomonas,* enterococcus or *Bacteroides fragilis.* The drug is administered every 6 to 8 hours parenterally and the dose is 100 to 200 mg/kg/day. It is sold under the brand name of Claforan.

Cefoperazone

Cefoperazone is the most active third generation cephalosporin against *Pseudomonas, Bacteroides fragilis* and Group D streptococci. The drug is primarily excreted in bile and therefore the dose only needs to be modified minimally in patients with renal dysfunction. Cefoperazone when combined with an aminoglycoside may be synergistic against *Pseudomonas aeruginosa.* Cefoperazone is, at this point, not approved for use in children. The dosage is given every 8 to 12 hours. The recommended dose is 100 to 150 mg/kg/day and it is sold under the brand name of Cefobid.

Ceftriaxone

Ceftriaxone is a third generation cephalosporin with a very long half-life. The elimination half-life in adults is felt to be between 6 and 9 hours and in children is approximately 4 to 7 hours. In adult patients this drug can be given once a day and in pediatrics it can be given every 12 hours. As with the other third generation cephalosporins, it lacks adequate activity against *Listeria monocytogenes* and enterococcus. Ceftriaxone is approved in pediatric patients for essentially all infections including meningitis. Ceftriaxone has been used effectively for significant staphylococcal infections including staphylococcal infections of the central nervous system. It, however, is not active against methicillin-resistant staphylococci, a property that it shares in common with the other cephalosporins. One of the advantages of this antibiotic over the other third generation cephalosporins is a lower minimal inhibitory concentration for most common pediatric pathogens, resulting in a greater than a 1000 fold level in the cerebrospinal fluid than is needed to eradicate the organisms. In contrast to moxalactam, ceftriaxone offers excellent coverage for Group B streptococcus, pneumococcus, and Group A streptococcus. This is an obvious advantage in treating neonatal meningitis as well as meningitis in infants and pediatric patients. Excretion of the drug is by both renal and biliary mechanisms. If either mechanism is dysfunctioning, it appears that the other can compensate making it unnecessary to adjust doses in patients with either renal or hepatitic dysfunction, and only in patients with severe combined dysfunction would alterations be needed. The drug crosses the placenta and is found in low levels in breast milk. Only minor adverse reactions have been reported with ceftriaxone and these include diarrhea, rash, fever and occasional local reactions. Thrombocytosis, elevated SGOT levels, eosinophilia, elevated SGPT, and leukopenia have all been reported, but these abnormalities are no more frequent than with other cephalosporins and are rapidly reversible. Ceftriaxone does not appear to be associated with bleeding problems or with platelet dysfunction. Ceftriaxone is sold under the brand name of Rocephin. In the treatment of pediatric patients without meningitis, the dosage is 50 to 75 mg/kg/day divided into one or two doses. In the treatment of meningitis, a daily dose of 100 mg/kg/day is given and is divided into two doses per day.

TETRACYCLINES

There are a few indications in pediatrics for the use of tetracyclines. Tetracyclines work by the inhibition of microbial proteins synthesis. They are excreted in the bile, stool and urine. Indications for the use of tetracyclines include: rickettsial diseases, infection by chlamydia, plague, brucellosis, chlorea gonococcal infection and acne. However, if given to pregnant mothers, infants, or young children, this can lead to brownish-yellow or greyish-black discoloration of the teeth. In addition, it is associated with inhibition of bone growth especially in premature infants, elevations of blood urea nitrogen, tubular damage and a Fanconi-like syndrome, especially with outdated preparations. Tetracycline is absorbed well after oral administration. Peak concentrations are achieved within 1 to 3 hours after the dose. Tetracycline is eliminated primarily by glomerular filtration. It is contraindicated in oliguria and anuria. The dose of tetracycline orally is 25 to 50 mg/kg/day divided into four doses. It is sold under a variety of trade names including Achromycin, Tetracyn and Panmycin. There are an intramuscular and intravenous preparation also available.

AMINOGLYCOSIDES

Aminoglycosides cause irreversible inhibition of protein synethesis. Preparations available include: streptomycin, kanamycin, gentamicin, tobramycin, amikacin, netilmicin, neomycin and spectinomycin. Resistance develops to the aminoglycosides through the appearance of extrachromosomally controlled enzymes called R-factors. These inactivate antibiotics by phosphorylation, acetylation and adenylylation.

Streptomycin

Streptomycin was originally primarily used in tuberculosis therapy. It is used now synergistically with penicillin against *Streptococcus viridans* and enterococcus especially in the treatment of endocarditis. It can be used in the therapy for tularemia and for the plague. The drug is poorly absorbed after oral administration and is given intramuscularly. Much resistance has developed to streptomycin and it is of less value now than it has been in the past. In addition, there is significant toxicities associated with the drug; both kidney and 8th nerve toxicity. The 8th nerve toxicity is both vestibular and auditory. The toxicities are greater with streptomycin than most of the other aminoglycosides and in most clinical situations streptomycin has been replaced by the other aminoglycosides.

Kanamycin

Kanamycin closely resembles neomycin. It is a safer drug when given parenterally. It is clinically used against enterobacteria like *E. coli* and *Klebsiella.* Its toxicities are less than streptomycin. Kidney toxicity occurs but is rare in infancy and 8th nerve toxicity occurs also. Resistance to kanamycin has also been increasing. Kanamycin is effective in urinary tract infections and works best in alkaline urine.

Gentamicin

Gentamicin very closely resembles kanamycin. Its inhibitory to almost all pseudomonas species. Many of the kanamycin resistance enterobacteria are still sensitive to gentamicin. Like kanamycin, it has both renal and 8th nerve toxicity. It causes destruction of cochlear hair cells and may lead to permanent deafness. It is therefore important to monitor gentamicin levels, both peaks and troughs, when the drug is prescribed; especially to infants and patients with renal compromise.

Neomycin

Neomycin is also closely related to kanamycin. It is not used parenterally because of severe 8th nerve toxicity and renal damage. It is poorly absorbed from the gastrointestinal tract, but in newborn babies as much as 10% can be absorbed and therefore if used orally in newborns must be used with extreme caution. Neomycin is occasionally used for sterilization of the gastrointestinal tract in patients who are undergoing bone marrow transplantation.

Spectinomycin

Spectinomycin is not really an aminoglycoside. It is really an aminocyclitol, but is lumped together with the other aminoglycosides in general. Its only real clinical application is for the treatment of acute uncomplicated gonococcal urethritis; cervitic and proctitis when penicillin cannot be used. The drug is not approved for use in children and it is not adequate therapy for syphilis.

Tobramycin

Tobramycin closely resembles gentamicin. Its toxicities are also similar. *Pseudomonas* appears to be somewhat more sensitive to tobramycin than to gentamicin. Again as with gentamicin, it is important to monitor drug levels especially in infants and patients with renal impairment to avoid toxicity.

Amikacin

Amikacin is similar to gentamicin microbiologically and similar to kanamycin pharmocologically. Most gentamicin and kanamycin resistant *Enterobacteriaceae* are susceptible to amikacin

Netilmicin

Netilmicin is a newer aminoglycoside antibiotic recently approved for parenteral treatment of susceptible bacteria. Its mode of action is similar to that of the other aminoglycosides in that it works by interference with bacterial protein synthesis. Netilmicin is active against a broad spectrum of bacteria including the Gram negative enteric organisms and *Pseudomonas aeruginosa.* In addition, some of the Gram negative organisms that are resistant to gentamicin and tobramycin are susceptible to netilmicin. Although netilmicin is active against *Pseudomonas,* it is less active than either tobramycin or gentamicin. Those organisms that are resistant to netilmicin, tobramycin and gentamicin are sometimes susceptible to amikacin. As with the other aminoglycosides, patients with renal insufficiency will need to have their dose of aminoglycoside changed in order to avoid an accumulation of drug resulting in toxicity. In animal models, netilmicin is less ototoxic and less nephrotoxic than gentamicin or tobramycin. Other side effects include elevations of SGOT, increased serum concentrations of bilirubin, thrombocytosis, prolonged prothombin time and, occasionally, rash and drug fever have been reported. It is important to remember that all aminoglycosides can probably cause neuromuscular blockade with respiratory paralysis and this certainly applies to netilmicin. As with other aminoglycosides, if they are given in conjunction with other nephrotoxic or ototoxic agents such as the cephalosporins or potent diuretics, the chances of nephrotoxicity or ototoxicity increases. Netilmicin is sold as Netromycin. The usual dose is 4 to 6.5 mg/kg/day divided into three doses. It can be given intramuscularly or intravenously. As with the other aminoglycosides, it is important to both monitor renal and auditory functions and to follow serum levels to make sure that the patient is not receiving toxic doses.

Traditionally in pediatrics, the aminoglycosides have played a major role in broad spectrum coverage during the neonatal period. The combination of ampicillin plus an aminoglycoside has provided routine broad spectrum coverage in newborn babies with suspected sepsis. Recently the role of the aminoglycoside has decreased somewhat as third generation cephalosporins appear to have taken up some of that role. The ultimate position of the third generation cephalosporins in the treatment of neonatal infection has not yet been determined and the aminoglycosides still continue to play a prominent role in broad spectrum coverage in the neonate. *REMEMBER:* It is essential in infants and patients with renal impairment to monitor peak and trough blood levels of gentamicin. In addition, it is important to monitor kidney function and to look for signs of ototoxicity in these patients. Patients who are expected to have prolonged therapy should have appropriate auditory testing done initially, during their therapy, and at the conclusion of their therapy.

The dosage of streptomycin is 20 to 30 mg/kg/day divided into twelve hour dosing and is given intramuscularly. The dosage of kanamycin is 15 to 30 mg/kg/day divided into three equal doses given IM or IV. It is sold under the brand names of Kantrex or Klebcil. An oral preparation is available for the suppression of bowel flora. Gentamicin is given intramuscularly or intravenously. The dose is 3 to 7.5 mg/kg/day. It is divided in three doses. In patients with cystic fibrosis the dose is usually increased. Gentamicin is sold under the brand name of Garamycin among others. Neomycin is sold under the name of Mycifradin. It is an oral preparation of 50 to 100 mg/kg/day divided into the three or four doses per day. Spectinomycin is a single dose of 30 to 40 mg/kg/day given intramuscularly but is not approved in pediatrics. The brand name is Trobicin. Tobramycin comes as an intravenous or intramuscular preparation. The dose is 3 to 6 mg/kg/day divided into three doses. The dose in cystic fibrosis patients is higher and it is sold as Nebcin. Amikacin is sold as Amikin. The drug is available either as an intramuscular or intravenous preparation. The dose is 15 to 30 mg/kg/day and is divided into three doses per day.

MONOBACTAMS

The first significant monobactam to be studied has been aztreonam. Aztreonam has no significant antimicrobial activity against Gram positive or anaerobic bacteria. This is because it does not bind to penicillin binding proteins in these bacteria. It is however effective against *Enterobacteriaceae, Pseudomonas* and other Gram negative aerobic bacteria. The drug is not well absorbed orally and is therefore administered intravenously. Urinary excretion is about 60% and the drug accumulates in the presence of renal failure. Serum half life is 1.7 hours but in renal failure may increase to as much as 6 hours. Adverse reactions to aztreonam include skin rashes and elevation in serum SGOT values, however, there have been no significant hematologic, gastrointestinal, nephrotoxic, or neurotoxic reactions to the agent. Anaphylaxis or skin rashes have not been seen in patients with positive skin tests to the penicillins. Clinical applications of aztreonam include treating serious infections due to *E. coli* and *Klebsiella, Serratia* and *Pseudomonas.* Because of their low level of toxicity, it is thought that perhaps the monobactams may serve as an appropriate alternative to the aminoglycosides for the treatment of Gram negative infection. As additional monobactams are synthesized and are clinically tested, it may be that the aminoglycosides will be used less frequently.

TRIMETHOPRIM-SULFAMETHOXAZOLE
(TMP-SMX)

This drug is a fixed combination of two drugs and is available in both oral and parenteral preparations. The combination inhibits sequential steps in the synthesis of tetrahydrofolic acid which is an essential part of the bacterial synthesis of purines and ultimately DNA. Individually they are both bacteriostatic, but as a combination, they exhibit some bactericidal activity. Since folic acid is not produced in mammalian cells, the sulfamethoxazole induced inhibition of folic acid does not take place in humans.

Except in life-threatening infections, trimethoprim-sulfamethoxazole is usually administered orally and achieves peak concentrations about one hour after administration. In adults, the elimination half-life of trimethoprim is between 8 and 16 hours and that of sulfamethoxazole is about 6 to 12 hours. Both are excreted primarily by the kidneys. The drug distributes particularly well to the liver and the biliary tract and about 40% of trimethoprim gets into the cerebrospinal fluid.

The antimicrobial spectrum of trimethoprim-sulfamethoxazole includes the facultative Gram negative bacilli of the *Enterobacteriacaea* family as well as many Gram positive bacteria such as *Staphylococcus, Streptococcus* and pneumococcus. It is important to keep in mind that many of the Gram positive bacteria are more susceptible *in vitro* than they are *in vivo* with the conventional doses that are given. In addition, resistant strains of *Streptococcus pneumoniae* have been reported. The susceptibility of *Streptococcus fecalis* is quite variable and resistance can develop even on therapy. Many salmonella species that are resistant to either ampicillin or chloramphenicol are susceptible to trimethoprim-sulfamethoxazole. Most *Proteus, Shigella, Vibrio cholera, Hemophilus, Neisseria* as well as *Yersinia pestis* are sensitive. Although *Neisseria meningitidis* is susceptible, TMP-SMX is not effective for the carrier state, nor is it recommended for the use of treatment of septicemia or meningitis due to meningococcus.

The major indications for the use of trimethoprim-sulfamethoxazole in children include the treatment of otitis media, the treatment of shigellosis, and for the treatment of urinary tract infections due to *E. coli, Klebsiella* and *Proteus.* In addition, trimethoprim-sulfamethoxazole is appropriate therapy for *Pneumocystis carinii.* The drug should be avoided in certain situations. These include patients who are suspected to have folic acid deficiency. This would be a particular concern in phenytoin use or with patients who are on folate antagonists. In addition, patients who have protein calorie malnutrition or prematurity are likely to be folate deficient, and unless they have been supplemented, should not be put on trimethoprim-sulfamethoxazole. The drug should be avoided in pregnancy as well as in patients who have the fragile X syndrome. Patients who have a known sensitivity to any of the sulfas should not be given trimethorpim-sulfamethoxazole. In addition, infants less than two months of age should not receive the drug. If patients develop a skin rash while on treatment, the drug should be discontinued and not used again. Those patients who are glucose-6-phosphate-dehydrogenase deficient should not receive trimethoprim-sulfamethoxazole. Trimethoprim-sulfamethoxazole is also used for prophylaxis in certain situations. The literature indicates that in adult women the use of trimethoprim-sulfamethoxazole can prevent recurring urinary tract infections and the same approach has been used in pediatric patients. Although it is controversial, some pediatricians use trimethoprim-sulfamethoxazole to prevent recurrences of otitis media in children with a history of frequent recurrences. In addition, children with biliary atresia who have an enterohepatic anastomosis are at risk for subsequent infections of the liver. Experience of the children who receive trimethoprim-sulfamethoxazole indicates an excellent response. Prophylaxis, especially during the first year following surgery, seems to prevent the majority of infectious problems. Patients with chronic granulomatous disease of childhood have a defect in their leukocyte killing capability and consequently develop recurrent abscesses at a variety of sights including the skin, liver, lungs and lymph nodes. Sulfas appear to increase leukocyte bactericidal capacity and patients who are put on continuous trimethoprim-sulfamethoxazole therapy have been reported to be freer of infection. Prophylaxis against *Pneumocystis carinii* pneumonia in the immunosuppressed child with trimethoprim-sulfamethoxazole has been studied well and has been proven to be effective, although these children may have a slightly increased incidence of fungal infection.

A variety of side effects have been associated with the use of trimethoprim-sulfamethoxazole. Skin rash is perhaps one of the most common seen. In addition, jaundice, anaphylaxis and hematologic depression have also been reported. Perhaps of most concern is the development of Stevens-Johnson Syndrome. Fatalities have been reported secondary to this complication. Neutropenia is seen with trimethoprim-sulfamethoxazole therapy. It appears to be more of a problem with prolonged use of the drug than in an acute short course therapy. Pancytopenia and thrombocytopenia have also been reported, but infrequently. It is important to remember that patients with glucose-6-phosphate-dehydrogenase deficiency may be predisposed to acute hemolytic events. Most rashes seen with the administration of trimethoprim-sulfamethoxazole are benign in nature and frequently are associated with pruritis. Nevertheless, once a skin reaction is seen, the drug should be discontinued to avoid progression to one of the more serious dermatologic responses such as Stevens-Johnson Syndrome. Thus, except for the two rare forms of adverse reactions to trimethoprim-sulfamethoxazole, namely the Stevens-Johnson Syndrome and the bone marrow depression, the drug otherwise is pretty well tolerated, and in the critical situations indicated earlier, is highly effective.

ANTIVIRAL THERAPY

The rapid and accurate diagnosis of viral infection has become increasingly important during the past decade as newer and more effective antiviral agents have become available. Because a variety of viral infections are treatable, it is important for the physician to be aware of the different clinical presentations that help distinguish between the variety of possible viral etiologies. In the immunocompromised patient, the rapid diagnosis of viral infections and the institution of therapy can be life-saving. This chapter will deal with four antiviral agents: adenine arabinoside, acyclovir, amantadine and ribovarine.

Adenine Arabinoside

Adenine arabinoside is also known by the names of vidarabine and Ara-A. Adenine arabinoside is a purine nucleotide which has been proven effective in the treatment of *Herpes simplex* virus infection as well as varicella-zoster infections. Specifically, it has been proven effective in ocular disease due to herpes, encephalitis, neonatal infection and in the immunocompromised patient with varicella infection. Approximately 60% of the drug, after an IV dose, is recovered in the urine within 24 hours. Prior to excretion, the drug is deaminated to a less active metabolite. The normal dose of Ara-A is 10 to 15 mg/kg/day infused over a 12 hour period. In neonates the dosage can go as high as 30 mg/kg/day also infused over 12 hours.

Ara-A initially was available as a topical ointment for the treatment of *Herpes simplex* virus keratitis. It was found to be as effective as idoxuridine and less toxic. It is effective against idoxuridine resistant strains of *Herpes simplex*. In addition, it has been proven effective in the treatment of herpes encephalitis, reducing mortality from around 70% to about 28%. The earlier the treatment is instituted, the better is the chance of survival. The drug also reduces the incidence of neurologic sequelae in those patients who survive. It is recommended that patients who receive Ara-A for the treatment of herpes encephalitis have a brain biospy to prove the diagnosis prior to the institution of therapy. This is because there are several diseases that can mimic herpes encephalitis, some of which are potentially treatable.

Examples would be either bacterial abscesses or CNS tuberculosis. Because Ara-A is relatively insoluble, it is administered in large doses of fluid which can produce fluid overload and cerebral edema problems for patients.

Neonatal herpes infection carries a very high mortality and in those patients who do survive, complications and sequelae are common. Neonates with central nervous system herpes infections treated with Ara-A have a significantly decreased mortality. Neurologic sequelae are less in patients that are treated. The drug is also effective in disseminated neonatal herpes, however, the outcome is still relatively poor in that group of patients. As many as 70% of babies who start off with localized skin lesions will progress to systemic disease due to herpes infection. It is therefore recommended that treatment with Ara-A should be initiated as early as possible if skin lesions are present and documented to be herpes. The presence of skin lesions is not necessary to make the diagnosis. It is therefore important to have a high index of suspicion about the possibility of neonatal herpes and to institute steps for diagnosis and treatment as soon as possible. Immunocompromised patients with mucocutaneous herpes lesions may also benefit from the use of Ara-A. Its primary effect seems to be in reducing the fever and decreasing the pain but there is no significant effect on the duration of viral shedding or on the time elapsed until the lesions are healed.

Ara-A has also been shown to be effective in the treatment of varicella infections in the immunocompromised patient. The use of the drug will decrease the incidence of pain and increase the rate of healing of the lesions. In addition, it will decrease the time span during which new vesicles may form. It will also result in quicker elimination of vesicle fluid virus and decrease the overall duration of the illness. The drug is also effective in reducing the incidence of complications and visceral dissemination. Those patients who should receive treatment include those that have either chickenpox or localized zoster and are immunocompromised. These include transplant patients, patients with primary immune deficiencies and those patients receiving chemotherapy for malignancies. The earlier that therapy is instituted, the more effective it appears to be.

Side effects from adenine arabinoside appear to be minimal. They are usually dose related and are usually reversible. In normal doses nausea and vomiting appear to be the major complication. At larger doses adult patients have experienced tremors, EEG abnormalities and megalobastic bone marrow changes. These were reversible when the drug was discontinued.

In patients with renal impairment, the dose of the drug should be adjusted. Patients who are receiving both adenine arabinoside and interferon appear to have increased risk of side effects.

Acyclovir

Acyclovir inhibits viral DNA polymerase and acts as a viral chain terminator. It is activated by thymidine kinase. The therapeutic-to-toxic ratio of acyclovir is very high due to the virus specific mechanism of action. Acyclovir is produced as a topical ointment, as an intravenous preparation, and an oral formulation. Acyclovir's primary value appears to be in the treatment of *Herpes simplex* infection and in the treatment of varicella zoster infection. Although other viruses of the herpes group appear to be inhibited with high doses of acyclovir, this does not appear to be of any clinical value. Acyclovir is given over a one hour period as 5-15 mg/kg/day divided into three doses. Peak levels after intravenous administration are about 10 times as high as when the drug is administered orally. Acyclovir appears to be a safe drug without teratogenic or mutagenic effects in animals. If the intravenous dose is infused too rapidly, reversible elevations of serum creatinine have been reported. Because acyclovir is eliminated by the kidney, dosage adjustment is required in patients with renal dysfunction. Uses of acyclovir include the treatment of mucocutaneous *Herpes simplex* infection and the prevention of reactivation and dissemination after bone marrow transplant. In patients undergoing transplantation or induction chemotherapy, the risk of reactivation of herpes infection in patients with positive antibody titers is 60 to 80%, thus prophylaxis may be of significant benefit to these patients. The use of acyclovir in the treatment of neonatal herpes and in herpes encephalitis appears to be effective, and at least preliminary studies suggest that its efficacy and safety are similar to those of Ara-A. One study from Sweden suggests that acyclovir may be superior to Ara-A in decreasing mortality and decreasing the incidence of sequelae. The outcome is clearly improved with early initiation of therapy.

Acyclovir has also been used for the treatment of genital herpes infection. A topical application of acyclovir shortens the clinical course of first episodes of genital herpes infection. Topical use does not appear to be effective for the recurrent infections nor in preventing recurrent infections. In addition, topical acyclovir is not effective in the treatment of oral herpes infections in normal hosts. The use of systemic therapy either orally or intravenously in patients with first episodes of genital herpes infection results in shortening the clinical course of infection, reducing the duration of shedding of virus, reducing the number of new lesions, and decreasing the systemic symptoms. Intermittent use of oral acyclovir reduces the duration of recurrent attacks but does not affect the rate of recurrent attacks. Topical application of acyclovir is also effective in the treatment of herpes keratitis and in patients with herpes lesions. In patients with herpes lesions close to the eye, prophylactic use of the ophthalmic ointment should be considered. The use of acyclovir should also be considered in patients with herpes infection who have underlying burns or skin disorders such as eczema.

In immunocompromised patients with varicella-zoster virus infections, acyclovir has been proven to be effective in treatment of the disease. Early institution of therapy with acyclovir reduces the spread of the skin lesions and decreases complications including both cutaneous and visceral dissemination. Again it needs to be emphasized that early institution of therapy is extremely important. The drug has also been proven effective when given intravenously to normal adult patients with zoster. Resistance by herpes and varicella virus to acyclovir occurs. It is therefore important that the use of the drug be limited to those situations where it is clearly clinically indicated.

Amantadine

Amantadine is an oral anti-viral drug which inhibits the uncoating of the influenzae A virus. Influenza is a significant cause of morbidity and mortality in infants and children and is also responsible for producing a picture that mimics bacterial sepsis in early infancy. Prevention of the disease is usually possible by immunization. Vaccines against influenza are safe and about 70 to 80% effective in preventing infection. Amantadine has been available in the United States for nearly 20 years. It probably has not been used as frequently as it should or could have been. This reluctance to use amantadine may be related to both inconvenience of taking prophylactic drugs and concern about side effects. The drug is 50 to 70% effective against influenzae A. It does not work against influenza B. Studies indicate that the use of amantadine within 48 hours of acute infection caused by influenza A will reduce fever within 24 hours and shorten the course of the illness. Peripheral airway dysfunction which can persist for weeks following acute infection with influenza is improved also with the use of amantadine. Side effects to amantadine do occur but are in general mild. Decreased concentration and dizziness have been reported. In addition, it has been suggested that amantadine may depress higher pyschomotor function but this appears to be of minimal significance. However, the use of amantadine and antihistamine together may potentiate anticholinergic and central nervous system effects. Amantadine is excreted in the urine and therefore side effects may increase in patients who have renal insufficiency. Amantadine can play a significant role in the prevention of influenza A if given to patients at the same time that they receive their immunization. The drug is taken until antibody develops which is usually two·weeks after booster vaccination. In addition, early treatment with amantadine of respiratory illness due to influenza A can significantly decrease associated morbidities. Amantadine may also be considered for prophylactic use in the prevention of nosocomial influenza A infection in hospitalized children during community outbreaks. Ideally, one should have available viral laboratories to make the definitive diagnosis of influenza A prior to institution of therapy. Where this is not available, it is probably reasonable to use amantadine for the treatment of severe respiratory illnesses in children during community influenza outbreaks.

Ribavirin

The drug inhibits a wide variety of both RNA and DNA viruses. It does not appear to be effective for certain single stranded RNA viruses such as enterovirus and rhinovirus. Ribavirin appears to work by alteration of nucleotide pools and messenger RNA formation. There is interference with the synthesis of guanine nucleotides and as a result with nucleic acid synthesis. In pediatrics, the drug's primary use is for the treatment of respiratory syncitial virus infections (RSV). The drug is administered by aerosol. The drug is associated with reductions in viral titers, duration of fever and systemic illness. Hospitalized infants with RSV pneumonia also demonstrate improved arterial oxygen saturation. Ribavirin is well tolerated. Some patients receiving the aerosal experience mild conjunctival injection. Because this drug is administered as an aerosal over 20 to 24 hours each day, it is only of value to hospitalized patients. Therefore, it is only practical for patients with moderate to severe illness. The cost of administration of the drug and the cost of hospitalization probably limits its usefulness in routine RSV bronchiolitis infections in children. Neonates and infants with severe RSV pneumonia may benefit from the use of ribavirin.

Interferon

In addition to the four viral agents previously discussed, interferon has proven to be effective in treatment of certain viral infections. Interferons do not directly inhibit viral replication, rather they induce an intracellular antiviral state in the host cells. They are nonspecifically effective against a variety of viruses. Interferons are species specific and those that are currently available for clinical investigation are produced in human cells. Interferons are proteins that exert virus nonspecific antiviral activity in cells through cellular metabolic processes that involve the synthesis of RNA and protein. Current classification of interferons include interferon alpha, interferon beta and interferon gamma. Most work with interferon has dealt with interferon alpha and its parenteral administration. If the drug is given intramuscularly, its half-life in the serum is 4 to 6 hours. The drug has been used in the treatment of herpes zoster infections. It has been used prophylactically in renal transplant patients and continued for up to 6 weeks post-operatively in order to delay the excretion of CMV and to decrease the cytomegalovirus viremia. Herpes keratitis may heal more rapidly with the topical application of interferon alpha. Interferon penetrates poorly into cerebrospinal fluid. Doses of interferon alpha greater than 10^4 units per kg/day can result in side effects including fever, nausea, vomiting, myalgias, chills and malaise. If given rapidly intravenously, hypotension has been reported. In addition, bone marrow supression has occurred. There are not any significant adverse effects associated with the topical application of interferon.

ANTIPARASITIC THERAPY

There is a large number of agents available for the treatment of parasitic disease. This section will only deal with some of the agents. Others have been discussed briefly in the chapter on parasitic diseases.

Chloroquine

Chloroquine is appropriate treatment for malaria. It is effective against the asexual erythrocytic forms of human plasmodia but not active against the hepatic forms of the parasite. The drug is absorbed well from the gastrointestinal tract. It is partly metabolized by the liver and both the unchanged drug and the metabolized drug are excreted in the urine. The half-life of the drug is 6 to 7 days, therefore, the drug is effective when taken weekly as antimalarial prophylaxis. When used for prophylaxis against malaria, side effects are extremely rare. Occasionally gastrointestinal intolerance to the drug occurs. This can be avoided by taking the drug with meals. In antimalarial treatment, chloroquine infrequently produces side effects. Those side effects that are seen include dizziness, headache, vomiting, and occasionally pruritis and rash.

Primaquine

This is a very safe drug against the liver stage of plasmodium. It is rapidly absorbed from the gastrointestinal tract and is metabolized. If given for fourteen days, it is usually successful in providing a radical cure for *Plasmodium vivax* and *Plasmodium malaria*. Patients with glucose-6-phosphate-dehydrogenase deficiency may experience problems with primaquine. These patients occasionally will have acute hemolysis that could be averted by altering the dosage schedule. Other side effects seen occasionally with primaquine include anorexia and abdominal pain.

Metronidazole

This is an effective drug in the treatment of amebic infection. It is also an effective drug in the treatment of anaerobic infection. It is considered the drug of choice in the treatment of amebic liver abscess and amebic dysentary. It can also be used for *Trichomonas vaginalis* and *Giardia lamblia.* The drug is available as both an oral preparation and a parenteral preparation. After oral administration, peak serum concentrations occur within one to three hours. The drug is about 20% bound to plasma proteins and distributes throughout the body. Much of the drug is metabolized in the liver and both the metabolized and the unchanged drug are excreted by the kidney. The half-life is about 8 to 9 hours. Side effects occur but are usually mild. They include nausea, vomiting, diarrhea and headache. Anorexia has been reported by some patients as has a metalic taste. Infrequently, central nervous system manifestations occur. These include weakness, vertigo and ataxia.

Mebendazole

It is sold under the brand name Vermox. It has broad spectrum antihelminthic activity. It is used for the treatment of trichuriasis and for ascariasis as well as hookworm infection. One dose of mebendazole is effective in curing pinworm in over 90% of the patients. After oral administration, less than 10% of the drug is absorbed from the intenstinal tract. Side effects from the drug are extremely rare. The drug is teratogenic in animals and is therefore not recommended for pregnant women.

Pyrantel Pamoate

This is sold under the brand name Antiminth and is effective as a single dose cure for the treatment of *Enterobius vermicularis* and *Ascaris lumbricoides.* The drug has low toxicity and poor absorption from the gastrointestinal tract. Gastrointestinal side effects are common. Because a small amount of the drug is absorbed, patients occasionally report dizziness, headache or drowziness.

Pyrvinium Pamoate

This is sold under the brand name Povan. It is a cyanide dye and is used to treat pinworms. The drug is not absorbed and therefore toxicity is primarily gastrointestinal. Patients should be warned that the drug will stain the stool red.

Niclosamide

Niclosamide is used for the treatment of tapeworn infections. A single dose will cure patients of *Taenia saginata, T. solium,* or *Diphyllobothrium latum* infection. The drug is also effective against *Hymenolepis nana* but requires at least 5 days of therapy. The preparation is an oral one and is not absorbed. Side effects are primarily those of gastrointestinal upset.

Praziquantel

Praziquantel has proven to be an effective treatment of liver and intestinal flukes. It is a highly effective anti-schistosomal agent. Praziquantel is active against all schistomes. It can be given as a single dose of 40 mg/kg for the treatment of *Schistoma mansoni* and *S. haematobium.* For the treatment of *S. japonicum* higher doses are required and it is recommended that 20 mg/kg be given three times at four hour intervals. Side effects usually begin within an hour of therapy and can last up to two days. These include nausea, vomiting and abdominal pain, all of which are relatively mild.

Furazolidone

This is an effective agent in the treatment of giardiasis. It is sold as Furoxone. It comes in tablet and liquid form. The liquid makes it useful in the treatment of infants and young children. In the United States, this is the only liquid anti-giardiasis medication available. This drug can produce a disulfiram-type reaction when taken with alcohol. Hypersensitivity reactions occasionally occur and these include hypotension, urticaria, fever, arthalgias, headache, vomiting and nausea. In patients with glucose-6-phosphate-dehydrogenase deficiency, there may be occasional mild hemolysis. The drug turns the urine brown color. Children should receive 1.25 mg/kg four times a day, but the drug should not be used under 1 month of age.

ANTIFUNGAL AGENTS

Amphotericin B

Amphotericin B remains the major cornerstone of antifungal therapy. It is effective against a variety of fungi that cause deep infection. It is an intravenous preparation. It can also be given intrathecally. The drug is a polyene antibiotic. It disrupts the integrity of the cellular membrane of those fungi and yeast that are susceptible. The drug has a very long half-life, about 24 hours. Penetration into body fluids including the cerebrospinal fluid is poor. Only a small part of the daily administered dose appears in the urine. In the urine, its concentration is approximately that of the serum. After therapy is discontinued, amphotericin B may be excreted in the urine for weeks. Among the organisms that amphotericin B treats are *Histoplasma capsulatum*, *Blastomyces*, *Cocciodioides*, *Cryptococcus*, *Candida*, *Torulopsis*, *Aspergillus* and mucor species.

Not all patients who have fungal infections require therapy. Patients with primary histoplasmosis, coccidiomycosis and blastomycosis usually resolve their infection spontaneously if they are not immunocompromised. When symptoms are severe however, treatment may be indicated. Treatment of localized cryptococcal pulmonary infection in patients who are otherwise healthy and have normal host defenses is not always necessary. However, the presence of underlying disease or evidence of dissemination necessitates treatment. *Aspergilla* may be a contaminate of sputum, may colonize the respiratory tract, may cause allergic aspergillosis or may cause an aspergilla fungus ball in pulmonary cavities. In addition, there is invasive pulmonary aspergillosis. Contamination or colonization does not usually need to be treated. Amphotericin B is not appropriate for allergic aspergillosis. *Candida* may contaminate sputum and is frequently found in urine cultures in patients with indwelling catheters. When the catheter is removed, the microorganisms usually are eliminated from the urine. Patients who persist with *Candida* despite the removal of the indwelling catheter, or are at risk for other reasons, require therapy. Systemic and disseminated candidal infection must be treated. In situations where there is an obvious source for the candidemia such as intravenous needles and catheters, often the removal of that source will lead to sterilization of the blood and in those situations treatment is not necessary. Amphotericin B is usually administered by first giving a test dose of the drug. If the test dose is tolerated, the therapy can begin. Regimes vary but one can start with .1 mg/kg/day and increase the dose. Maximum dosage varies between .5 mg/kg up to 1 mg/kg/day. Once the maximum dose is reached, the patient can then be started on every other day therapy or occasionally less frequently. There is a long list of side effects associated with amphotericin B. Children and infants, in general, tolerate the drug reasonably well. Side effects include: anorexia, nausea, vomiting, headache, fever, thrombophlibitis, hypomagnesemia, anemia, leukopenia, thrombocytopenia, hepatic dysfunction and anaphylaxis. Nephrotoxicity is frequently seen, especially in adults. This can take the form of azotemia, renal tubular acidosis or hypokalemia. Azotemia is usually reversible. In adults when the total dose of amphotericin B exceeds 4 grams, persistent renal damage may ensue.

Flucytosine

This is also known as 5-flurocytosine. The drug is absorbed from the gastrointestinal tract extremely well and is excreted unchanged in the urine. The drug penetrates well into cerebrospinal fluid to as much as 70% of the serum level. *Candida, Torulopsis* and *Cryptococcus* are frequently sensitive to flucytosine. The drug has been particularly effective in patients with cryptococcal meningitis, invasive pulmonary cryptococcosis and disseminated candidias. Resistance of *Candida* to flucytosine has been reported as high as 50%. The drug is frequently used in combination with amphotericin B. The drug is sold under the brand name Ancobon. The dosage in children is 150 mg/kg/day. It is usually given in four divided doses each day. Adverse effects are not common but occur. Mild nausea and diarrhea may occur. In addition, patients may develop rash, bone marrow supression and elevated liver function enzymes. Rarely cases of fatal leukopenia and thrombocytopenia have been reported. When given in combination with amphotericin B, one must monitor very closely for the possibility of renal failure.

Griseofulvin

This is effective against intradermal dermatophytoses including onychomycosis. Griseofulvin is not effective against *Candida*. The drug is given orally and the dosage in children is 10 mg/kg/day as a single daily dose of the microcrystalline form. *REMEMBER:* Dermatophyte infections may take 4 to 6 weeks of therapy in order to be cured and onychomycosis infections may take several months. Occasionally in stubborn infections it is beneficial to use both oral and topical antifungal agents. It is recommended that the dose of medication be given with the largest meal. Side effects do occur and they include: gastrointestinal disturbances, rash, and photosensitivity; and less frequently blood dyscrasias, peripheral neuritis, confusion, proteinuria and estrogen-like effects in children.

Miconazole

Miconazole is sold under the name of Monistat and appears to be effective against *Cryptococcus, Coccidioidomycosis, Candida* and *Histoplasmosis.* In addition, *Paracoccidioides brasiliensis,* which causes South American blastomycosis, is also sensitive. Doses in pediatrics are 20 to 40 mg/kg/day usually divided into three doses. Duration of therapy depends on the disease but 20 weeks and longer is not uncommon. Adverse reactions include: phlebitis, pruritis, nausea, vomiting, fever, drowziness, chills, aggregation of erythrocytes, anemia, thrombocytopenia, elevated levels of lipids in the blood, hyponatremia and skin rashes. If the drug is infused too rapidly, tachycardia and other arrythmias may occur.

Ketoconazole

Ketoconazole achieves satisfactory serum levels when administered orally. It acts like the other imidazole derivitives. *In vitro* it is active against dermatophytes, *Candida, Coccidioides, Histoplasma,* and many of the *Aspergilla. In vivo* the drug has worked effectively in disseminated candidiases, mucocutaneous candidiases, cryptococcal infection, coccidioidomycosis, and blastomycosis. It has been used with dermatophytosis and histoplasmosis. Although it is effective in these situations, amphotericin B remains the agent of choice in most situations for disseminated candidiasis, coccidioidomycosis and possibly blastomycosis. Ketoconazole is given orally in a dose of 10 mg/kg/day. It is absorbed best when gastric acidity is sufficient. Therefore it should not be given to patients with achlorhydria or patients who are on antacids or cimetidine. Patients with coccidioidomycosis meningitis have been treated successfully with a combination of high dose oral ketoconazole and interventricular miconazole. Side effects include nausea, vomiting, abdominal pain, skin rash, itchiness and diarrhea. Hepatotoxicity has been reported. In addition, interference with synthesis of cortisol and testosterone occurs. Gynecomastia has been reported.

Nystatin

Nystatin is effective against candidal infections of skin, mucus membranes, GI tract and the vagina. It comes in an oral form, a topical form and an intravaginal form. Dosage of suspension in children is 4 to 6 ml four times daily in which the patient swirls it around in his mouth for monilia infections. Topical nystatin is applied twice a day and the intravaginal form is 1 or 2 tablets daily for two weeks. Occasionally there are side effects which include nausea and vomiting after the oral administration.

Tolnaftate

Tolnaftate is sold under the brand name of Tinactim. It is effective against intradermal dermatophytic infections and is a non-prescription drug. It comes in a topical form including cream, powder and solution and it is applied to the affected area twice daily for several weeks. No significant side effects are seen.

ANTITUBERCULOSIS THERAPY

There is an ever increasing list of drugs available to treat tuberculosis. Streptomycin and rifamprin have been discussed earlier in this chapter and will not be discussed here. Three others will be discussed here.

Isoniazid (INH)

INH is a bacteriocidal agent. It is available in both oral and parenteral forms. It is well absorbed after an oral dose and peak blood levels occur within two hours of oral administration. It is distributed throughout the body including the cerebrospinal fluid. The drug is acetylated in the liver and is renally excreted unchanged and as a metabolite. People are either slow or rapid acetylaters. It is genetically controlled. Both groups respond well to the usual doses of INH.

Most strains of *Mycobacterium tuberculosis* are INH sensitive. This is not the case for many of the atypical mycobacterial strains. Most strains of *M. marinum* and *M. avium* are resistant. In children the dose is 10 to 20 mg/kg/day. It is relatively inexpensive. It can be given as a single daily dose. Side effects are not common, but can be severe. Hepatitis is the most serious complication of therapy and is age related. Older patients are at increased risk. The incidence in children is very low. Some patients will develop isolated elevations in SGOT or SGPT. In general, if the levels remain below three times normal, the therapy can be continued. In patients taking INH and rifampin, the incidence of hepatic side effects may be increased. Other side effects associated with INH include pyridoxine deficiency resulting in symptoms of pellegra (rash, anemia and peripheral neuritis) and hypersensitivity reactions. INH interacts with alcohol to cause increased metabolism of INH. Aluminum containing antacids will decrease absorption of INH. Phenytoin plus INH will result in increased levels of phenytoin and possible phenytoin toxicity.

Pyrazinamide

This drug is well absorbed and is well distributed throughout the body.

It is bacteriocidal to actively dividing organisms. Peak levels occur about two hours after the oral dose is administered. The dose is 20 to 30 mg/kg/day. Hepatic toxicity occurs. Nausea, vomiting, fever and arthralgias can occur.

Ethambutol

This oral agent is less active than INH, rifampin or streptomycin. Safety of the drug in young children is not known. The drug is effective against actively dividing cells. Peak concentrations occur 2 to 4 hours after an oral dose. The dosage is 15 mg/kg/day. Side effects include ocular toxicity which is usually reversible if the drug is promptly withdrawn. Manifestations include decreased activity, central scotomas, loss of green color vision and decreased peripheral fields. Rash, anaphylaxis, gastrointestinal disturbances and increased urate have also been reported.

KEY POINTS

1. Chloramphenicol is bacteriostatic for a wide spectrum of organisms. It is an important drug in pediatrics because of its bactericidal activity against *H. influenzae, St. pneumoniae* and *N. meningitidis.*
2. Rifampin has a wide spectrum of antimicrobial activity, is highly effective against staphylococci, and is well tolerated. Rapid emergence of resistance develops when it is used alone.
3. Vancomycin can be useful in patients with penicillin or cephalosporin allergy, in beta-lactamase resistant infections, in patients who respond poorly to other agents with organisms sensitive to vancomycin, in ventricular shunt infections, and when given orally for pseudomembranous colitis.
4. Clindamycin is effective against most anaerobic and many staphylococci.
5. The penicillins have a wide spectrum of activity. Penicillin allergy occurs in about 5 percent of patients. Although a much larger percent give a history of penicillin allergy, many of these patients will be penicillin skin test negative.
6. Erythromycin is a good broad spectrum antibiotic with few side effects. It is particularly valuable for non-life-threatening infections and is usually used as an outpatient antibiotic.

7. The cephalosporins are a large class of antibiotics. First generation cephalosporins are effective primarily against Gram positive organisms. Second generation cephalosporins increase the Gram negative coverage and the third generation drugs have improved CNS penetration.
8. The aminoglycosides provide good Gram negative coverage but may cause significant ototoxicity and nephrotoxicity.
9. The monobactams are a new class of antibiotics which have good Gram negative coverage and appear to be relatively safe.
10. Trimethoprim-sulfamethoxazole is the treatment of choice for *Pneumocystis carinii* infection.
11. Ara-A and acyclovir have proven to be effective antiviral drugs against herpes and varicella in certain situations.
12. Amantadine is effective prophylaxis against influenzae A, and if instituted early is also effective therapy.
13. Ribavirin in aerosolized form may be valuable in serious RSV infections.
14. Most antiparasitic agents are effective against specific parasites and have a low level of toxicity in appropriate doses.
15. Antifungal therapy usually requires a long duration of treatment and has side effects which need to be monitored closely.

REFERENCES

1. Aronoff SC, Reed MD, O'Brien CA, et al: Comparison of the efficacy and safety of ceftriaxone to ampicillin/chloramphenicol in the treatment of childhood meningitis. J. Antimicrob. Chemother. 1984; 13:-143–151.
2. Aronoff SC, Thomford W, Bertino JS, et al: Development of meningitis during therapy with cefamandole. Pediatrics 1981; 67:727–728.
3. Borelli D, Fuentes J. Leiderman E, et al: Ketoconazole, an oral antifungal: laboratory and clinical assessment of imidazole drugs. Postgraduate Medical Journal 1979; 55:657–661.
4. Bryson YJ: Clinical Aspects of Antiviral Therapy. In Nelson JD McCracken GH (eds) *Clinical Reviews in Pediatric Infectious Disease;* Philadelphia: B.C. Decker, Inc, 1985; 117–128.
5. Dambro N, Friedman AD, Alexander ER, et al: Augmentin therapy for urinary tract infections in children. Post Graduate Medicine. (supple), Sept/Oct 1984; pp 263–266.

6. Eichenwald HF: Antimicrobial therapy in infants and children: Update 1976–1985. J. Pediatr 1985; 107:161–167, 331–345.

7. Eichenwald HF, McCracken GH: Antimicrobial therapy in infants and children. J Pediatr 1978; 93:337–377.

8. Epstein JS, Hasselquist SM, Simon GL: Efficacy of ceftriazone in serious bacterial infections. Antimicrob. Agents Chemother. 1982; 21:402–406.

9. Farr B, Mandell G: Rifampin. Cuba BA, eds. The Medical Clinics of North America. Philadelphia: WB Saunders Co.; 1982; 66 (1):157–168.

10. Gribble MJ, Chow AW: Erythromycin. Cunha BA, eds. The Medical Clinics of North America. Philadelphia: WB Saunders Co.; 1982: 66 (1) 79–90.

11. Gutman LT: The use of trimethoprim-sulfamethoxazole in Children. Pediatric Infectious Diseases 1984; 3:349–357.

12. Harrison HR, Galgiani JN, Reynolds AF, et al: Coccidioidal meningitis in young children: Experience with amphoteracin B and imidazole therapy. Pediatric Infectious Diseases, 1983; 148–332.

13. Hermans PE, Keys TF: Antifungal agents used in deep-seated mycotic infections. Mayo Clin Proc, 1983; 58:223–231.

14. Katz M: Treatment of protozoan infections: Malaria. Pediatric Infectious Diseases, 1983; 2:475–480.

15. Marks MI, Laferriere CI: Chloramphenicol: Properties and Clinical Use. In: Nelson JD, McCracken GH, eds. *Clinical Reviews in Pediatric Infectious Diseases.* Philadelphia: BC Decker, Inc, 1985: 97–106.

16. McCracken GH, Nelson JD: The third generation cephalosporins and the pediatric practitioner. In: Nelson JD, McCracken GH, eds. *Clinical Reviews in Pediatric Infectious Diseases.* Philadelphia: BC Decker, Inc, 1985: 79–84.

17. Medoff G, Kobayashi GS: Strategies in the treatment of systemic fungal infections. N Engl J. Med, 1980; 302:145–155.

18. Nelson JD, Kusmiesz H, Shelton S: Cefuroxime therapy for pneumonia in infants and children. Pediatric Infectious Diseases, 1982; 1:159–163.

19. Ogawara H: Antibiotic resistance in pathogenic and producing bacteria, with special reference to beta-lactam antibiotics, Microbiol Revs, 1981; 45:591–619.

20. Pancost S, Price AS, Francke EL, et al: Clinical evaluation of piperacillin therapy for infection. Arch Intern Med, 1981; 141:1447–1450.

21. Sheld WM: Rationale for antibiotic therapy of bacterial meningitis. Pediatric Infectious Diseases, 1985; 4:74–83.
22. Steele RW: Ceftriaxone. Pediatric Infectious Diseases, 1985; 4:188–191.
23. Sullivan TJ: Allergic reactions to penicillin and other beta-lactam antibiotics. In: Nelson JD, McCracken GH, eds. *Clinical Reviews in Pediatric Infectious Diseases.* Philadelphia: BC Decker, Inc, 1985: 89–96.
24. Thompson RL, Wright AJ: Cephalosporin antibiotics. Mayo Clin Proc, 1983; 58:79–87.
25. Van Scoy RE, Wilkowske CJ: Antituberculous agents. Mayo Clin Proc, 1983; 58:233–245.
26. Washington JA, Wilson WR: Erythromycin: A microbial and clinical perspective after 30 years of clinical use. Mayo Clin Proc, 1985; 60:1889–2003.
27. Wiser D, Dyas A, Hegarty A, et al: Pharmocokinetics and tissue penetration of Azthreonam. Antimicrob Agents Chemother., 1982; 22:969–971.
28. Wright AJ, Wilkowske CJ: The penicillins. Mayo Clin Proc, 1983; 58:21–32.

REVIEW QUESTIONS

Match the drugs in Column A with their characteristics in Column B.

A

1.) Vancomycin
2.) Amoxicillin
3.) Cefuroxime
4.) Rifampin
5.) Clindamycin
6.) Furazolidone
7.) Procaine penicillin
8.) Chloramphenicol
9.) Acyclovir
10.) Erythromycin
11.) Amphoteracin B

B

A. Aplastic anemia, good penetration into CSF and into WBCs.
B. Inhibits RNA synthesis, excellent antistaphylococcal drug, rapid emergence of resistance.
C. Treats pseudomembranous colitis, may cause neurotoxicity in high doses.
D. Effective anaerobic and antistaphylococcal drug associated with the development of *Clostridium difficile* overgrowth.
E. Oral therapy with similar spectrum to ampicillin.
F. Hoigne Syndrome.
G. May increase theophylline level.
H. Second generation cephalosporin with good CNS penetration.
I. Oral antiviral effective against genital herpes.
J. Treats *Giardia*
K. Drug of choice for serious *Candida* infection.

21

IMMUNOLOGIC ASPECTS OF INFECTIOUS DISEASES

An intact immune system is essential for the body to adequately control and eliminate infection. The two principal parts of the immune system are the cell mediated immunity and the humoral mediated immunity. Cell mediated immunity includes T-lymphocyte cells, monocytes, basophils, and eosinophils. The humoral mediated immunity includes complement, immune globulins, polymorphonuclear leukocytes and B-cells. The purpose of this chapter is to briefly discuss aspects of immunity in order to give you a better understanding of its role in fighting infection.

Immune globulins serve the purpose of attaching to organisms and then to phagocytize them. Essentially, they help direct the phagocyte to the pathogen. The antigen-antibody complex formed by the antibody can then activate the complement system. The antigen-antibody-complement complex is more efficient in phagocytosis of the pathogen than the antigen-antibody complex alone. The immune globulins include IgG, IgM, IgA, IgE, and IgD. IgA interferes with the microorganism's ability to adhere to a surface. They are predominant in mucous secretions, colostrum and milk. Immune globulin M is the first antibody to appear after an infection and is followed usually by IgG. IgE mediates hypersensitivity and is also important in the defense against parasites. IgG plays a broad role in defense. Low levels of IgG are associated with high rates of infections. The basic role of antibody is to stimulate the immune system. Complement is activated by antibody. Antibody binds antigen. Antibody increases phagocytosis and the binding to receptors on cell surfaces and has a suppression affect on the immune system. That is, it activates suppressor T-lymphocyte cells, suppresses helper T-lymphocyte cells, inhibits antibody function, and it inactivates B-cells. This stimulation and suppression activity related to antibodies keeps the immune system in balance so that neither role becomes too extensive nor inappropriate. IgA appears to have both antiviral and antitoxin effect. It also inhibits bacterial adherence, it inhibits antigen absorption and it suppresses inflammatory responses. It is important to remember that IgG does not reach adults levels until a patient is about 10 years of age and levels are lowest around 9 months of age.

T-lymphocyte cells also play a major role in the immune system. T cells recognize foreign matter. In addition, T cells remember previous encounters with foreign matter and prepare for a second encounter with what is foreign. T cells also destroy or inactivate foreign substances. Effector T cells are cytotoxic and they are lymphokine producing, resulting in activation of macrophages. Helper T cells interact with B cells resulting in the production of antibody. Suppressor T cells inhibit the helper-effector function thus keeping things in balance. Phagocytes also play a major role in fighting infection. By chemotaxis, phagocytes go to the site of the foreign matter, they bind to foreign substances and they ingest and kill them. Defects in any of these steps can result in phagocytic abnormalities and deficiencies in the immune system.

ABNORMALITIES OF IMMUNE SYSTEM

There are several ways that increased susceptibility to infection can present. Patients with immune dysfunction may have increased numbers of infections or they may have normal numbers of infections but increased severity of infections. That is to say, normal infections which are routine in most patients become serious in these patients. In addition, some patients may have normal number of infections and appropriate degree of severity of the illness but the infection may be unusually prolonged. Other patients with immune dysfunctions have infections with unusual organisms or opportunistic organisms. In evaluating a patient with suspected immune dysfunction, several important points of history need to be elicited. History should include facts relating to the frequency of the infections, the type of infections the patient gets, and whether or not the patient is described as always sick. History of persistent or recurrent thrush, severe recurrent or unusual presentations of impetigo, or history of malabsorption or diarrhea all are suggestive of possible immune dysfunction. Patients who have persistent recurrent or unexplained lymphadenitis also are candidates for an evaluation for immune dysfunction. All children who have functional or anatomical splenectomy are at risk for being immune deficient. It is important to carefully check for a family history of immune problems. Relatives with a history of chronic infections, unusually severe infections, or dying from what would be considered normal routine infections, should be suspect for possible immune abnormalities. Immune deficiencies can be divided into primary and secondary. Primary immune deficiencies are rare and are unlikely to be the cause of immune dysfunction in most patients. Secondary immune deficiencies are relatively more common.

Deficiencies in B cells may present in one of several ways. Patients with a history of recurrent infections or patients with history of frequent acute bacterial infections should be evaluated for B cell dysfunction. Patients with chronic sinopulmonary disease are also patients in which the possibility of B cell abnormalities should be considered. Children that have persistent giardiasis or persistent enteroviral infection including polio should be evaluated for B cell dysfunction. Most patients with B cell dysfunction will survive to adulthood. Complement dysfunction may present as recurrent bacterial infections or frequent acute bacterial infections. In addition, patients with chronic sinopulmonary disease may also be complement deficient. While it is not unusual to have one *Neisseria* infection, any child that has more than one *Neisseria* infection (for example, meniningococcal meningitis, gonococcal arthritis) should be suspected of having either a complement dysfunction and/or B cell deficiency. Patients with collagen-vascular disease should be evaluated for complement deficiency. Complement deficiency is usually compatible with survival into adulthood. Patients with T cell deficiency may present with recurrent fungal, viral or pneumocystis infection. These patients often have delayed cutaneous anergy and may have no reaction to things like poison ivy. These patients characteristically have serious systemic abnormalities including growth retardation, diarrhea, wasting or malabsorption. These patients may present with graft-versus-host abnormalities and there are reports of fatal reactions to live vaccines in patients with T cell deficiency. Finally, patients with T cell deficiency have a high incidence of malignancy and need to be evaluated very closely for the possibility of cancer. Patients with phagocytic deficiencies often have recurrent infections with very pathogenic organisms like *Staphylococcus*. They will classically have splenomegaly, hepatomegaly and lymphadenopathy. In addition, they may present with a history of recurrent aphthous ulcers or periodontitis. Their immune glogulin levels may be normal or slightly elevated.

As previously mentioned, primary immune dysfunctions are relatively rare. One primary immune deficiency occasionally seen is severe combined immunodeficiency. These patients have absence of both T and B lymphocytes and usually symptoms appear when the child is 5 to 6 months of age. Classically these children present with severe recurrent infections. Common variable immune deficiency is described by low levels of immune globulin. In addition, they may have T cell defects. This abnormality occurs both in children and in adults, and its inheritance pattern is poorly defined. Patients with DiGeorge syndrome often have abnormal facies, hypocalcemia secondary to hypoparathyroidism, congenital heart disease, decreased cellular immunity, lymphopenia and abnormal third and fourth pharyngeal pouches. Wiskott-Aldrich syndrome is characterized by thrombocytopenia, eczema, frequent infections, and is a T and B cell deficiency. This disease is x-linked recessive. Other immune deficiencies seen in children include chronic granulomatous disease which is usually an x-linked disease in which there is abnormal oxidative metabolism. Diagnosis is made by doing the nitroblue tetrazolium test (NBT). Unfortunately AIDS (Acquired Immune Deficiency Syndrome) is increasingly seen in pediatric patients. This illness may present atypically as compared to the classic adult presentation but needs to be considered in patients who do not fit into other categories of immune deficiency.

WORKUP OF IMMUNE DEFICIENCY IN CHILDREN

Children who present with histories or physical examination compatible with immune deficiency need to be worked up to further define the type of immune deficiency that the patient has. Often based on historical data or physical exam, one can narrow down the differential diagnosis to one or the other parts of the immune system. Generally, in children with suspected immune deficiency, a battery of initial screening tests should be done to better define the abnormality. While there are a variety of initial screening tests available, one approach includes obtaining blood for a complete blood count including differential; protein electrophoresis; quantitative immunoglobulins; isohemaglutinins; specific antibody titers against infections such as rubella, diphtheria or tetanus; erythrocycte sedimentation rates; sinus and chest x-rays and if the patient is actively infected, appropriate cultures should be obtained. Generally, in pediatrics, if a quantitative immunoglobulin panel is obtained, protein electrophoresis is not necessary. The rationale for this initial screening test is that the CBC will provide information about white cell numbers and morphology, the quantitative immunoglobulins will provide information related to adequate amounts of immunoglobulins, isohemagglutinins will test IgM function, specific antibody titers will test IgG function, and the sedimentation rate, x-rays and cultures will evaluate for potential infection. Once the initial screening is done, a decision needs to be made related to further screening. This decision should be based on the severity of illness in the child and the potential benefit of a more exhausted and expensive workup to the child.

In general, after the initial tests for antibody immunodeficiency are done; (that is the immunoglobulin levels, the isohemagglutinins, and the specific antibody titers) further workup should include B cell innumeration by surface immunoglobulin staining, specific antibody responses, and IgG subclass levels. These tests are not necessarily available at every medical center, but in the child where further evaluation is necessary these tests should be sought. In patients where cellular T cell immunodeficiency is suspected, lymphocyte counts and morphology, delayed hypersensitivity skin testing, and thymus x-rays in infants should be considered initially. When further workup is indicated, T cell innumeration, E-rosettes, T-subsets, lymphocyte proliferation to mitogens and antigens, and lymph node biopsy should be considered. Phagocytic deficiencies can initially be evaluated by the granulocyte count and morphology, the nitroblue tetrazolium test, and IgE levels. Further workup can include white cell response to epinephrine and steroids, phagocytic and bactericidal assays and chemotaxis studies. Complement is best initially evaluated by obtaining C3 and C4 levels as well as a CH50 assay. The C3 and C4 levels primarily tell whether complement is present and a CH50 assay is essentially a functional assay for the classical pathway of complement. Beyond the tests mentioned here, in general, a consultation with a subspecialist is necessary for additional evaluation.

ACQUIRED IMMUNE DEFICIENCY SYNDROME IN CHILDREN

As mentioned previously, acquired immune deficiency syndrome in children often does not present in the same way as it presents in adults. It has been suggested that the diagnosis of AIDS in children can be based on major and minor criteria. The major criteria include interstitial pneumonia, oral thrush, salivary gland enlargement, bacterial sepsis and meningitis, and a history of AIDS or the AIDS related virus in the mother. Minor criteria include lymphadenopathy, failure-to-thrive, diarrhea, hepatosplenomegaly, and recurrent bacterial infections. It has been suggested that children with two major and two minor criteria will fit the diagnosis of AIDS. In addition, now that the organism responsible for AIDS has been identified, evidence for the virus in the patient is also helpful in making the diagnosis. AIDS remains an untreatable disease with a poor prognosis although several antivirals are currently under investigation. Nevertheless, pediatric patients appear to have a slightly better prognosis than do adult patients.

Treatment of Immune Deficiencies

The diagnosis of immunodeficiency is not just of academic interest. Increasingly, we are able to control or treat immune deficiencies in many patients. B cell disorders can frequently be treated with the use of gammaglobulin which comes in both intramuscular and intravenous preparations. Gammaglobulin is effective in x-linked hypogammaglobulinemia. It is also effective in acquired hypogammaglobulinemia, as well as secondary hypogammaglobulinemia when associated with infection. Its value in T cell disorders is limited to those patients who also have absent antibody response.

Hyperimmune globulins exist to rabies, hepatitis, varicella, and tetanus and in those specific illnesses, hyperimmune globulin may be very useful. Frozen plasma has been given intravenously in patients with x-linked hypogammaglobulinemia and in acquired hypogammaglobulinemia.

Treatments exist for patients with T cell disorders also. Bone marrow transplantation has increasingly been used in patients who have impaired T cell function, for example those patients with severe combined immune deficiency and those patients with Wiskott-Aldrich syndrome. Fetal thymic transplant has been used with some degree of success in DiGeorge syndrome and in severe combined immunodeficiencies when no suitable bone marrow donor has been found. Cultured thymus epithelium has been used in selected cases of T-cell disorders where no suitable marrow donor is available. Transfer factor has been successful in chronic candidiasis when used in association with appropriate antifungal therapy. Other therapies including fetal liver transplantation and thymic factors, have been used occasionally with some degree of success.

There has been some controversy about the value and appropriate use of intravenous gammaglobulin. While no rigid rule should apply, in general, IV gammaglobulin may be of value in patients with the acquired immune deficiency syndrome, Kawaski disease, autoimmune neutropenia, and idiopathic thrombocytopenia purpura, especially those cases which are chronic or refractory to steroids. As previously mentioned, in certain primary immune deficiencies, IV gammaglobulin is appropriate therapy.

KEY POINTS

1. Most immunologic deficiencies in children are secondary. Primary immune dysfunctions are relatively rare.
2. In evaluating the immune system, remember to consider the B cell system, the T cell system and the complement and neutrophil function.
3. Children with unusual numbers of infection, unusually severe infections, or unusual pathogens should be evaluated for immune dysfunction.

REFERENCES

1. Albrecht RM, Hong R: Basic and clinical considerations of the monocyte-macrophage system in man. J Pediatr 1976; 88:751–760.
2. Dannenberg AM: Macrophages in inflammation and infection. N Engl J Med 1975; 293:489–493.
3. MacKianess GB: Cellular resistance to infection. J Exp Med 1962; 116:381–406. Ruddy S, Gigli I, Austen KF: The complement system of Man. N Engl J Med 1972; 287:489-496.

REVIEW QUESTIONS

1.) A history of recurrent bacterial infections in a patient may suggest a dysfuncton of___________ (T or B) cells.

2.) _________________syndrome is often characterized by abnormal facies, hypocalcemia secondary to hypo parathyroidism, congenital heart disease, decreased cellular immunity, lymphopenia and abnormal third and fourth pharyngeal pouches.

3.) Characteristics of Wisckott-Aldrich syndrome includes_______________ (4).

4.) Patients with recurrent *Neisseria* infections should be evaluated for____________and__________.

REVIEW QUESTION ANSWERS

Chapter 1

1.) Neonatal otitis
Immunocompromised child
Otitis unresponsive to routine therapy
Child with otitis and serious complications

2.) Red or yellow-white TM
Inability to see boney landmarks behind TM
Bulging of TM
Decreased mobility of TM

3.) 1. False
2. True
3. False
4. False
5. False

4.) 1. True
2. True
3. True
4. False

5.) Adenovirus
Streptococcus
Epstein-Barr virus
Para influenzae (and influenzae) viruses

6.) a, c, d

7.) A. 3
B. 2
C. 1
D. 4

8.) A. 1
B. 2
C. 3
D. 4

9.) A. 1
B. 4
C. 3
D. 2

Chapter 2

1.)   A. 5
         B. 4
         C. 1
         D. 2
         E. 3
         F. 6

2.)   A. 3
         B. 4
         C. 5
         D. 1
         E. 2

Chapter 3

1.)   A. 3
         B. 4
         C. 8
         D. 6
         E. 5
         F. 2
         G. 7
         H. 1

2.)   1. True
         2. False
         3. True
         4. True
         5. False

3.)   Catarrhal (prodrome)
         Paroxysmal (cough)
         Convalescent (recovery)

4.)   1. Keep child calm, do not agitate.
         2. Arrange for direct visualization of epiglottis with ENT and/or anesthesia backup-(lateral x-ray of neck is alternative if visualization is delayed).
         3. Intubation (or tracheotomy), culture of epiglottis.
         4. Blood culture.

Chapter 3 (Continued)

5. Intravenous antibiotics.
6. Evaluation for possible other sites of infection.

Chapter 4

1.) 1. False
     2. True
     3. True
     4. False
     5. True
     6. True

2.) A. 3
     B. 2
     C. 6
     D. 7.
     E. 8
     F. 1
     G. 4
     H. 5

Chapter 5

1.) 90 days (40-180 days)
2.) liver function tests (SGPT/SGOT)
    HB_sAg
    HB_eAg
3.) HB_sAg
4.) immune globulins (HBIG or ISG)
5.) 15 - 50 days
6.) Fecal-oral route
7.) ISG
8.) Non-A, Non-B
9.) Hepatitis B

Chapter 6

1.) *H. influenzae*
    N. meningitidis
    Str. pneumoniae
2.) glucose
    protein
    cell count
    differential
    Gram stain (or acridine orange stain)
    culture
    (Additional tubes may be used for antigen detection, viral cultures, fungal, or tuberculosis cultures).
3.) Inappropriate anti-diuretic hormone syndrome.
4.) 1. False
    2. False
    3. False
    4. False
    5. True
    6. True

Chapter 7

1.) fever, chills, CVA tenderness.
2.) Feeding problems, vomiting, poor weight gain, fever.
3.) *E. coli*
4.) Pyelonephritis
5.) red or reddish orange
6.) greater than 100,000
7.) acidic

Chapter 8

1.) 1. B
    2. F
    3. E
    4. D
    5. F

Chapter 8 (Continued)

6.	B
7.	A
8.	C
9.	G
10.	G

2.)　A.　3
　　　B.　6
　　　C.　5
　　　D.　4
　　　E.　1
　　　F.　2

3.)　1.　False
　　　2.　True
　　　3.　False
　　　4.　True
　　　5.　True
　　　6.　True
　　　7.　True

Chapter 9

1. True
2. False
3. True
4. True
5. True
6. False
7. False
8. True

Chapter 10

1.) *Pasteurella multocida*
2.) Cats
3.) Water moccasins
Rattle Snakes
Copperheads
4.) Coral
5.) Coral
6.) Non-poisonous
7.) Winter
8.) *Salmonellae*

Chapter 11

1.) respiratory distress and sepsis
2.) rarely
3.) Herpes
4.) Endometritis
UTI
bacteremia
Colonization with pathogens
Lack of antibody to specific pathogens
prolonged rupture of membranes
premature labor, fever
5.) invasive fetal monitoring
congenital anomalies
asphyxia
prematurity
hyperalimentation

Chapter 12

1.) B
2.) C
3.) A
4.) D
5.) E
6.) H
7.) G
8.) D
9.) A
10.) F

Chapter 13

A. 5
B. 2
C. 3
D. 1
E. 4
F. 6

Chapter 14

1.) A. 5
     B. 4
     C. 1
     D. 6
     E. 2
     F. 3

2.) 1. False
     2. True
     3. True
     4. True

Chapter 15

1.) D
2.) C
3.) F
4.) C
5.) A
6.) B
7.) E
8.) A

Chapter 16

1.) G
2.) F
3.) B
4.) C
5.) E
6.) D
7.) H
8.) A
9.) E
10.) C

Chapter 17

1.) H
2.) D
3.) B
4.) A
5.) C
6.) E
7.) F
8.) I
9.) J
10.) G

Chapter 18

1.) 1. B
    2. F
    3. C
    4. E
    5. E
    6. A
    7. D

2.) Tetanus
    Hepatitis B
    Rabies
    Varicella

3.) *H. influenzae*
    N. meningitidis

4.) A. 1
    B. 4
    C. 2
    D. 3
    E. 5
    F. 6

Chapter 19

1.) Antigen or antibody
2.) Enrichment, Selective, Differential
3.) CPE (cytopathic effect)
4.) Neutrophil dysfunction (chronic granulomatous disease)
5.) Limulus lysate
6.) A. Increase
    B. Increase
    C. Decrease
    D. Increase
    E. Increase
    F. Decrease

Chapter 19 (Continued)

7.) A. 3
    B. 2
    C. 5
    D. 1
    E. 7
    F. 6
    G. 4

Chapter 20

1.) C
2.) E
3.) H
4.) B
5.) D
6.) J
7.) F
8.) A
9.) I
10.) G
11.) K

Chapter 21

1.)   B
2.)   Di George
3.)   Thrombocytopenia, eczema, frequent infections, T and B
       cell deficiency.
4.)   Complement deficiency, B cell deficiency.

INDEX